T0184279

Lecture Notes in Computer Science   **11255**

Commenced Publication in 1973
Founding and Former Series Editors:
Gerhard Goos, Juris Hartmanis, and Jan van Leeuwen

More information about this series at http://www.springer.com/series/7411

Reneta P. Barneva · Valentin E. Brimkov
João Manuel R. S. Tavares (Eds.)

Combinatorial
Image Analysis

19th International Workshop, IWCIA 2018
Porto, Portugal, November 22–24, 2018
Proceedings

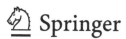 Springer

Editors
Reneta P. Barneva
State University of New York at Fredonia
Fredonia, NY, USA

João Manuel R. S. Tavares ⓘ
University of Porto
Porto, Portugal

Valentin E. Brimkov
State University of New York
Buffalo, NY, USA

and

Institute of Mathematics and Informatics
Bulgarian Academy of Sciences
Sofia, Bulgaria

ISSN 0302-9743   ISSN 1611-3349 (electronic)
Lecture Notes in Computer Science
ISBN 978-3-030-05287-4   ISBN 978-3-030-05288-1 (eBook)
https://doi.org/10.1007/978-3-030-05288-1

Library of Congress Control Number: 2018962921

LNCS Sublibrary: SL5 – Computer Communication Networks and Telecommunications

This Springer imprint is published by the registered company Springer Nature Switzerland AG
The registered company address is: Gewerbestrasse 11, 6330 Cham, Switzerland

Preface

This volume contains the proceedings of the 19th International Workshop on Combinatorial Image Analysis (IWCIA 2018) held in Porto, Portugal, November 22–24, 2018.

Image analysis provides theoretical foundations and methods for solving real-life problems arising in various areas of human practice, such as medicine, robotics, defense, and security. Since typically the input data to be processed are discrete, the "combinatorial" approach to image analysis is a natural one and therefore its applicability is expanding. Combinatorial image analysis often provides advantages in terms of efficiency and accuracy over the more traditional approaches based on continuous models that require numeric computation.

The IWCIA workshop series provides a forum for researchers throughout the world to present cutting-edge results in combinatorial image analysis, to discuss recent advances and new challenges in this research area, and to promote interaction with researchers from other countries. IWCIA had successful prior meetings in Paris (France) 1991, Ube (Japan) 1992, Washington DC (USA) 1994, Lyon (France) 1995, Hiroshima (Japan) 1997, Madras (India) 1999, Caen (France) 2000, Philadelphia, PA (USA) 2001, Palermo (Italy) 2003, Auckland (New Zealand) 2004, Berlin (Germany) 2006, Buffalo, NY (USA) 2008, Playa del Carmen (Mexico) 2009, Madrid (Spain) 2011, Austin, TX (USA) 2012, Brno (Czech Republic) 2014, Kolkata (India) 2015, and Plovdiv (Bulgaria) 2017. The workshop in Porto retained and enriched the international spirit of these workshops. The IWCIA 2018 Program Committee members are renowned experts coming from 17 different countries in Asia, Europe, North and South America, and the authors come from 12 different countries.

Each submitted paper was sent to at least three reviewers for a double-blind review. EasyChair provided a convenient platform for smoothly carrying out the rigorous review process. The most important selection criterion for acceptance or rejection of a paper was the overall score received. Other criteria included: relevance to the workshop topics, correctness, originality, mathematical depth, clarity, and presentation quality. We believe that as a result only papers of high quality were accepted for presentation at IWCIA 2018 and for publication in this volume.

The program of the workshop included presentations of contributed papers and keynote talks by three distinguished scientists. The talk of José M. Bioucas-Dias (University of Lisbon, Portugal) presented methods for solving certain inverse problems of interferometric phase imaging, aimed at the estimation of phase from sinusoidal and noisy observations. He proposed characterizations of the obtained estimates and illustrated their effectiveness by results of extensive experiments with simulated and real data. Jan Kratochvil (Charles University, Czech Republic) reviewed various problems on intersection, contact, or visibility representations of graphs, which are a natural way of graph and network visualization. He surveyed known results on these classes of graphs and discussed new as well as persisting open problems. Nicolai

Petkov (University of Groningen, The Netherlands) presented novel trainable filters as an alternative to deep networks for the extraction of effective representations of data for the purposes of pattern recognition. He discussed the advantages of this approach and illustrated it on handwritten digit images, traffic signs, and sounds in audio signals.

The contributed papers are grouped into two sections. The first one includes nine papers devoted to theoretical foundations of combinatorial image analysis, including digital geometry and topology, array grammars, tilings and patterns, discrete geometry in non-rectangular grids, and other technical tools for image analysis. The second part includes nine papers presenting application-driven research on topics such as discrete tomography, image segmentation, texture analysis, and medical imaging. We believe that many of these papers would be of interest to a broader audience, including researchers in scientific areas such as computer vision, shape modeling, pattern analysis and recognition, and computer graphics.

A special session provided some authors with the opportunity to present their ongoing research projects and original works in progress. The texts of these works are not included in this volume.

Many individuals and organizations contributed to the success of IWCIA 2018. The editors are indebted to IWCIA's Steering Committee for endorsing the candidacy of Porto for the 19th edition of the workshop. We wish to thank everybody who submitted their work to IWCIA 2018; thanks to their contributions, we succeeded in having a technical program of high scientific quality. We are grateful to all participants and especially to the contributors of this volume. Our most sincere thanks go to the IWCIA 2018 Program Committee whose cooperation in carrying out high-quality reviews was essential in establishing a strong scientific program. We express our sincere gratitude to the keynote speakers, José M. Bioucas-Dias, Jan Kratochvil, and Nicolai Petkov for their excellent talks and overall contribution to the workshop program.

The success of the workshop would not be possible without the hard work of the local Organizing Committee. We are grateful to our partners: FEUP – Faculdade de Engenharia da Universidade do Porto; LABIOMEP: Laboratório de Biomecânica do Porto; APMTAC – Associação Portuguesa de Mecânica Teórica, Aplicada e Computacional; FCT – Fundação para a Ciência e a Tecnologia; INEGI – Instituto de Ciência e Inovação em Engenharia Mecânica e Engenharia Industrial; ITHEA ISS – International Scientific Society; and Taylor & Francis Group. Finally, we wish to thank Springer, and especially Alfred Hofmann and Anna Kramer, for their efficient and kind cooperation in the timely production of this book.

October 2018

Reneta P. Barneva
Valentin E. Brimkov
João Manuel R. S. Tavares

Organization

The 19th International Workshop on Combinatorial Image Analysis, IWCIA 2019 was held in Porto, Portugal, November 22–24, 2018.

General Chair

João Manuel R. S. Tavares   University of Porto, Portugal

Chairs

Reneta P. Barneva	SUNY Fredonia, USA
Valentin E. Brimkov	SUNY Buffalo State, USA
Renato M. Natal Jorge	University of Porto, Portugal

Steering Committee

Bhargab B. Bhattacharya	Indian Statistical Institute, Kolkata, India
Valentin E. Brimkov	SUNY Buffalo State, Buffalo, USA
Gabor Herman	CUNY Graduate Center, USA
Kostadin Korutchev	Universidad Autonoma, Spain
Josef Slapal	Technical University of Brno, Czech Republic

Invited Speakers

José M. Bioucas-Dias	University of Lisbon, Portugal
Jan Kratochvil	Charles University, Czech Republic
Nicolai Petkov	University of Groningen, The Netherlands

Program Committee

Eric Andres	Université de Poitiers, France
Peter Balazs	University of Szeged, Hungary
Jacky Baltes	University of Manitoba, Canada
George Bebis	University of Nevada at Reno, USA
Bhargab B. Bhattacharya	Indian Statistical Institute, India
Partha Bhowmick	IIT Kharagpur, India
Arindam Biswas	IIEST Shibpur, India
Peter Brass	City College, City University of New York, USA
Boris Brimkov	Rice University, USA
Srecko Brlek	Université du Quebec a Montreal, Canada
Alfred M. Bruckstein	Technion, I.I.T, Israel

Jean-Marc Chassery	Université de Grenoble, France
Li Chen	University of the District of Columbia, USA
David Coeurjolly	Université de Lyon, France
Rocio Gonzalez-Diaz	University of Seville, Spain
Mousumi Dutt	St. Thomas College of Engineering and Technology, India
Fabien Feschet	Université d'Auvergne, France
Leila De Floriani	University of Genova, Italy and University of Maryland, USA
Chiou-Shann Fuh	National Taiwan University, Taiwan
Edwin Hancock	University of York, UK
Fay Huang	National Ilan University, Taiwan
Krassimira Ivanova	Bulgarian Academy of Sciences, Bulgaria
Atsushi Imiya	IMIT, Chiba University, Japan
Maria Jose Jimenez	University of Seville, Spain
Kamen Kanev	Shizuoka University, Japan
Yung Kong	CUNY Queens College, USA
Vladimir Kovalevski	Technische Fachhochschule Berlin, Germany
Walter G. Kropatsch	Vienna University of Technology, Austria
Longin Jan Latecki	Temple University, USA
Jerome Liang	SUNY Stony Brook, USA
Joakim Lindblad	Uppsala University, Sweden
Benedek Nagy	Eastern Mediterranean University, Cyprus
Gregory M. Nielson	Arizona State University, USA
Janos Pach	EPFL Lausanne, Switzerland and Renyi Institute Budapest, Hungary
Kalman Palagyi	University of Szeged, Hungary
Petra Perner	Institute of Computer Vision and Applied Computer Sciences, Germany
Nicolai Petkov	University of Groningen, The Netherlands
Hemerson Pistori	Dom Bosco Catholic University, Brazil
Ioannis Pitas	University of Thessaloniki, Greece
Konrad Polthier	Freie Universität Berlin, Germany
Hong Qin	SUNY Stony Brook, USA
Paolo Remagnino	Kingston University, UK
Ralf Reulke	Humboldt University, Germany
Bodo Rosenhahn	MPI Informatik, Germany
Arun Ross	Michigan State University, USA
Nikolay Sirakov	Texas A&M University - Commerce, USA
Rani Siromoney	Madras Christian College, India
Wladyslaw Skarbek	Warsaw University of Technology, Poland
Ali Shokoufandeh	Drexel University, USA
K. G. Subramanian	Madras Christian College, India
Gnanaraj Thomas	Madras Christian College, India
Peter Veelaert	University of Gent, Belgium

Petra Wiederhold   CINVESTAV-IPN, Mexico
Jinhui Xu   SUNY University at Buffalo, USA

Local Organizing Committee

Jessica Delmoral   University of Porto, Portugal
Marco Marques   University of Porto, Portugal
João Nunes   University of Porto, Portugal
André Luiz Pilastri   University of Porto, Portugal
Domingos Vieira   University of Porto, Portugal

Additional Reviewers

Chouaib Moujahdi
Tin Nguyen
Ali Erol
Jiri Hladuvka
Minwei Ye
Xiangyu Wang
Ulderico Fugacci
Paola Magillo
Ziyun Huang
Federico Iuricich

Contents

Theoretical Contributions

On Gaps in Digital Objects

Lidija Čomić[(✉)]

Faculty of Technical Sciences, University of Novi Sad, Novi Sad, Serbia
comic@uns.ac.rs

Abstract. Different formulae were proposed in the literature for the number of gaps in digital objects. We give several new formulae for the number of 0-gaps in 2D, based on the known connection between the number of 0-gaps and the Euler characteristic of 2D digital objects. We also present two new, short and intuitive proofs of one of the two known equivalent formulae for the number of $(n-2)$-gaps in nD digital objects.

Keywords: Digital objects · Digital topology · Gaps
Euler characteristic

1 Introduction

Topological analysis of images and shapes is an active research field, important in many application domains. Two numerical topological descriptors of digital objects, the number of gaps and the Euler characteristic, have been widely investigated in the literature. Establishing the relations between these descriptors and the number of cells of different types in the decomposition of the digital object O into a cell complex Q enables a better understanding and a deeper insight into the topological structure of the object O and complex Q.

Intuitively, gaps in a digital object O are locations in O through which a discrete curve can penetrate [6]. They play an important role in ray-casting based rendering of digital curves and surfaces [15,46], and in particular of digital planes [1,24,30]. The notion of a gap is closely related to the notion of well-composedness [4,35,36]. The number of gaps characterizes the topological structure of the object [10]. The Euler characteristic is another basic, locally computable topological descriptor. In 2D, it is equal to the number of connected components of the object O minus the number of holes in O.

Several different formulae for the number of 0-gaps in a 2D [9,10] and 1-gaps in a 3D digital object O [38] have been proposed, in terms of the number of cells in the cubical complex Q associated with the object O (and the Euler characteristic of O [9]).

For the number of $(n-2)$-gaps in an nD digital object O, there are two such formulae. One [6,11], expresses the number of gaps in O through the total number of cells of dimension n, $n-1$ and $n-2$, and the number of interior cells of dimension $n-2$ in the cubical complex Q associated with O. This formula was used to obtain some combinatorial relations for digital curves [6,11]. Relations

© Springer Nature Switzerland AG 2018
R. P. Barneva et al. (Eds.): IWCIA 2018, LNCS 11255, pp. 3–16, 2018.
https://doi.org/10.1007/978-3-030-05288-1_1

between the dimension of a hypersurface (and in particular a digital hyperplane) and the types of gaps the hypersurface may possess [6,8], and good pairs of adjacency relations in nD [8] were established.

The other formula [39] expresses the number of $(n-2)$-gaps in O through the number of boundary cells in Q of dimension $n-1$ and $n-2$. It is obtained by defining several new notions in the discrete space and deriving many interesting relations between various types of cells in Q. The number of 0-gaps in 2D, obtained through the 2D specialization of this formula, together with the number of 2-, 1- and 0-cells in Q, was related to the dimension of the 2D digital object O [40]. A relation between the dimension and the Euler characteristic of 2D digital objects was also established [12].

The contributions of this paper are:

- Several new formulae for the number of 0-gaps in 2D, obtained from the known formulae for the Euler characteristic of a 2D digital object O [25,43,45] and the relation [9] between the number of gaps in O and its Euler characteristic.
- Two alternative, short and intuitive proofs for one [39] of the two equivalent formulae for the number of $(n-2)$-gaps in nD digital objects. One proof is combinatorial, and the other is graph theoretical.

2 Preliminaries

We introduce some basic notions on the cubical grid [31,32], on gaps in digital objects in the cubical grid [6,9,24,38] and on the Euler characteristic of such objects in 2D [32].

2.1 The Cubical Grid

Definition 1. *An nD cubical grid is a set of closed unit n-cubes (voxels) centered at points in $\mathbb{Z}^n$, with faces parallel to the coordinate planes. The naturally associated (cubical) cell complex is composed of all voxels, and all their k-faces (k-cells), $0 \leq k \leq n-1$.*

Different types of adjacency relation are defined between the voxels (n-cells) in the grid, depending on their intersection.

Definition 2. *Two voxels are k-adjacent if they share a common k-cell. They are strictly k-adjacent if they are k-adjacent but not $(k+1)$-adjacent.*

In 2D, two pixels (2-cells) that share an edge or a vertex are 1- or 0-adjacent, respectively. In 3D, two voxels that share a square face, an edge or a vertex are 2-, 1- or 0-adjacent, respectively.

Combinatorial coordinate system is naturally defined for the cubical grid [33]. It addresses grid cells of all dimensions and enables easy navigation between them through integer arithmetics. We give some basic properties of cell coordinates and examples of the topological relations that will be used in the sequel. To obtain integer coordinate values for all cells, the grid is rescaled by factor 2 in all coordinate directions.

Definition 3. *Each cell in the cubical grid is assigned the combinatorial coordinates equal to the double of the Cartesian coordinates of its (bary)center.*

A k-cell has k even and $n - k$ odd coordinates. A voxel (n-cell) has n even, and a vertex (0-cell) has n odd coordinates.

The dimension, spatial position and relative orientation of a cell are encoded in its coordinates. For example, an n-tuple consisting of one even and $n - 1$ odd numbers represents an edge in the combinatorial coordinate system. The Cartesian coordinates of its center are obtained by dividing the n-tuple by 2. If the ith coordinate is even, the edge is parallel to the ith coordinate axis.

Topological incidence and adjacency relations between cells can be easily retrieved from the coordinate values.

Proposition 1. *Each k-cell e is bounded by $2^{k-i}\binom{k}{i}$ i-cells, $0 \leq i \leq k$, and bounds $2^{j-k}\binom{n-k}{j-k}$ j-cells, $k \leq j \leq n$.*

The boundary cells are obtained by changing $k - i$ even coordinates of e by ± 1. The coboundary cells are obtained by changing $j - k$ odd coordinates of e by ± 1. For example, a voxel is bounded by $2n$ $(n - 1)$-cells, that are obtained by changing one of the voxel coordinates by ± 1, and fixing the remaining $n - 1$ coordinates.

An $(n-1)$-cell is bounded by $2(n-1)$ $(n-2)$-cells, that are obtained by fixing the odd coordinate and changing one of the remaining $n - 1$ even coordinates by ± 1. It bounds two voxels, that are obtained by changing the odd coordinate of the $(n - 1)$-cell by ± 1.

An $(n - 2)$-cell has two odd coordinates and $n - 2$ even ones. It is incident to four voxels, that are obtained by changing each of the two odd coordinates by ± 1, and to four $(n - 1)$-cells, that are obtained by changing by ± 1 one and keeping the other of the two odd coordinates.

2.2   Gaps in Digital Objects

Definition 4. *An nD digital object O is a finite set of voxels in the cubical grid. The associated cubical complex is denoted as Q. It consists of all voxels in O and all their k-dimensional faces.*

The number of k-faces (k-cells) in Q is denoted as c_k. The voxels in O are called black (object) voxels. The voxels in the complement O^c of O are called white (background).

A $2^{n-k} \times 1^k$ block of voxels is called a $2^{n-k}1^k$-block, $0 \leq k \leq n$. The $2^{n-k}1^k$-block $B_k(e)$ centered at a k-cell e consists of 2^{n-k} voxels incident to e.

Definition 5. *A pair of strictly k-adjacent voxels through a k-cell e is called a k-tandem over e, $0 \leq k \leq n - 1$.*

Definition 6. *An nD digital object O has a k-gap at a k-cell e if $B_k(e) \backslash O$ is a k-tandem over e.*

An object O has an $(n-2)$-gap at an $(n-2)$-cell e if two (out of four) voxels incident to e (in the $2^2 1^{n-2}$-block $B_{n-2}(e)$) are black and strictly $(n-2)$-adjacent through e (and the other two are white and strictly $(n-2)$-adjacent through e). Thus, the black and white voxels alternate cyclically around the $(n-2)$-gap e.

In 2D, a 0-gap occurs at a vertex that is incident to two strictly 0-adjacent white pixels (and two black ones). In 3D, a 1-gap occurs at an edge incident to two strictly 1-adjacent white voxels (and two black ones). A 0-gap occurs at a vertex incident to two strictly 0-adjacent white voxels (and to six black ones). The number of k-gaps in an object is denoted as g_k.

Definition 7. *A boundary (free) k-cell in Q, $0 \le k \le n-1$, is a k-cell incident both to a voxel in O and a voxel in O^c. An interior cell is incident to voxels in O only.*

A k-cell e in Q is interior if the $2^{n-k}1^k$-block $B_k(e)$ centered at e is contained in O. Otherwise, e is a boundary k-cell [10,39]. The number of interior and boundary k-cells in Q is denoted as c'_k and c^*_k, respectively, and

$$c_k = c'_k + c^*_k.$$

If an nD object O has an $(n-2)$-gap at an $(n-2)$-cell e, then e is a boundary $(n-2)$-cell in Q, and all four $(n-1)$-cells incident to e are boundary $(n-1)$-cells in Q. For a non-gap boundary $(n-2)$-cell e in Q, two out of four incident $(n-1)$-cells are boundary $(n-1)$-cells in Q. These claims can be verified by examining the possible configurations of the four voxels in the block $B_{n-2}(e)$ [11,39], or by inspecting the combinatorial coordinates of the involved cells (see Sect. 2.1).

2.3   The Euler Characteristic of 2D Digital Objects

The Euler characteristic is one of the basic topological descriptors of a shape. It can be defined in two equivalent ways: through the topological properties related to the connectedness of O and through the number of cells in the cubical complex Q associated with O. In either case, its value depends on the chosen adjacency relation. We define it here for 2D digital objects.

Two pixels (2-cells) p and q in a 2D object O are k-connected in O, $k = 0, 1$, if there is a sequence of pixels in O, starting at p and ending at q, such that any two consecutive pixels in the sequence are k-adjacent. Connected k-components of O are maximal subsets of O with respect to k-connectedness. Their number is denoted as c^k. A hole is a finite connected component of the complement O^c of O. If connected components of O are counted with respect to 0-adjacency, then holes are counted with respect to 1-adjacency and vice versa. The number of holes with k-adjacency for O and $(1-k)$-adjacency for O^c is denoted as h^{1-k}. We denote as $\chi^k(O)$ the Euler characteristic with k-adjacency for black pixels and $(1-k)$-adjacency for white pixels, $k = 0, 1$.

Definition 8. *The Euler characteristic $\chi^k(O)$, $k = 0, 1$, of a 2D digital object O is equal to the number of connected components of O minus the number of holes in O, i.e.,*

$$\chi^k(O) = c^k - h^{1-k}.$$

For a 2D digital object with 0-adjacency, i.e., for the associated cubical complex Q, the Euler characteristic can be computed as the alternating sum of the number c_i of i-cells in Q, $i = 0, 1, 2$. For 1-adjacency, vertices exhibiting a 0-gap are duplicated. Thus,

$$\chi^0(O) = c_0 - c_1 + c_2,$$
$$\chi^1(O) = (c_0 + g_0) - c_1 + c_2.$$

The computation of the Euler characteristic of a 2D object O is a widely investigated research field. Many algorithms, and the corresponding formulae, were proposed in the literature, both for 0- and for 1-adjacency relation.

Some algorithms are based on relations between the Euler characteristic and the number of cells of various types in the complex Q [5,42,43,45] or in the dual complex [14,28,48]. Some algorithms examine the boundary curve C (composed of edges and vertices) of Q, and count the number of convex and concave vertices in C [13,25,29,43,44]. Others are based on counting different pixel configurations around the vertices in Q [25,47], or on the divide and conquer strategy [20,21]. Some are adapted to a specific data structure encoding the complex Q, such as quad-tree [23], skeleton [22] or run-length encoding [2,3,20,21,37,41,48,49]. Some algorithms adopt the topological definition of the Euler characteristic, and use a connected component labeling algorithm for counting the number of connected components and the number of holes [26,27].

3   Related Work

We review the formulae proposed in the literature for the number of 0-gaps in 2D, 1-gaps in 3D and $(n-2)$-gaps in nD digital objects.

3.1   0-Gaps in 2D Objects

Two equivalent [40] formulae were proposed for the number g_0 of 0-gaps in a 2D digital object O.

One [9] states that

$$g_0 = c_0 - 2(c_2 + c^0 - h^1) + c'_0,$$

where c^0 is the number of 0-components (maximal connected components of black pixels with respect to 0-adjacency), and h^1 is the number of 1-holes (maximal finite connected components of white pixels with respect to 1-adjacency).

The proof is by induction on the number of pixels. For the base case, the gap-free object O consists of a single black pixel, and $c_0 = 4$, $c_2 = 1$, $c^0 = 1$, $h^1 = 0$, $c'_0 = 0$. For the inductive step, all possible configurations of black and white pixels are examined in a 3×3 neighborhood of a pixel added to a digital object with n pixels for which the formula is valid.

An alternative formula for the number of gaps in 2D [10] expresses g_0 in terms of boundary cells in Q as

$$g_0 = c_1^* - c_0^* = c_1 - c_1' - c_0 + c_0'.$$

The proof is by induction on the number of pixels, and is based on examining the possible 3×3 configurations of pixels.

Another proof [7,12] of the formula

$$g_0 = c_1^* - c_0^*$$

uses the fact that the graph composed of boundary vertices and edges of O is Eulerian, and that each gap vertex is incident to four, and each non-gap vertex is incident to two edges. Since edges and vertices alternate on the Eulerian cycle,

$$c_1^* = c_0^* + g_0.$$

Using the Euler formula

$$c_0 - c_1 + c_2 = c^0 - h^1,$$

it follows that

$$g_0 = h^1 - c^0 + c_2 - c_1' + c_0'.$$

This relation was obtained independently in the context of calculating the number of holes in a 2D binary image [42]. The number of 0-gaps in 2D was related to the dimension of a digital object O [40].

3.2   1-Gaps in 3D Objects

One formula was proposed [38] for the number g_1 of 1-gaps in a 3D digital object O, namely

$$g_1 = 2c_2^* - c_1^*.$$

The proof is based on constructing a graph $G = (N, A)$, and using that the sum of vertex degrees is equal to twice the number of arcs. The nodes in N correspond to the boundary 2-cells in Q, and two nodes in N are connected through an arc in A if the corresponding 2-cells (square faces) share a common 1-cell (edge). Each non-gap boundary 1-cell is incident to two boundary 2-cells, and contributes $\binom{2}{2} = 1$ arc in A. Each 1-gap is incident to four boundary 2-cells, and contributes $\binom{4}{2} = 6$ arcs. The degree of a node depends on whether the corresponding 2-cell is incident to a 1-gap or not.

3.3 $(n-2)$-Gaps in nD Objects

Two formulae were proposed in the literature for the number g_{n-2} of $(n-2)$-gaps in an nD digital object O.

One [6,11] expresses the number of gaps through the total number of n-, $(n-1)$- and $(n-2)$-cells, and the number of interior $(n-2)$-cells in Q as

$$g_{n-2} = -2n(n-1)c_n + 2(n-1)c_{n-1} - c_{n-2} + c'_{n-2}. \tag{1}$$

The other [39] expresses this number in terms of boundary $(n-1)$- and $(n-2)$-cells in Q as

$$g_{n-2} = (n-1)c^*_{n-1} - c^*_{n-2}. \tag{2}$$

The proofs of both formulae rely on the regular structure of the cubical grid, in which the number of cells in the boundary and coboundary of a given k-cell is constant: each n-cell in Q is incident to $2n$ $(n-1)$-cells in Q; each $(n-1)$-cell is incident to one or two n-cells, depending if it is a boundary or interior $(n-1)$-cell in Q; each $(n-2)$-cell in Q is incident to 0 (if it is an interior cell), 2 (if it is a non-gap cell) or 4 (if it is an $(n-2)$-gap) boundary $(n-1)$-cells.

The equivalence of the two formulae was established [39], based on the following relation:

$$2nc_n = c_{n-1} + c'_{n-1}.$$

The relation follows from the fact that each of the c_n n-cells (voxels) in Q is bounded by $2n$ $(n-1)$-cells. Each boundary $(n-1)$-cell is incident to one voxel, and each interior $(n-1)$-cell is incident to two voxels [6,11] (see also Sect. 2.1). Thus, boundary $(n-1)$-cells are counted once, and interior $(n-1)$-cells are counted two times in $2nc_n$, i.e.,

$$2nc_n = c^*_{n-1} + 2c'_{n-1} = c^*_{n-1} + c'_{n-1} + c'_{n-1} = c_{n-1} + c'_{n-1}, \tag{3}$$

or equivalently

$$2nc_n = 2c_{n-1} - c^*_{n-1}.$$

4   Some New Formulae for the Number of 0-Gaps in 2D

We propose several new formulae for the number of 0-gaps in 2D digital objects.

(1) We obtain the first one from the known formula [43]

$$\chi^1 = \frac{1}{4}(c^*_1 - 2c'_1) + c'_0$$

for the Euler characteristic χ^1, proposed as an extension to arbitrary objects of the formula [5] valid for unit-width (without inner vertices) objects with 1-adjacency.

Let us consider a multigraph $G = (N, A)$, whose nodes correspond to maximal connected 1-components of O, and the arcs correspond to gaps at which such components are (0-)connected. Let us denote as $\chi^1(O_j)$ the Euler characteristic of such component O_j. If we iteratively add the arcs in A to the nodes in N, then each arc either connects two different connected components of nodes in N, or it creates a loop connecting two nodes from the same connected component of nodes in N (it creates a hole in G). In either case, each arc (each 0-gap) decreases the Euler characteristic by 1. The final graph G has the same Euler characteristic as the object O with 0-adjacency, i.e.,

$$\chi(G) = \sum_j \chi^1(O_j) - g_0 = \chi^0(O),$$

and

$$g_0 = \sum_j \chi^1(O_j) - \chi^0(O).$$

We use the Euler characteristic formula $\chi^1 = \frac{1}{4}(c_1^* - 2c_1') + c_0'$, and apply it on each connected component O_j. Using the fact that each inner or boundary cell in O is inner or boundary cell in some component O_j, we have

$$g_0 = \sum_j (\frac{1}{4}(c_1^*(O_j) - 2c_1'(O_j)) + c_0'(O_j)) - \chi^0(O) = \frac{1}{4}c_1^* - \frac{1}{2}c_1' + c_0' - \chi^0(O).$$

Using the definition of χ^0 as the alternating sum of i-cells, $i = 0, 1, 2$, we get

$$g_0 = \frac{1}{4}c_1^* - \frac{1}{2}c_1' + c_0' - c_0 + c_1 - c_2 = \frac{5}{4}c_1 + \frac{1}{2}c_1' - c_0^* - c_2.$$

The same formula follows from $g_0 = h^1 - c^0 + c_2 - c_1' + c_0'$ [7,12] and $4c_2 = c_1^* + 2c_1'$ (obtained by letting $n = 2$ in (3)).

(2) If we combine formula $g_0 = c_0 - 2(c_2 + c^0 - h^1) + c_0'$ for the number of 0-gaps in 2D with the definition of the Euler characteristic with 0-adjacency as an alternating sum of the number of i-cells in O, $i = 0, 1, 2$, we obtain

$$g_0 = 2c_1 - c_0^* - 4c_2.$$

(3) One of the first algorithms [25] for the computation of the Euler characteristic of a 2D digital object O counts the number of different pixel configurations in the 2×2 blocks around the grid vertices. The configurations Q_1, Q_3 and Q_D that affect the Euler characteristic are those having exactly one black (exactly one white) pixel, with other three pixels being white (black), and those having exactly two diagonally placed black pixels (and two white ones), respectively. The former two configurations correspond to convex and concave vertices in the boundary of O, respectively, and the latter ones correspond to 0-gaps, i.e., $|Q_D| = g_0$. The Euler characteristic is computed as follows:

$$\chi^0(O) = \frac{1}{4}|Q_1| + \frac{1}{4}|Q_3| - \frac{1}{2}g_0,$$

$$\chi^1(O) = \frac{1}{4}|Q_1| + \frac{1}{4}|Q_3| + \frac{1}{2}g_0.$$

From this, we get

$$g_0 = \frac{1}{2}|Q_1| + \frac{1}{2}|Q_3| - 2\chi^0(O),$$

$$g_0 = 2\chi^1(O) - \frac{1}{2}|Q_1| - \frac{1}{2}|Q_3|,$$

and the obvious relation

$$g_0 = \chi^1(O) - \chi^0(O).$$

The same relation can be obtained from $\chi^0(O) = c_0 - c_1 + c_2$ and $\chi^1(O) = (c_0 + g_0) - c_1 + c_2$ (see Sect. 2.3).

(4) Using the formula [45]

$$\chi^1(O) = c_0' - c_1' + c_2,$$

we obtain

$$g_0 = c_0' - c_1' + c_2 - \chi^0(O).$$

This is equivalent to the well-known expression of the Euler characteristic as the alternating sum of the number of i-cells in a complex, i.e.,

$$\chi^0(O) = c_0 - c_1 + c_2,$$

because $c_i = c_i' + c_i^*$, $i = 0, 1$, and $g_0 = c_1^* - c_0^*$ [10].

5   Two Alternative Proofs of Formula (2)

We give two new short proofs of formula (2), i.e., of the formula

$$c_{n-2}^* + g_{n-2} = (n-1)c_{n-1}^*.$$

The first proof is combinatorial, the second one is based on graph theory. Both proofs use the information on the number of incident cells of various dimensions for a given cell, obtained in a straightforward manner from the combinatorial coordinates, as detailed in Sect. 2.1.

(**First Proof**)

Note that c_{n-2}^* is the number of boundary $(n-2)$-cells that may or may not be $(n-2)$-gaps. Thus,

$$c_{n-2}^* = \bar{g}_{n-2}^* + g_{n-2},$$

where we denoted as $\bar{g}_{n-2}^*$ the number of non-gap boundary $(n-2)$-cells (called also totally boundary cells [6,11] or nubs [39]).

Let us consider the set of all ordered pairs (f, e), where f is a boundary $(n-1)$-cell and e is a boundary $(n-2)$-cell (non-gap or gap) incident to f. There are c_{n-1}^* cells f and $c_{n-2}^* = \bar{g}_{n-2}^* + g_{n-2}$ cells e.

Each boundary $(n-1)$ cell is incident to $2(n-1)$ boundary $(n-2)$-cells [6,11,39]. Each boundary non-gap $(n-2)$-cell is incident to two, and each $(n-2)$-gap is incident to four boundary $(n-1)$-cells. Consequently, each boundary $(n-1)$ cell is in $2(n-1)$, each boundary non-gap $(n-2)$-cell is in two and each $(n-2)$-gap is in four such pairs (f, e). Thus

$$2(n-1)c_{n-1}^* = 2\bar{g}_{n-2}^* + 4g_{n-2},$$
$$(n-1)c_{n-1}^* = \bar{g}_{n-2}^* + g_{n-2} + g_{n-2},$$
$$(n-1)c_{n-1}^* = c_{n-2}^* + g_{n-2}.$$

The existing proof [39] of formula (2) in essence reduces to this one. It uses various interesting relations between different types of cells in Q obtained by defining some new notions in the cubical grid.

(Second Proof)

Let us consider the graph $G = (N, A)$, where the nodes in N correspond to the boundary $(n-1)$-cells. There are two types of arcs in A. The first type is associated with non-gap boundary $(n-2)$-cells, and the second is associated with $(n-2)$-gaps. Each non-gap boundary $(n-2)$-cell is incident to two, and each $(n-2)$-gap is incident to four boundary $(n-1)$-cells. The two black and two white voxels incident to an $(n-2)$-gap e in the block $B_{n-2}(e)$ alternate cyclically around e. Thus, two of the four boundary $(n-1)$-cells incident to e are both incident to one of the two white voxels, and the other two of the four boundary $(n-1)$-cells are incident to the other white voxel.

We connect two nodes in N through an arc in A if the corresponding two boundary $(n-1)$-cells share a common boundary non-gap $(n-2)$-cell, or if they share a common $(n-2)$-gap and they are both incident to the same white voxel. Thus, each non-gap boundary $(n-2)$-cell generates one arc in A, and each $(n-2)$-gap generates two arcs in A. Each boundary $(n-1)$-cell is connected to exactly one $(n-1)$-cell across each of its $2(n-1)$ incident $(n-2)$-cells.

There are c_{n-1}^* nodes in N and $\bar{g}_{n-2}^* + 2g_{n-2}$ arcs in A. The degree of each node in N is equal to $2(n-1)$ (the number of non-gap or gap $(n-2)$-cells in the boundary of the $(n-1)$-cell corresponding to the node).

The sum of degrees of the nodes in N is equal to twice the number of arcs in A, i.e.,

$$2(n-1)c_{n-1}^* = 2(\bar{g}_{n-2}^* + 2g_{n-2}),$$
$$(n-1)c_{n-1}^* = \bar{g}_{n-2}^* + g_{n-2} + g_{n-2},$$
$$(n-1)c_{n-1}^* = c_{n-2}^* + g_{n-2}.$$

A similar idea of constructing the dual graph from boundary 2- and 1-cells was used in the proof of the formula in the special case $n = 3$ [38]. The difference is that in our graph $G = (N, A)$, each $(n-2)$-gap contributes only two (and not six, as in the 3D case) arcs to A, and each node in N has degree $2(n-1)$ independently of whether the corresponding boundary $(n-1)$-cell is incident to some $(n-2)$-gaps or not.

6 Conclusion and Future Work

Two research fields in the area of topological image analysis, namely the computation of the number of 0-gaps and the computation of the Euler characteristic of 2D digital objects, are closely related. This is demonstrated by an expression [9] that links the number of 0-gaps in a 2D digital object with its Euler characteristic.

Using this connection, we give several new formulae for the number of 0-gaps in 2D, obtained from some known formulae for the Euler characteristic of a 2D digital object O [25,43,45]. Alternatively, the formulae for the number of 0-gaps can be used to obtain new relations between the Euler characteristic and the number of cells of various types in the associated cubical complex.

We give two new short and intuitive proofs of one [39] of the two known formulae for the number of $(n-2)$-gaps in nD digital objects. The two proofs rely on the information on the number of cells in the boundary and coboundary of a given cell, readily obtained from the cell coordinates (see Sect. 2.1). Combinatorial coordinates were defined recently for some nontraditional 3D grids (such as body centered cubic, face centered cubic and the diamond grids) [16–19], alternative to the traditional cubic one, and were proven useful for standard image processing tasks such as boundary extraction and computation of the Euler characteristic [16,34].

The number of 1-gaps in 3D digital objects is well-understood, due to the fact that each edge exhibiting a 1-gap is incident to exactly four boundary faces, and all other boundary edges are incident to exactly two such faces. The computation of the number of 0-gaps in 3D digital objects does not lend itself to a straightforward generalization, as vertices exhibiting a 0-gap are not uniquely characterized by the number of incident boundary cells. It would be interesting to investigate the connection between the Euler characteristic and the number of 0-gaps in 3D digital objects.

Acknowledgement. This work has been partially supported by the Ministry of Education and Science of the Republic of Serbia within the Project No. 34014.

References

1. Andres, E., Acharya, R., Sibata, C.H.: Discrete analytical hyperplanes. CVGIP: Graph. Model Image Process. **59**(5), 302–309 (1997)
2. Bishnu, A., Bhattacharya, B.B., Kundu, M.K., Murthy, C.A., Acharya, T.: On-chip computation of Euler number of a binary image for efficient database search. In: Proceedings of the 2001 International Conference on Image Processing, ICIP, pp. 310–313 (2001)
3. Bishnu, A., Bhattacharya, B.B., Kundu, M.K., Murthy, C.A., Acharya, T.: A pipeline architecture for computing the Euler number of a binary image. J. Syst. Archit. **51**(8), 470–487 (2005)
4. Boutry, N., Géraud, T., Najman, L.: How to make nD images well-composed without interpolation. In: 2015 IEEE International Conference on Image Processing, ICIP 2015, pp. 2149–2153 (2015)

5. Bribiesca, E.: Computation of the Euler number using the contact perimeter. Comput. Math. Appl. **60**(5), 1364–1373 (2010)
6. Brimkov, V.E.: Formulas for the number of $(n-2)$-gaps of binary objects in arbitrary dimension. Discrete Appl. Math. **157**(3), 452–463 (2009)
7. Brimkov, V.E., Barneva, R.: Linear time constant-working space algorithm for computing the genus of a digital object. In: Bebis, G., et al. (eds.) ISVC 2008. LNCS, vol. 5358, pp. 669–677. Springer, Heidelberg (2008). https://doi.org/10.1007/978-3-540-89639-5_64
8. Brimkov, V.E., Klette, R.: Border and surface tracing - theoretical foundations. IEEE Trans. Pattern Anal. Mach. Intell. **30**(4), 577–590 (2008)
9. Brimkov, V.E., Maimone, A., Nordo, G.: An explicit formula for the number of tunnels in digital objects. CoRR abs/cs/0505084 (2005). http://arxiv.org/abs/cs/0505084
10. Brimkov, V.E., Maimone, A., Nordo, G.: Counting gaps in binary pictures. In: Reulke, R., Eckardt, U., Flach, B., Knauer, U., Polthier, K. (eds.) IWCIA 2006. LNCS, vol. 4040, pp. 16–24. Springer, Heidelberg (2006). https://doi.org/10.1007/11774938_2
11. Brimkov, V.E., Moroni, D., Barneva, R.: Combinatorial relations for digital pictures. In: Kuba, A., Nyúl, L.G., Palágyi, K. (eds.) DGCI 2006. LNCS, vol. 4245, pp. 189–198. Springer, Heidelberg (2006). https://doi.org/10.1007/11907350_16
12. Brimkov, V.E., Nordo, G., Barneva, R.P., Maimone, A.: Genus and dimension of digital images and their time- and space-efficient computation. Int. J. Shape Model. **14**(2), 147–168 (2008)
13. Chen, L.: Determining the number of holes of a 2D digital component is easy. CoRR abs/1211.3812 (2012)
14. Chen, M., Yan, P.: A fast algorithm to calculate the Euler number for binary images. Pattern Recogn. Lett. **8**(5), 295–297 (1988)
15. Cohen-Or, D., Kaufman, A.E.: 3D line voxelization and connectivity control. IEEE Comput. Graph. Appl. **17**(6), 80–87 (1997)
16. Čomić, L., Magillo, P.: Repairing 3D binary images using the BCC grid with a 4-valued combinatorial coordinate system. Inf. Sci., to appear
17. Čomić, L., Nagy, B.: A topological coordinate system for the diamond cubic grid. Acta Crystallogr. Sect. A **72**(5), 570–581 (2016)
18. Čomić, L., Nagy, B.: A combinatorial coordinate system for the body-centered cubic grid. Graph. Models **87**, 11–22 (2016)
19. Čomić, L., Nagy, B.: A topological 4-coordinate system for the face centered cubic grid. Pattern Recogn. Lett. **83**, 67–74 (2016)
20. Dey, S., Bhattacharya, B.B., Kundu, M.K., Acharya, T.: A Fast algorithm for computing the euler number of an image and its VLSI implementation. In: 13th International Conference on VLSI Design (VLSI Design 2000), pp. 330–335 (2000)
21. Dey, S., Bhattacharya, B.B., Kundu, M.K., Bishnu, A., Acharya, T.: A Co-processor for computing the Euler number of a binary image using divide-and-conquer strategy. Fundam. Inf. **76**(1–2), 75–89 (2007)
22. Díaz-de-León S., J.L., Sossa-Azuela, J.H.: On the computation of the Euler number of a binary object. Pattern Recognit. **29**(3), 471–476 (1996)
23. Dyer, C.R.: Computing the Euler number of an image from Its quadtree. Comput. Graph. Image Process. **13**, 270–276 (1980)
24. Françon, J., Schramm, J.-M., Tajine, M.: Recognizing arithmetic straight lines and planes. In: Miguet, S., Montanvert, A., Ubéda, S. (eds.) DGCI 1996. LNCS, vol. 1176, pp. 139–150. Springer, Heidelberg (1996). https://doi.org/10.1007/3-540-62005-2_12

25. Gray, S.: Local properties of binary images in two dimensions. IEEE Trans. Comput. **20**, 551–561 (1971)
26. He, L., Chao, Y.: A very fast algorithm for simultaneously performing connected-component labeling and Euler number computing. IEEE Trans. Image Process. **24**(9), 2725–2735 (2015)
27. He, L., Chao, Y., Suzuki, K.: An algorithm for connected-component labeling, hole labeling and Euler number computing. J. Comput. Sci. Technol. **28**(3), 468–478 (2013)
28. He, L., Yao, B., Zhao, X., Yang, Y., Chao, Y., Ohta, A.: A graph-theory-based algorithm for Euler number computing. IEICE Trans. **98**–D(2), 457–461 (2015)
29. Imiya, A., Eckhardt, U.: The Euler characteristic of discrete object. In: Ahronovitz, E., Fiorio, C. (eds.) DGCI 1997. LNCS, vol. 1347, pp. 161–174. Springer, Heidelberg (1997). https://doi.org/10.1007/BFb0024838
30. Kenmochi, Y., Imiya, A.: Combinatorial topologies for discrete planes. In: Nyström, I., Sanniti di Baja, G., Svensson, S. (eds.) DGCI 2003. LNCS, vol. 2886, pp. 144–153. Springer, Heidelberg (2003). https://doi.org/10.1007/978-3-540-39966-7_13
31. Klette, R., Rosenfeld, A.: Digital Geometry. Geometric Methods for Digital Picture Analysis. Morgan Kaufmann Publishers, San Francisco (2004)
32. Kong, T.Y., Rosenfeld, A.: Digital topology: introduction and survey. Comput. Vis. Graphi. Image Process. **48**(3), 357–393 (1989)
33. Kovalevsky, V.A.: Geometry of Locally Finite Spaces (Computer Agreeable Topology and Algorithms for Computer Imagery). Editing House Dr. Bärbel Kovalevski, Berlin (2008)
34. Lachaud, J.-O.: Coding cells of digital spaces: a framework to write generic digital topology algorithms. Electron. Notes Discrete Math. **12**, 337–348 (2003)
35. Latecki, L.J.: 3D well-composed pictures. CVGIP: Graph. Model Image Process. **59**(3), 164–172 (1997)
36. Latecki, L.J., Eckhardt, U., Rosenfeld, A.: Well-composed sets. Comput. Vis. Image Underst. **61**(1), 70–83 (1995)
37. Lin, X., Sha, Y., Ji, J., Wang, Y.: A proof of image Euler number formula. Sci. China Ser. F: Inf. Sci. **49**(3), 364–371 (2006)
38. Maimone, A., Nordo, G.: On 1-gaps in 3D digital objects. Filomat **22**(3), 85–91 (2011)
39. Maimone, A., Nordo, G.: A formula for the number of $(n - 2)$-gaps in digital n-objects. Filomat **27**(4), 547–557 (2013)
40. Maimone, A., Nordo, G.: A note on dimension and gaps in digital geometry. Filomat **31**(5), 1215–1227 (2017)
41. Rosenfeld, A., Kak, A.C.: Digital Picture Processing. Academic Press, London (1982)
42. Sossa, H.: On the number of holes of a 2-D binary object. In: 14th IAPR International Conference on Machine Vision Applications, MVA, pp. 299–302 (2015)
43. Sossa-Azuela, J.H., Cuevas-Jiménez, E.B., Zaldivar-Navarro, D.: Alternative way to compute the Euler number of a binary image. J. Appl. Res. Technol. **9**, 335–341 (2011)
44. Sossa-Azuela, J., Santiago-Montero, R., Pérez-Cisneros, M., Rubio-Espino, E.: Computing the Euler number of a binary image based on a vertex codification. J. Appl. Res. Technol. **11**(3), 360–370 (2013)
45. Sossa-Azuela, J., Santiago-Montero, R., Pérez-Cisneros, M., Rubio-Espino, E.: Alternative formulations to compute the binary shape Euler number. IET Comput. Vis. **8**(3), 171–181 (2014)

46. Yagel, R., Cohen, D., Kaufman, A.E.: Discrete ray tracing. IEEE Comput. Graph. Appl. **12**(5), 19–28 (1992)
47. Yao, B., et al.: An efficient strategy for bit-quad-based Euler number computing algorithm. IEICE Trans. Inf. Syst. **E97.D**(5), 1374–1378 (2014)
48. Zenzo, S.D., Cinque, L., Levialdi, S.: Run-based algorithms for binary image analysis and processing. IEEE Trans. Pattern Anal. Mach. Intell. **18**(1), 83–89 (1996)
49. Zhang, Z., Moss, R.H., Stoecker, W.V.: A novel morphological operator to calculate Euler number. In: Medical Imaging and Augmented Reality: First International Workshop, MIAR, pp. 226–228 (2001)

Fixpoints of Iterated Reductions
with Equivalent Deletion Rules

Kálmán Palágyi$^{(\boxtimes)}$ and Gábor Németh

Department of Image Processing and Computer Graphics,
University of Szeged, Szeged, Hungary
{palagyi,gnemeth}@inf.u-szeged.hu

Abstract. A reduction transforms a binary picture only by deleting
some black points to white ones. Sequential reductions traverse the black
points of a picture, and focus on the actually visited point for possible deletion, while parallel reductions delete all 'deletable' black points
simultaneously. Two reductions are called equivalent if they produce the
same result for each input picture. A deletion rule is said to be equivalent if it provides a pair of equivalent sequential and parallel reductions.
Thinning and shrinking algorithms iterate reductions until no points are
deleted. If a black point is not deleted in an iteration step, it is taken
into consideration again in the next step. This work examine fixpoints of
iterated reductions with equivalent deletion rules, i.e., 'survival' points
whose rechecking is not needed in the remaining iterations.

Keywords: Digital geometry and topology · Equivalent reduction
Thinning

1   Introduction

A *digital binary picture* [5,9] on a grid is a mapping that assigns a color of
black or *white* to each grid element that is called a *point*. A *reduction* [2] transforms a binary picture only by changing some black points to white ones, which
is referred to as *deletion*. *Sequential reductions* focus on a single black point
for possible deletion at a time as it is illustrated in Algorithm 1, while *parallel
reductions* can delete all black points from a picture that satisfy their deletion
rules simultaneously, see Algorithm 2. Iterated reductions play a key role in various topological algorithms, e.g. *thinning* [3,7,17] (i.e., a layer-by-layer erosion
for approximating *skeleton-like features* in a topology–preserving way) or *reduc-
tive shrinking* [2] (i.e., that is capable of producing a minimal structure that is
topologically equivalent to the original object).

Reductions generally classify the set of black points B into two subsets:
elements of the *constraint set* $C(B) \subseteq B$ may not be deleted, and the set of
interesting points $X = B \setminus C(B)$ are formed by the potentially deletable points.
The deletion rule R associated with the reduction in question is evaluated only
for the elements in X, and black points in $C(B)$ are not taken into consideration.

© Springer Nature Switzerland AG 2018
R. P. Barneva et al. (Eds.): IWCIA 2018, LNCS 11255, pp. 17–27, 2018.
https://doi.org/10.1007/978-3-030-05288-1_2

Algorithm 1. Sequential reduction (thinning/shrinking iteration step)

Input: set of black points B,
            constraint set $C(B)$,
            permutation Π of set $B \setminus C(B)$, and
            deletion rule R
Output: set of black points SB
`// specifying the set of interesting points` X
$X = B \setminus C(B)$
`// initializing the set` SB
$SB = B$
`// traversal of set` X `according to permutation` Π
foreach $p \in X$ **do**
  if R $(SB \cap S_{\mathsf{R}}(p),\ C(B) \cap S_{\mathsf{R}}(p)\ ) =$ **true** **then**
    `// deletion of the single point` p
    $SB = SB \setminus \{p\}$

Algorithm 2. Parallel reduction (thinning/shrinking iteration step)

Input: set of black points B,
            constraint set $C(B)$, and
            deletion rule R
Output: set of black points PB
`// specifying the set of interesting points` X
$X = B \setminus C(B)$
`// specifying the set of deletable points` D
$D = \{\, p \mid p \in X$ and R $(B \cap S_{\mathsf{R}}(p),\ C(B) \cap S_{\mathsf{R}}(p)\ ) =$ **true** $\}$
`// simultaneous deletion of all points in` D
$PB = B \setminus D$

A sequential reductions (see Algorithm 1) requires a permutation of the interesting points, since the produced output may depend on the order in which the points are selected by the **foreach** loop. In contrast, the output picture produced by a parallel reduction is uniquely determined by Algorithm 2. For practical purposes it is assumed that all input pictures are *finite* (i.e., they contain finitely many black points).

A *deletion rule* R is a mapping that assigns a value of **true** or **false** to all possible point configurations in the support of R. The *support* [3] of R applied at a point p is a minimal set of points whose values determine whether p is deleted by R. In Algorithms 1 and 2, the support of deletion rule R with respect to an interesting point p is denoted by $S_{\mathsf{R}}(p)$. Note that all existing thinning and shrinking algorithms use local supports with 'small' diameters.

An interesting point $p \in X$ is *deletable* by deletion rule R from the set of points $Y \subseteq B$ with the constraint set $C(B)$, if R$(Y \cap S_{\mathsf{R}}(p), C(B) \cap S_{\mathsf{R}}(p)) =$ **true**. If R$(Y \cap S_{\mathsf{R}}(p), C(B) \cap S_{\mathsf{R}}(p)) =$ **false**, then point p is called *non-deletable* by R. Note that $Y = B$ in parallel reductions (see Algorithm 2), and $Y = SB \subseteq B$ in the sequential case (see Algorithm 1). By comparing the two approaches, we can state that in the parallel case the initial set of black points B is examined when the deletion rule is evaluated for elements in X. In contrast, when a sequential reduction is performed, the set of black points SB is dynamically altered. Constraints of existing thinning algorithms contain the set of *interior points* [5] (i.e., black points that are not *border points* [5]). Since thinning differs from shrinking, *endpoints* [3] (i.e., some border points that provide important geometrical information relative to the shape of the objects) or accumulated *isthmuses* [1] (i.e., generalization of curve and surface interior points) are preserved. Thinning algorithms that do not delete *endpoints* are said to be *endpoint-based* ones.

Sequential reductions with the same deletion rule may produce different results for different visiting orders (raster scans) of the interesting points. A sequential reduction is called *order-independent* if the result of Algorithm 1 does not depend on the selected permutation Π [16]. Two reductions are said to be *equivalent* if they produce the same result for any input pictures [13]. A deletion rule is called *equivalent* if it provides a pair of equivalent parallel and sequential reductions [13].

If an interesting point is not deleted in a phase of an iterated reduction, it may be interesting in the next iteration step. Thus the deletability of all 'survival' points are to be checked again in the next iteration. In their previous work [15], the authors characterized 'safe' points that are in the skeleton-like feature produced by any endpoint-based sequential 2D and 3D thinning algorithm, and they reported a computationally efficient implementation scheme for these algorithms.

Here, our attention is focussed on equivalent deletion rules, and we examine fixpoints of iterated pairs of equivalent sequential and parallel reductions. Rechecking of these points are not needed, as they must remain black in the forthcoming iteration step. An implementation scheme for iterated pairs of equivalent sequential and parallel reductions is also presented.

2   Basic Notions and Results

Next, we apply the fundamental concepts of digital topology as reviewed by Kong and Rosenfeld [5]. Despite the fact that there are other approaches based on cellular/cubical complexes [6], here we shall consider the 'conventional paradigm' of digital topology.

For the sake of brevity, the expression $\mathsf{R}(X \cap S_{\mathsf{R}}(p), C(Y) \cap S_{\mathsf{R}}(p))$ is simply replaced by $\mathsf{R}_p(X, C(Y))$ in the rest of this paper (i.e., indication of the support of a deletion rule is omitted).

A $(k, \bar{k})$ *(binary digital) picture* on a grid $\mathcal{V}$ is a quadruple $(\mathcal{V}, k, \bar{k}, B)$ [5], where $B \subseteq \mathcal{V}$ denotes the set of *black points*, and each point in $\mathcal{V} \setminus B$ is said to be a *white point*; adjacency relations k and $\bar{k}$ are assigned to B and $\mathcal{V} \setminus B$, respectively. In order to avoid connectivity paradoxes, it is generally assumed that $k \neq \bar{k}$ [5,9]. Since all studied relations are reflexive and symmetric, their transitive closure form equivalence relations, and their equivalence classes are said to be *components*. A *black component* or an *object* is a k-component of B, while a *white component* is a $\bar{k}$-component of $\mathcal{V} \setminus B$.

A point $p \in B$ is an *interior point* if all further points being $\bar{k}$-adjacent to p are in B. Let $I(B)$ denote the set of all interior points in B. A black point is said to be a *border point* if it is not an interior point. A black point is a *curve-endpoint* if it is k-adjacent to exactly one further black point.

A reduction in a 2D picture is *topology-preserving* if each object in the input picture contains exactly one object in the output picture, and each white component in the output picture contains exactly one white component in the input picture [5]. There is an additional concept called *tunnel* (which doughnuts have) in 3D pictures [5]. Topology preservation implies that eliminating or creating any tunnel is not allowed.

A black point is said to be *simple* for a set of black points (or in a picture) if its deletion is a topology-preserving reduction [4,5]. Note that simplicity is a local property, and only border points may be simple.

One of the authors gave a sufficient condition for deletion rules that provide pairs of equivalent and topology-preserving sequential and parallel reductions [13]. The following definitions and theorems are to summarize the corresponding results:

Definition 1 [13]. *Let* R *be a deletion rule, let B be the set of black points in a picture, let $p \in B \setminus C(B)$ be an interesting point with respect to the constraint set $C(B)$, and let us now assume that $\mathsf{R}_p(B, C(B)) = \mathbf{true}$. Then* R *is general if $\mathsf{R}_q(B, C(B)) = \mathsf{R}_q(B \setminus \{p\}, C(B))$ for any point $q \in B \setminus (C(B) \cup \{p\})$.*

Theorem 1 [13]. *A deletion rule* R *is order-independent if and only if* R *is general.*

Theorem 2 [13]. *A deletion rule* R *is equivalent if* R *is general.*

Definition 2 [13]. *A deletion rule* R *is* general-simple *if* R *is general, and it deletes only simple points.*

Theorem 3 [13]. *A (sequential or parallel) reduction is topology-preserving if its deletion rule is general-simple.*

3   Characterization of Fixpoints

Let us define a fixpoint in a picture with respect to an iterated reduction.

Definition 3. *Let B be the set of black points in a picture, let* R *be the deletion rule assigned to an iterated reduction, and let $C(B)$ be the constraint. Then an interesting point $p \in B \setminus C(B)$ is called a* fixpoint *if*

$$\mathsf{R}_p(B, C(B)) = \mathsf{R}_p(B \setminus Q, C(B \setminus Q)) = \mathbf{false},$$

where $Q = \{\, q \mid q \in B \setminus C(B) \text{ and } \mathsf{R}_q(B, C(B)) = \mathbf{true} \,\}$.

The following lemma states a useful property of general deletion rules:

Lemma 1. *Let B be the set of black points in a picture, let R be a general deletion rule with respect to the constraint $C(B)$, and let $p \in B \setminus C(B)$ be any interesting point. Then*

$$\mathsf{R}_p\left(B, C(B)\right) = \mathsf{R}_p\left(B \setminus Q, C(B)\right),$$

where $Q = \{\, q \mid q \in B \setminus C(B) \text{ and } \mathsf{R}_q(B, C(B)) = \textbf{true} \,\} \setminus \{p\}$.

Proof. Since R is general, by Theorem 2, deletion rule R provides a pair of equivalent sequential and parallel reductions. Now let us examine the sequential case (see Algorithm 1).

If $\mathsf{R}_p(B, C(B))$ is evaluated, p's turn comes before visiting any point in Q. Similarly, if $\mathsf{R}_p(B \setminus Q, C(B))$ is taken into consideration, the deletability of point p is evaluated after the deletion of set Q. Since R is general, by Theorem 1, deletion rule R is order-independent.

Thus $\mathsf{R}_p(B, C(B)) = \mathsf{R}_p(B \setminus Q, C(B))$. □

Let us now introduce the concepts of a descendent constraint set and a narrows point.

Definition 4. *Let $C(B)$ be the constraint with respect to the set of black points B in a picture. Then that constraint is called a* descendent *if $C(B') \subseteq C(B)$ for any $B' \subset B$.*

Definition 5. *Let B be the set of black points in a picture, let R be a deletion rule with respect to the constraint $C(B)$. Then a point $p \in B \setminus C(B)$ is said to be a* narrows point *if $S_\mathsf{R}(p) \cap C(B) = \emptyset$.*

Now let us state a characterization of fixpoints for general deletion rules.

Theorem 4. *Let B be the set of black points in a picture, let R be a general deletion rule with respect to the descendent constraint $C(B)$, and let $p \in B \setminus C(B)$ be a point such that $\mathsf{R}_p\left(B, C(B)\right) = \textbf{false}$. Then p is a fixpoint if it is a narrows point.*

Proof. Let $p \in B \setminus C(B)$ be a narrows point.

Since R is general, by Lemma 1, $\mathsf{R}_p(B, C(B)) = \mathsf{R}_p(B \setminus Q, C(B))$, where $Q = \{\, q \mid q \in B \setminus C(B) \text{ and } \mathsf{R}_q(B, C(B)) = \textbf{true} \,\} \setminus \{p\}$.

As the given constraint is descendent, $C(B \setminus Q) \subseteq C(B)$. Therefore, $C(B \setminus Q) \cap S_\mathsf{R}(p) \subseteq C(B) \cap S_\mathsf{R}(p)$.

Since p is a narrows point, by Definition 5, $S_\mathsf{R}(p) \cap C(B) = \emptyset$. Thus $C(B \setminus Q) \cap S_\mathsf{R}(p) = C(B) \cap S_\mathsf{R}(p)$.

Consequently, $\mathsf{R}_p(B \setminus Q, C(B)) = \mathsf{R}_p(B \setminus Q, C(B \setminus Q))$.

As p is undeletable, $\mathsf{R}_p(B, C(B)) = \textbf{false}$. Thus, $\mathsf{R}_p(B \setminus Q, C(B \setminus Q)) = \textbf{false}$.

Hence, by Definition 3, p is a fixpoint. □

Let us state the following proposition as an immediate consequence of Theorem 4.

Proposition 1. *Narrows points are fixpoints of iterated reductions with general deletion rules and descendent constraints.*

The following proposition designates a descendent constraint:

Proposition 2. *The set of interior points $I(B)$ in a picture forms a descendent constraint for arbitrary reductions.*

Proof. Recall that a point $p \in B$ is an interior point in picture $(\mathcal{V}, k, \bar{k}, B)$ if all points that are $\bar{k}$-adjacent to p are in B, and it is a border point if it is not an interior point. It is obvious that any reduction can change some interior points into border points, but it cannot produce an interior point from a border point. Thus $I(B') \subseteq I(B)$ for any $B' \subset B$. □

4 Implementing Equivalent Thinning Algorithms

One of the authors proposed a computationally efficient implementation scheme for arbitrary thinning algorithms [10,11]. His 'blanket' method utilizes the followings:

- Only border points in the current picture can be deleted in each iteration step (i.e., we do not have to evaluate the deletion rules for interior points). Thus the set of interior points may be viewed as constraint.
- Only some simple points in the current picture may be deleted (since topology preservation is the most important requirement to be complied with).

The 'blanket' implementation is described by Algorithm 3. It uses a list named *border_list* for storing the border points in the input and the interim pictures, thus the repeated scans of the entire (actual) array storing the picture are avoided. In input array A, the value '1' corresponds to black points in the picture to be thinned, and the value '0' is assigned to white ones. In order to avoid storing more than one copy of a border point in *border_list*, A is a three-value array in which value of '2' corresponds to border points to be checked.

If a border point is deleted, all interior points that are 'adjacent' to it become border points. These brand new border points of the resulted picture are added to the *border_list*. It is assumed that the given thinning algorithms act on $(k, \bar{k})$ pictures, thus 'adjacent' means $\bar{k}$-adjacent. Note that some thinning algorithms do not apply the same deletion rule at each iteration [3,10,12].

The thinning process terminates when no more points are deleted (i.e., stability is reached). After thinning, all points having a nonzero value in array A belong to the produced skeleton-like feature.

With the help of Propositions 1 and 2, we can propose an advanced implementation scheme for thinning algorithms with general(-simple) deletion rules and interior points as constraint (see Algorithm 4). In this case, array A represents a four-color picture, where

---

Algorithm 3. 'Blanket' Sequential Thinning

Input: array A storing the picture to be thinned
Output: array A storing the picture with the produced skeleton-like feature
`// collecting border points`
$border\_list \leftarrow$ < empty list >
foreach element p in array A **do**
    if $A[p] = 1$ and p is a border point **then**
        $border\_list \leftarrow border\_list + <p>$
        $A[p] \leftarrow 2$

`// thinning process`
repeat
    $number\_of\_deleted\_points \leftarrow 0$
    foreach point p in $border\_list$ **do**
        if p is 'deletable' **then**
            `// deletion`
            $border\_list \leftarrow border\_list - <p>$
            $A[p] \leftarrow 0$
            $number\_of\_deleted\_points \leftarrow number\_of\_deleted\_points +1$
            `// list updating`
            foreach point q being 'adjacent' to p **do**
                if $A[q] = 1$ **then**
                    $A[q] \leftarrow 2$
                    $border\_list \leftarrow border\_list + <q>$

until $number\_of\_deleted\_points > 0$;

- a value of '0' corresponds to white points,
- a value of '1' is assigned to interior points,
- a value of '2' corresponds to border points to be checked (i.e., elements of the current $border\_list$), and
- a value of '3' is assigned to each detected fixpoint (see Definition 3).

5 Efficiency of Selecting Fixpoints

In [14], one of the authors proved that the deletion rule of the 2D parallel thinning algorithm proposed by Manzanera et al. [8] called **MBPL2002** is general-simple. Thus, by Theorem 2, the reduction (and the entire algorithm) with that deletion rule is equivalent. Note that algorithm **MBPL2002** acts on $(8, 4)$ pictures on grid $\mathbb{Z}^2$ (i.e., the planar square grid).

The efficiency of the proposed implementation scheme (see Algorithm 4) over the 'blanket' one (see Algorithm 3) is illustrated in Table 1 for eight test images. The examined algorithm **MBPL2002** was run on a usual PC under Linux (Fedora 27–64 bit), using a 3.30 GHz 4x Intel Core i5-2500 CPU. (Note that just the iterative thinning process itself was considered here; reading the input volume, the look-up-table associated to the deletion rule, and writing the

---

Algorithm 4. Equivalent Thinning with Selecting Fixpoints

Input: array A storing the $(k, \bar{k})$ picture to be thinned
general-simple deletion rule R
Output: array A storing the picture with the produced skeleton-like feature
// collecting border points
$border\_list \leftarrow <$ empty list $>$
foreach element p in array A **do**
$\quad$ **if** $A[p] = 1$ and p is a border point **then**
$\quad\quad$ $border\_list \leftarrow border\_list + < p >$
$\quad\quad$ $A[p] \leftarrow 2$

// thinning process
repeat
$\quad$ $number\_of\_deleted\_points \leftarrow 0$
$\quad$ **foreach** point p in $border\_list$ **do**
$\quad\quad$ **if** p is 'deletable' by R **then**
$\quad\quad\quad$ // deletion
$\quad\quad\quad$ $border\_list \leftarrow border\_list - < p >$
$\quad\quad\quad$ $A[p] \leftarrow 0$
$\quad\quad\quad$ $number\_of\_deleted\_points \leftarrow number\_of\_deleted\_points + 1$
$\quad\quad\quad$ // list updating
$\quad\quad\quad$ **foreach** point q being $\bar{k}$-adjacent to p **do**
$\quad\quad\quad\quad$ **if** $A[q] = 1$ **then**
$\quad\quad\quad\quad\quad$ $A[q] \leftarrow 2$
$\quad\quad\quad\quad\quad$ $border\_list \leftarrow border\_list + < q >$
$\quad\quad$ **else if** there is no interior point in $S_R(p)$ **then**
$\quad\quad\quad$ // designating a fixpoint
$\quad\quad\quad$ $border\_list \leftarrow border\_list - < p >$
$\quad\quad\quad$ $A[p] \leftarrow 3$
until $number\_of\_deleted\_points > 0$;

---

output image were not taken into account but the processing involved is not excessive.)

If a test image contains a black disk, all border points have interior neighbors. Thus there are no narrows points in this picture. That is why we selected test images containing objects with some 'slim' and some 'fat' parts. After a few iterations, 'slim' parts are reduced into sets of fixpoints, hence the residues of these parts are not investigated in the remaining thinning phases.

We can state that the proposed implementation scheme (see Algorithm 4) can be twice or more times as fast as the 'blanket' approach (see Algorithm 3). Note that in their recent work, the authors reported an advanced method for implementing sequential endpoint-based thinning algorithms [15]. Combining the previously proposed implementation scheme with Algorithm 4 provide a computationally more efficient implementation of endpoint-based equivalent thinning algorithms. (Note that algorithm **MBPL2002** [8] falls into this category.)

Table 1. Computation times (in sec.) of algorithm **MBPL2002** for eight test images. The 'blanket' and the 'proposed' implementation schemes are under comparison.

test image	size	number of object points	number of skeletal points	'blanket' comp. time **A**	'proposed' comp. time **B**	speed-up **A/B**
	1212×902	219 051	3 669	0.104	0.045	**2.322**
	2300×1422	888 734	8 467	0.461	0.182	**2.529**
	800×753	140 482	4 355	0.078	0.030	**2.617**
	800×800	182 972	3 803	0.101	0.038	**2.647**
	624×700	108 871	3 299	0.067	0.023	**2.935**
	1000×1011	154 104	4 284	0.126	0.033	**3.831**
	2050×2050	1 040 892	14 159	1.004	0.219	**4.592**
	1266×1269	268 560	8 342	0.284	0.057	**4.980**

6   Conclusions

In this paper, fixpoints of iterated reductions with equivalent deletion rules are examined. The presented characterization of these fixpoints provides a computationally efficient implementation scheme for equivalent thinning algorithms. It is to be emphasized that the reported results are absolutely general, as they are valid for arbitrary equivalent reductions acting on any digital binary pictures.

Acknowledgments. This research was supported by the project "Integrated program for training new generation of scientists in the fields of computer science", no EFOP-3.6.3-VEKOP-16-2017-0002. The project has been supported by the European Union and co-funded by the European Social Fund.

References

1. Bertrand, G., Couprie, M.: Transformations topologiques discrètes. In: Coeurjolly, D., Montanvert, A., Chassery, J-M. (eds.) Géométrie discrète et images numériques, pp. 187–209. Hermès Science Publications (2007)
2. Hall, R.W., Kong, T.Y., Rosenfeld, A.: Shrinking binary images. In: Kong, T.Y., Rosenfeld, A. (eds.) Topological Algorithms for Digital Image Processing, pp. 31–98. Elsevier Science, Amsterdam (1996)
3. Hall, R.W.: Parallel connectivity-preserving thinning algorithms. In: Kong, T.Y., Rosenfeld, A. (eds.) Topological Algorithms for Digital Image Processing, pp. 145–179. Elsevier Science, Amsterdam (1996)
4. Kong, T.Y.: On topology preservation in 2-D and 3-D thinning. Int. J. Pattern Recognit. Artif. Intell. **9**, 813–844 (1995). https://doi.org/10.1142/S0218001495000341
5. Kong, T.Y., Rosenfeld, A.: Digital topology: introduction and survey. Comput. Vis. Graph. Image Process. **48**, 357–393 (1989). https://doi.org/10.1016/0734-189X(89)90147-3
6. Kovalevsky, V.A.: Geometry of Locally Finite Spaces. Publishing House, Berlin (2008). https://doi.org/10.1142/S0218654308001178
7. Lam, L., Lee, S.-W., Suen, C.Y.: Thinning methodologies - a comprehensive survey. IEEE Trans. Pattern Anal. Mach. Intell. **14**, 869–885 (1992). https://doi.org/10.1109/34.161346
8. Manzanera, M., Bernard, T.M., Pretêux, F., Longuet, B.: n-dimensional skeletonization: a unified mathematical framework. J. Electron. Imaging **11**, 25–37 (2002). https://doi.org/10.1117/1.1506930
9. Marchand-Maillet, S., Sharaiha, Y.M.: Binary Digital Image Processing: A Discrete Approach. Academic Press, Cambridge (2000). https://doi.org/10.1117/1.1326456
10. Palágyi, K., Tschirren, J., Hoffman, E.A., Sonka, M.: Quantitative analysis of pulmonary airway tree structures. Comput. Biol. Med. **36**, 974–996 (2006). https://doi.org/10.1016/j.compbiomed.2005.05.004
11. Palágyi, K.: A 3D fully parallel surface-thinning algorithm. Theor. Comput. Sci. **406**, 119–135 (2008). https://doi.org/10.1016/j.tcs.2008.06.041
12. Palágyi, K., Németh, G., Kardos, P.: Topology preserving parallel 3D thinning algorithms. In: Brimkov, V.E., Barneva, R.P. (eds.) Digital Geometry Algorithms: Theoretical Foundations and Applications to Computational Imaging. LNCVB, vol. 2, pp. 165–188. Springer, Dordrecht (2012). https://doi.org/10.1007/978-94-007-4174-4_6
13. Palágyi, K.: Equivalent sequential and parallel reductions in arbitrary binary pictures. Int. J. Pattern Recognit. Artif. Intell. **28**, 1460009-1–1460009-16 (2014). https://doi.org/10.1142/S021800141460009X
14. Palágyi, K.: Equivalent 2D sequential and parallel thinning algorithms. In: Barneva, R.P., Brimkov, V.E., Šlapal, J. (eds.) IWCIA 2014. LNCS, vol. 8466, pp. 91–100. Springer, Cham (2014). https://doi.org/10.1007/978-3-319-07148-0_9
15. Palágyi, K., Németh, G.: Endpoint-based thinning with designating safe skeletal points. In: Barneva, R.P., Brimkov, V.E., Kulczycki, P., Tavares, J.M.R.S. (eds.) CompIMAGE 2018. LNCS. Springer, Heidelberg (2018). In press

16. Ranwez, V., Soille, P.: Order independent homotopic thinning for binary and grey tone anchored skeletons. Pattern Recognit. Lett. **23**, 687–702 (2002). https://doi.org/10.1016/S0167-8655(01)00146-5

17. Suen, C.Y., Wang, P.S.P. (eds.): Thinning Methodologies for Pattern Recognition. Series in Machine Perception and Artificial Intelligence, vol. 8. World Scientific, Singapore (1994). https://doi.org/10.1142/9789812797858_0009

Parallel Contextual Array Insertion Deletion Grammar

D. G. Thomas[1(✉)], S. James Immanuel[2], Atulya K. Nagar[3],
and Robinson Thamburaj[2]

[1] Department of Science and Humanities, Saveetha School of Engineering, SIMATS,
Chennai 602 105, India
dgthomasmcc@yahoo.com
[2] Department of Mathematics, Madras Christian College,
Tambaram, Chennai 600 059, India
james_imch@yahoo.co.in, robinson@mcc.edu.in
[3] Department of Mathematics and Computer Science, Liverpool Hope University,
Liverpool, UK
nagara@hope.ac.uk

Abstract. We introduce a new grammar, called parallel contextual array insertion deletion grammar and show that it has a strictly higher generative power than a system generating recognizable 2D-picture language and Siromoney context-sensitive matrix grammar.

Keywords: Rectangular array · Parallel contextual array grammar
Insertion and deletion

1 Introduction

A study on two-dimensional languages or picture languages, which are the extensions of string language theory is of current interest. The techniques related to the formal string languages are being adapted for developing methods to study the problem of picture generation and description, where pictures are considered as connected, digitized finite arrays in the two-dimensional plane. Over the past several years this literature on array grammars and array acceptors has seen a steady growth.

In [17,18], the need for array rewriting rules for picture languages has been investigated for the isometric array generation. For generalizing the Chomsky grammars to arrays, we have rewriting rules that allow replacement of a sub-array of a picture with another sub-array. In [19], Siromoney et al. has proposed a simple generative model to describe digital pictures, viewed as rectangular arrays of terminals, called as two-dimensional matrix grammar.

While Chomsky grammars are the origin for the study of formal language theory, but in 1969 Marcus [11] introduced another class of grammars, called contextual grammars. Contextual grammars offer novel insight to a number of

R. P. Barneva et al. (Eds.): IWCIA 2018, LNCS 11255, pp. 28–42, 2018.
https://doi.org/10.1007/978-3-030-05288-1_3

issues central to formal language theory and hence have been intensively investigated by formal language theorists. A contextual grammar produces a language by starting from a given finite set of strings and adding, iteratively, pairs of strings(called as contexts), associated to sets of strings(called selectors) to the string already obtained. Many variants of contextual grammars have been considered in the literature and investigated from a mathematical point of view [1, 13].

Extension of these grammars to 2-dimensional array structures has been attempted in [4,5,8,10,16]. In [5] a new and simple approach is considered for description of array, generalizing the concept of contextual grammars. In [16] a model of external array column contextual grammar generating arrays has been considered. In [10] another model of array contextual grammars is introduced. But these models are different from parallel contextual array grammars, in [8]. In the former model [16], only column contexts are considered although arrays generated can be non-rectangular. In the latter model [10], instead of a finite set of contextual rules, a language of arrays, which may be an infinite set, is used for choosing the contexts. In the parallel contextual array grammars, row as well as column contexts are allowed and the contextual rules are finite.

In the study of two dimensional languages as there is no definite hierarchy in analogy with Chomskian hierarchy for string languages, we are motivated to look for a powerful two dimensional grammar than the existing grammars. In this paper, we introduce one such grammar, using two operations array insertion and array deletion, called parallel contextual array insertion deletion grammar, based on the modified contextual style of internal parallel contextual array grammars considered in [8,21] which has applications in floor designing and kolam pattern generation. In Sect. 2, we define parallel contextual array insertion deletion grammar and give an example. In Sect. 3, we give the comparison of the family of picture languages generated by this new grammar with the families of local languages, recognizable languages and Siromoney matrix languages, thus bringing out their generative powers.

2   The New Grammar

In this section we define parallel contextual array insertion deletion grammar and give an example.

Let V be a finite alphabet, V^* be the set of words over Σ including the empty word λ. $V^+ = V^* - \{\lambda\}$. For $w \in V^*$ and $a \in V$, $|w|_a$ denotes the number of occurrences of a in w. An array consists of finitely many symbols from V that are arranged as rows and columns in some particular order and is written in the form,

$$A = \begin{matrix} a_{11} & \cdots & a_{1n} \\ \vdots & \ddots & \vdots \\ a_{m1} & \cdots & a_{mn} \end{matrix} \quad \text{or in short } A = [a_{ij}]_{m \times n}, \text{ for all } a_{ij} \in \Sigma, i = 1, 2, \ldots, m \text{ and}$$

$j = 1, 2, \ldots, n$. The set of all arrays over V is denoted by V^{**} which also includes the empty array Λ (zero rows or zero columns). $V^{++} = V^{**} - \{\Lambda\}$. For $a \in V$, $|A|_a$ denotes the number of occurrences of a in A. The column concatenation of $A = \begin{matrix} a_{11} & \cdots & a_{1p} \\ \vdots & \ddots & \vdots \\ a_{m1} & \cdots & a_{mp} \end{matrix}$, and $B = \begin{matrix} b_{11} & \cdots & b_{1q} \\ \vdots & \ddots & \vdots \\ b_{n1} & \cdots & b_{nq} \end{matrix}$, defined only when $m = n$, is given

by $A \oplus B = \begin{matrix} a_{11} & \cdots & a_{1p} & b_{11} & \cdots & b_{1q} \\ \vdots & \ddots & \vdots & \vdots & \ddots & \vdots \\ a_{m1} & \cdots & a_{mp} & b_{n1} & \cdots & b_{nq} \end{matrix}$. As $1 \times n$-dimensional arrays can be easily

interpreted as words of length n (and vice versa), we will then write their column catenation by juxtaposition (as usual). Similarly, the row concatenation of A

and B, defined only when $p = q$, is given by $A \ominus B = \begin{matrix} a_{11} & \cdots & a_{1p} \\ \vdots & \ddots & \vdots \\ a_{m1} & \cdots & a_{mp} \\ b_{11} & \cdots & b_{1q} \\ \vdots & \ddots & \vdots \\ b_{n1} & \cdots & b_{nq} \end{matrix}$. The empty

array acts as the identity for column and row catenation of arrays of arbitrary dimensions.

Definition 1. *Let V be a finite alphabet. A column array context over V is of the form $c = \dfrac{u_1}{u_2} \in V^{**}$, u_1, u_2 are of size $1 \times p$, $p \geq 1$.*

A row array contexts over V is of the form, $r = u_1 \, u_2 \in V^{**}$, u_1, u_2 are of size $p \times 1$, $p \geq 1$.

Definition 2. *The parallel column contextual insertion operation is defined as follows: Let V be an alphabet, C be a finite subset of V^{**} whose elements are the column array contexts and $\varphi_c^i : V^{**} \times V^{**} \to 2^C$ be a choice mapping. For arrays, $A = \begin{matrix} a_{1j} & \cdots & a_{1(k-1)} \\ \vdots & \ddots & \vdots \\ a_{mj} & \cdots & a_{m(k-1)} \end{matrix}, B = \begin{matrix} a_{1k} & \cdots & a_{1(l-1)} \\ \vdots & \ddots & \vdots \\ a_{mk} & \cdots & a_{m(l-1)} \end{matrix}, j < k < l, a_{ij} \in V$, we define*

$\hat{\varphi}_c^i : V^{**} \times V^{**} \to V^{**}$ such that, $I_c \in \hat{\varphi}_c^i(A, B)$, $I_c = \begin{matrix} u_1 \\ u_2 \\ \vdots \\ u_m \end{matrix}$ if $c_i = \dfrac{u_i}{u_{i+1}} \in$

$\varphi_c^i \begin{pmatrix} a_{ij} & \cdots & a_{i(k-1)} & a_{ik} & \cdots & a_{i(l-1)} \\ a_{(i+1)j} & \cdots & a_{(i+1)(k-1)} & a_{(i+1)k} & \cdots & a_{(i+1)(l-1)} \end{pmatrix}, c_i \in C, 1 \leq i \leq m-1$, not all need to be distinct.

Given an array $W = [a_{ij}]_{m \times n}, a_{ij} \in V$ such that $W = X_1 \oplus A \oplus B \oplus X_2$,

$X_1 = \begin{matrix} a_{11} & \cdots & a_{1(j-1)} \\ \vdots & \ddots & \vdots \\ a_{m1} & \cdots & a_{m(j-1)} \end{matrix}, A = \begin{matrix} a_{1j} & \cdots & a_{1(k-1)} \\ \vdots & \ddots & \vdots \\ a_{mj} & \cdots & a_{m(k-1)} \end{matrix}, B = \begin{matrix} a_{1k} & \cdots & a_{1(l-1)} \\ \vdots & \ddots & \vdots \\ a_{mk} & \cdots & a_{m(l-1)} \end{matrix}, X_2 =$

$$a_{1l} \cdots a_{1n}$$
$$\vdots \quad \ddots \quad \vdots \quad , 1 \le j \le k < l \le n+1 \ (or) \ 1 \le j < k \le l \le n+1, \ we \ write \ W \Rightarrow_i Z$$
$$a_{ml} \cdots a_{mn}$$

if $Z = X_1 \oplus A \oplus I_c \oplus B \oplus X_2$, such that $I_c \in \hat{\varphi}_c^i(A, B)$. I_c is called as the inserted column context. We say that Z is obtained from W by parallel column contextual insertion operation. The following 4 special cases for $W = X_1 \oplus A \oplus B \oplus X_2$ are also considered,

1. For $j = 1$, we have $X_1 = \Lambda$.
2. For $j = k = 1$, we have $X_1 = \Lambda$ and $A = \Lambda$.
3. For $l = n + 1$, we have $X_2 = \Lambda$.
4. For $k = l = n + 1$, we have $B = \Lambda$ and $X_2 = \Lambda$.

The case $j = k = l$ is not possible for performing parallel column contextual insertion operation.

Similarly we can define parallel row contextual insertion operation also.

Definition 3. *The parallel column contextual deletion operation is defined as follows: Let V be an alphabet, C be a finite subset of V^{**} whose elements are the column array contexts and $\varphi_c^d : V^{**} \times V^{**} \to 2^C$ be a choice mapping. For*

$$arrays, \ A = \begin{matrix} a_{1j} & \cdots & a_{1(k-1)} \\ \vdots & \ddots & \vdots \\ a_{mj} & \cdots & a_{m(k-1)} \end{matrix} \ , B = \begin{matrix} a_{1(k-p)} & \cdots & a_{1(l-1)} \\ \vdots & \ddots & \vdots \\ a_{m(k-p)} & \cdots & a_{m(l-1)} \end{matrix} \ , j < k < l, a_{ij} \in V, \ we$$

$$define \ \hat{\varphi}_c^d : V^{**} \times V^{**} \to V^{**} \ such \ that, \ D_c \in \hat{\varphi}_c^d(A, B), \ D_c = \begin{matrix} u_1 \\ u_2 \\ \vdots \\ u_m \end{matrix} \ if \ c_i = \begin{matrix} u_i \\ u_{i+1} \end{matrix} \in$$

$$\varphi_c^d \begin{pmatrix} a_{ij} & \cdots & a_{i(k-1)} & a_{i(k+p)} & \cdots & a_{i(l-1)} \\ a_{(i+1)j} & \cdots & a_{(i+1)(k-1)} & a_{(i+1)(k+p)} & \cdots & a_{(i+1)(l-1)} \end{pmatrix}, c_i \in C, 1 \le i \le m-1, \ not$$

all need to be distinct.

Given an array $W = [a_{ij}]_{m \times n}, a_{ij} \in V$ such that $W = X_1 \oplus A \oplus D_c \oplus B \oplus X_2$,

$$X_1 = \begin{matrix} a_{11} & \cdots & a_{1(j-1)} \\ \vdots & \ddots & \vdots \\ a_{m1} & \cdots & a_{m(j-1)} \end{matrix} \ , A = \begin{matrix} a_{1j} & \cdots & a_{1(k-1)} \\ \vdots & \ddots & \vdots \\ a_{mj} & \cdots & a_{m(k-1)} \end{matrix} \ , B = \begin{matrix} a_{1(k+p)} & \cdots & a_{1(l-1)} \\ \vdots & \ddots & \vdots \\ a_{m(k+p)} & \cdots & a_{m(l-1)} \end{matrix} \ , X_2 =$$

$$a_{1l} \cdots a_{1n}$$
$$\vdots \quad \ddots \quad \vdots \quad , 1 \le j \le k < l \le n+1, \ we \ write \ W \Rightarrow_d Z \ if \ Z = X_1 \oplus A \oplus B \oplus X_2,$$
$$a_{ml} \cdots a_{mn}$$

such that $D_c \in \hat{\varphi}_c^d(A, B)$. D_c is called as the deleted column context. We say that Z is obtained from W by parallel column contextual deletion operation. The following 4 special cases for $W = X_1 \oplus A \oplus D_c \oplus B \oplus X_2$ are also considered,

1. For $j = 1$ we have $X_1 = \Lambda$.
2. For $j = k = 1$, we have $X_1 = \Lambda$ and $A = \Lambda$.
3. For $l = n + 1$, we have $X_2 = \Lambda$.

4. For $k + p = l = n + 1$, we have $B = \Lambda$ and $X_2 = \Lambda$.

Similarly we can define parallel row contextual deletion operation also.

Definition 4. *A parallel contextual array insertion deletion grammar is defined as $G = (V, T, M, C, R, \varphi_c^i, \varphi_r^i, \varphi_c^d, \varphi_r^d)$, where V is an alphabet, $T \subseteq V$ is a terminal alphabet, M is a finite subset of V^{**} called the base of G, C is a finite subset of V^{**} called column array contexts, R is a finite subset of V^{**} called row array contexts, $\varphi_c^i : V^{**} \times V^{**} \to 2^C$, $\varphi_r^i : V^{**} \times V^{**} \to 2^R$, $\varphi_c^d : V^{**} \times V^{**} \to 2^C$, $\varphi_r^d : V^{**} \times V^{**} \to 2^R$, are the choice mappings which perform the parallel column contextual insertion, row contextual insertion, column contextual deletion and row contextual deletion operations, respectively.*

The insertion derivation with respect to G is a binary relation $\Rightarrow_i$ on V^{**} and is defined as $W \Rightarrow_i Z$, where $W, Z \in V^{**}$ if and only if $W = X_1 ⓧ A ⓧ B ⓧ X_2$, $Z = X_1 ⓧ A ⓧ I_c ⓧ B ⓧ X_2$ or $W = X_3 ⊖ A ⊖ B ⊖ X_4$, $Z = X_3 ⊖ A ⊖ I_r ⊖ B ⊖ X_4$ for some $X_1, X_2, X_3, X_4 \in V^{**}$ and I_c, I_r are inserted column and row contexts obtained by the parallel column or row contextual insertion operations according to the choice mappings.

The deletion derivation with respect to G is a binary relation $\Rightarrow_d$ on V^{**} and is defined as $W \Rightarrow_d Z$, where $W, Z \in V^{**}$ if and only if $W = X_1 ⓧ A ⓧ D_c ⓧ B ⓧ X_2$, $Z = X_1 ⓧ A ⓧ B ⓧ X_2$ or $W = X_3 ⊖ A ⊖ D_r ⊖ B ⊖ X_4$, $Z = X_3 ⊖ A ⊖ B ⊖ X_4$ for some $X_1, X_2, X_3, X_4 \in V^{**}$ and D_c, D_r are deleted column and row contexts with respect to the parallel column or row contextual deletion operations according to the choice mappings.

The direct derivation with respect to G is a binary relation $\Rightarrow_{i,d}$ on V^{**} which is either $\Rightarrow_i$ or $\Rightarrow_d$.

Definition 5. *Let $G = (V, T, M, C, R, \varphi_c^i, \varphi_r^d, \varphi_c^d, \varphi_r^d)$ be a parallel contextual array insertion deletion grammar. The language generated by G, denoted by $L(G)$ is defined as,*

$$L(G) = \{ Z \in T^{**} | \exists W \in M \text{ with } W \Rightarrow_{i,d}^* Z \}.$$

The family of all array languages generated by parallel contextual array insertion deletion grammar is denoted by PCAIDG.

We now give an example.

Example 1. Let $G = (V, T, M, C, R, \varphi_c^i, \varphi_r^d, \varphi_c^d, \varphi_r^d)$ be a parallel contextual array insertion deletion grammar where,

$$V = \{X, Y, \bullet\}, \ T = \{X, \bullet\}, \ M = \left\{ \begin{matrix} \bullet & X & \bullet \\ X & X & \bullet \\ \bullet & \bullet & \bullet \end{matrix} \right\},$$

$$C \quad = \quad \left\{ \begin{matrix} \bullet \ Y \ X \\ \bullet \ Y \ X \end{matrix}, \quad \begin{matrix} \bullet \ Y \ X \\ X \ Y \ X \end{matrix}, \quad \begin{matrix} X \ Y \ X \\ X \ Y \ X \end{matrix}, \quad \begin{matrix} X \ Y \ X \\ \bullet \ Y \ \bullet \end{matrix}, \quad \begin{matrix} \bullet \ Y \ \bullet \\ \bullet \ Y \ \bullet \end{matrix}, \right.$$

$$\left. \begin{matrix} Y \ \bullet \ Y \\ Y \ \bullet \ Y \end{matrix} \right\},$$

$$R \quad = \quad \left\{ \begin{matrix} \bullet\ \bullet \\ Y\ Y \\ X\ X \end{matrix},\ \begin{matrix} \bullet\ Y \\ Y\ Y \\ X\ Y \end{matrix},\ \begin{matrix} Y\ X \\ Y\ Y \\ Y\ X \end{matrix},\ \begin{matrix} X\ X \\ Y\ Y \\ X\ X \end{matrix},\ \begin{matrix} X\ Y \\ Y\ Y \\ X\ Y \end{matrix},\ \begin{matrix} Y\ \bullet \\ Y\ Y \\ Y\ \bullet \end{matrix}, \right.$$

$$\left. \begin{matrix} \bullet\ \bullet \\ Y\ Y \\ \bullet\ \bullet \end{matrix},\ \begin{matrix} Y\ Y \\ \bullet\ \bullet \end{matrix},\ \begin{matrix} Y\ Y \\ \bullet\ Y \end{matrix},\ \begin{matrix} Y\ Y \\ Y\ \bullet \end{matrix},\ \begin{matrix} Y\ Y \\ Y\ Y \end{matrix} \right\}.$$

$$\varphi_c^i \begin{bmatrix} \bullet\ X \\ \bullet'\,X \end{bmatrix} = \left\{ \begin{matrix} \bullet\ Y\ X \\ \bullet\ Y\ X \end{matrix} \right\},\ \varphi_c^i \begin{bmatrix} \bullet\ X \\ X'\,X \end{bmatrix} = \left\{ \begin{matrix} \bullet\ Y\ X \\ X\ Y\ X \end{matrix} \right\},\ \varphi_c^i \begin{bmatrix} X\ X \\ X'\,X \end{bmatrix} =$$

$$\left\{ \begin{matrix} X\ Y\ X \\ X\ Y\ X \end{matrix} \right\},\ \varphi_c^i \begin{bmatrix} X\ X \\ \bullet',\bullet \end{bmatrix} = \left\{ \begin{matrix} X\ Y\ X \\ \bullet\ Y\ \bullet \end{matrix} \right\},\ \varphi_c^i \begin{bmatrix} \bullet\ \bullet \\ \bullet',\bullet \end{bmatrix} = \left\{ \begin{matrix} \bullet\ Y\ \bullet \\ \bullet\ Y\ \bullet \end{matrix},\ \begin{matrix} Y\ \bullet \\ Y\ \bullet \end{matrix} \right\},$$

$$\varphi_c^i \begin{bmatrix} X\ \bullet \\ X'\,\bullet \end{bmatrix} = \left\{ \begin{matrix} Y\ \bullet \\ Y\ \bullet \end{matrix} \right\},\ \varphi_c^i \begin{bmatrix} X\ \bullet \\ \bullet',\bullet \end{bmatrix} = \left\{ \begin{matrix} Y\ \bullet \\ Y\ \bullet \end{matrix} \right\}$$

$$\varphi_r^i \left[\bullet\ \bullet, X\ X \right] = \left\{ \begin{matrix} \bullet\ \bullet \\ Y\ Y \\ X\ X \end{matrix} \right\},\ \varphi_r^i \left[\bullet\ Y, X\ Y \right] = \left\{ \begin{matrix} \bullet\ Y \\ Y\ Y \\ X\ Y \end{matrix} \right\},\ \varphi_r^i \left[Y\ X, Y\ X \right] =$$

$$\left\{ \begin{matrix} Y\ X \\ Y\ Y \\ Y\ X \end{matrix} \right\},\ \varphi_r^i \left[X\ X, X\ X \right] = \left\{ \begin{matrix} X\ X \\ Y\ Y \\ X\ X \end{matrix} \right\},\ \varphi_r^i \left[X\ Y, X\ Y \right] = \left\{ \begin{matrix} X\ Y \\ Y\ Y \\ X\ Y \end{matrix} \right\},$$

$$\varphi_r^i \left[Y\ \bullet, Y\ \bullet \right] = \left\{ \begin{matrix} Y\ \bullet \\ Y\ Y \\ Y\ \bullet \end{matrix},\ \begin{matrix} Y\ Y \\ Y\ \bullet \end{matrix} \right\},\ \varphi_r^i \left[\bullet\ \bullet, \bullet\ \bullet \right] = \left\{ \begin{matrix} \bullet\ \bullet \\ Y\ Y \\ \bullet\ \bullet \end{matrix},\ \begin{matrix} Y\ Y \\ \bullet\ \bullet \end{matrix} \right\},$$

$$\varphi_r^i \left[X\ X, \bullet\ \bullet \right] = \left\{ \begin{matrix} Y\ Y \\ \bullet\ \bullet \end{matrix} \right\},\ \varphi_r^i \left[X\ Y, \bullet\ Y \right] = \left\{ \begin{matrix} Y\ Y \\ \bullet\ Y \end{matrix} \right\},\ \varphi_r^i \left[Y\ X, Y\ \bullet \right] =$$

$$\left\{ \begin{matrix} Y\ Y \\ Y\ \bullet \end{matrix} \right\}$$

$$\varphi_c^d \begin{bmatrix} \bullet\ X \\ \bullet'\,X \end{bmatrix} = \left\{ \begin{matrix} Y \\ Y \end{matrix} \right\},\ \varphi_c^d \begin{bmatrix} \bullet\ X \\ Y'\,Y \end{bmatrix} = \left\{ \begin{matrix} Y \\ Y \end{matrix} \right\},\ \varphi_c^d \begin{bmatrix} Y\ Y \\ X'\,X \end{bmatrix} = \left\{ \begin{matrix} Y \\ Y \end{matrix} \right\},\ \varphi_c^d \begin{bmatrix} X\ X \\ X'\,X \end{bmatrix} =$$

$$\left\{ \begin{matrix} Y \\ Y \end{matrix} \right\},\ \varphi_c^d \begin{bmatrix} X\ X \\ Y'\,Y \end{bmatrix} = \left\{ \begin{matrix} Y \\ Y \end{matrix} \right\},\ \varphi_c^d \begin{bmatrix} Y\ Y \\ \bullet',\bullet \end{bmatrix} = \left\{ \begin{matrix} Y \\ Y \end{matrix} \right\},\ \varphi_c^d \begin{bmatrix} \bullet\ \bullet \\ \bullet',\bullet \end{bmatrix} = \left\{ \begin{matrix} Y \\ Y \end{matrix} \right\},$$

$$\varphi_c^d \begin{bmatrix} X\ \bullet \\ X'\,\bullet \end{bmatrix} = \left\{ \begin{matrix} Y \\ Y \end{matrix} \right\},\ \varphi_c^d \begin{bmatrix} X\ \bullet \\ Y'\,Y \end{bmatrix} = \left\{ \begin{matrix} Y \\ Y \end{matrix} \right\},\ \varphi_c^d \begin{bmatrix} Y\ Y \\ X'\,\bullet \end{bmatrix} = \left\{ \begin{matrix} Y \\ Y \end{matrix} \right\}.$$

$$\varphi_r^d \left[\bullet\ \bullet, X\ X \right] = \{ Y\ Y \},\ \varphi_r^d \left[\bullet\ X, X\ X \right] = \{ Y\ Y \},\ \varphi_r^d \left[X\ X, X\ X \right] =$$
$$\{ Y\ Y \},\ \varphi_r^d \left[X\ \bullet, X\ \bullet \right] = \{ Y\ Y \},\ \varphi_r^d \left[\bullet\ \bullet, \bullet\ \bullet \right] = \{ Y\ Y \},\ \varphi_r^d \left[X\ X, \bullet\ \bullet \right] =$$
$$\{ Y\ Y \},\ \varphi_r^d \left[X\ \bullet, \bullet\ \bullet \right] = \{ Y\ Y \}.$$

$$L(G) = \left\{ \begin{pmatrix} (\bullet)_n \\ (X)_n \\ (\bullet)_n \end{pmatrix}^n \begin{pmatrix} (X)_n \\ (X)_n \\ (\bullet)_n \end{pmatrix}^n \begin{pmatrix} (\bullet)_n \\ (\bullet)_n \\ (\bullet)_n \end{pmatrix}^n \middle| n \geq 1 \right\}.$$

In fact $L(G)$ contains pictures which are the reflections of L's with respect to a vertical line with arms of same proportion. ie.,
$$X\ X\ \bullet,$$

with illustrations:

```
          • • X X • •
          • • X X • •
      • X • X X X X • •
  X X • X X X X • •
  • • •   • • • • • •
          • • • • • •
```

```
• • • X X X • • •
• • • X X X • • •
• • • X X X • • •
X X X X X X • • •
X X X X X X • • • , . . .
X X X X X X • • •
• • • • • • • • •
• • • • • • • • •
• • • • • • • • •
```

3   Results

In this section we compare the generative power of $PCAIDG$ with that of other families of picture languages available in the literature [6,7,19].

Definition 6 (Local Two-dimensional Languages). *Given a picture A of size $m \times n$, we denote by $B_{h,k}(A)$, for $h \leq m, k \leq n$, the set of all sub-pictures of A of size $h \times k$. We call a square picture of size 2×2 as a tile. Given a picture A of size $m \times n$, $\hat{A}$ denotes a picture of size $(m+2) \times (n+2)$ obtained by surrounding A with a special boundary symbol $\# \notin V$.*

A two-dimensional language $L \subseteq V^{**}$ is **local** *if there exists a finite set T of tiles over the alphabet $V \cup \{\#\}$ such that $L = \{A \in V^{**} | B_{2,2}(\hat{A}) \subseteq T\}$.*

We consider the set T as the set of possible blocks of size 2×2 of pictures that belong to L. The language L is local if, given such a set T, we can exactly retrieve the language L and we write $L = L(T)$. The empty picture Λ belongs to L if and only if T contains the tile with four $\#$ symbols. The family of local picture languages is denoted by LOC.

Definition 7 (Tiling Recognizable Languages). *A tiling system (TS) is a 4-tuple $T_S = (\Sigma, V, T, \pi)$, where Σ and V are two finite alphabets, T is the finite set of tiles over the alphabet $V \cup \{\#\}$ and $\pi : V \to \Sigma$ is a projection. The tiling system T_S defines a language L over the alphabet Σ as follows: $L = \pi(L')$ where $L' = L(T)$ is the local language over V corresponding to the set of tiles T. We write $L = L(T_S)$. A language $L \subseteq \Sigma^{**}$ is recognizable by tiling systems (or tiling recognizable) if there exists a tiling system $T_S = (\Sigma, V, T, \pi)$*

such that $L = L(T_S)$. *REC* denotes the family of all two-dimensional languages recognizable by tiling system. In other words, $L \in REC$ if it is a projection of some local language.

Theorem 1. *PCAIDG is closed under projection.*

Proof. We consider a parallel contextual array insertion deletion grammar $G = (V, T, M, C, R, \varphi_c^i, \varphi_r^i, \varphi_c^d, \varphi_r^d)$ generating L. Let $\pi : T \to \Gamma$ be a projection such that $\pi(a) = \alpha, a \in T, \alpha \in \Gamma$. Without loss of generality, we consider that $T \cap \Gamma = \emptyset$. We can construct a parallel contextual array insertion deletion grammar $G_p = (V', \Gamma, M, C, R', \varphi_c^i, \varphi_r^i, \varphi_c^d, \varphi_r^d)$ such that $L(G_p) = L$, where
$$V' = V \cup \Gamma,$$
$$R' = R \cup \{a\ b | a, b \in T\} \cup \{\pi(a)\ \pi(b) | \pi(a), \pi(b) \in \Gamma\}, \quad \varphi_r^i : (V'^{**}, V'^{**}) \to$$
$2^{R'}$ where in addition to the contextual insertion rules of φ_r^i we also have the following rules for $a, b, c, d \in T$, $\varphi_r^i [\Lambda, a\ b] = \{\pi(a)\ \pi(b)| $

$\pi(a), \pi(b) \in \Gamma\}$, $\varphi_r^i [a\ b, c\ d] = \{\pi(c)\ \pi(d) | \pi(c), \pi(d) \in \Gamma\}$,

$\varphi_r^d : (V'^{**}, V'^{**}) \to 2^{R'}$ where in addition to the contextual deletion rules of φ_r^d we also have the following rules for $\pi(a), \pi(b), \pi(c), \pi(d) \in \Gamma$, $\varphi_r^d [\pi(a)\ \pi(b),$ $\pi(c)\ \pi(d)] = \{a\ b \mid a, b \in T\}$, $\varphi_r^d [\pi(a)\ \pi(b), \Lambda] = \{a\ b \mid a, b \in T\}$.

Hence we can clearly see that PCAIDG is closed under projection.

Theorem 2. $LOC \subsetneq PCAIDG$.

Proof. Every *LOC* language can be easily generated by some *PCAIDG*. Let L be a language over Γ in *LOC* with a finite set of tiles, Θ such that $L = L(\Theta)$. Consider the *PCAIDG*, $G = (V, T, M, C, R, \varphi_c^i, \varphi_r^i, \varphi_c^d, \varphi_r^d)$ with $V = \Gamma \cup$
$\{\#, Y\}$, $T = \Gamma$, $M = \left\{ \begin{matrix} \# & \# & Y \\ \# & a & Y \end{matrix} \middle| \begin{matrix} \# & \# \\ \# & a \end{matrix} \in \Theta \right\}$, $C = \left\{ \begin{matrix} \# \\ b \end{matrix} \middle| \begin{matrix} \# & \# \\ a & b \end{matrix} \in \Theta \right\} \cup \left\{ \begin{matrix} \# & Y \\ \#' & Y \end{matrix} \right\}$,
$R = \left\{ \begin{matrix} \# & b \\ Y & Y \end{matrix}, \# \ b \middle| \begin{matrix} \# & a \\ \# & b \end{matrix} \in \Theta \right\} \cup \left\{ \begin{matrix} c & d \\ Y & Y \end{matrix}, c\ d \middle| \begin{matrix} a & b \\ c & d \end{matrix} \in \Theta \right\} \cup \left\{ \begin{matrix} b & \# \\ Y & Y \end{matrix}, b\ \# \middle| \begin{matrix} a & \# \\ b & \# \end{matrix} \in \Theta \right\}$
$\cup \{\# \ \#, Y\ Y\}$.

For all $\begin{matrix} \# & \# \\ \# & a \end{matrix} \in \Theta$, we define

$\varphi_c^i \begin{bmatrix} \# & \# & Y \\ \# & a \end{bmatrix}, Y \end{bmatrix} = \left\{ \begin{matrix} \# \\ b \end{matrix} \middle| \begin{matrix} \# & \# \\ a & b \end{matrix} \in \Theta \right\}$, $\varphi_r^i \begin{bmatrix} \# & \# \\ \# & a \end{bmatrix}, \Lambda \end{bmatrix} = \left\{ \begin{matrix} \# & b \\ Y & Y \end{matrix} \middle| \begin{matrix} \# & a \\ \# & b \end{matrix} \in \Theta \right\}$,
$\varphi_c^d \begin{bmatrix} \Lambda, \begin{matrix} \# \\ a \end{matrix} \end{bmatrix} = \left\{ \begin{matrix} \# \\ \# \end{matrix} \right\}$
For all $\begin{matrix} \# & \# \\ a & b \end{matrix} \in \Theta$, we define

$\varphi_c^i \begin{bmatrix} \# & \# & Y \\ a & b \end{bmatrix}, Y \end{bmatrix} = \left\{ \begin{matrix} \# \\ c \end{matrix} \middle| \begin{matrix} \# & \# \\ b & c \end{matrix} \in \Theta \right\} \cup \left\{ \begin{matrix} \# \\ \# \end{matrix} \middle| \begin{matrix} \# & \# \\ b & \# \end{matrix} \in \Theta \right\}$, $\varphi_r^i \begin{bmatrix} \# & \# \\ a & b \end{bmatrix}, \Lambda \end{bmatrix} = \left\{ \begin{matrix} c & d \\ Y & Y \end{matrix} \middle| \begin{matrix} a & b \\ c & d \end{matrix} \in \right.$
$\left. \Theta \right\}$, $\varphi_r^d [\Lambda, a\ b] = \left\{ \# \ \# \right\}$

For all $\begin{smallmatrix} \# & \# \\ a & \# \end{smallmatrix} \in \Theta$, we define

$$\varphi_r^i \begin{bmatrix} \# & \# \\ a & \# \end{bmatrix}, \Lambda \end{bmatrix} = \left\{ \begin{smallmatrix} b & \# \\ Y & Y \end{smallmatrix} \,\middle|\, \begin{smallmatrix} a & \# \\ b & \# \end{smallmatrix} \in \Theta \right\}, \quad \varphi_c^d \begin{bmatrix} \# \\ a \end{bmatrix}, \Lambda \end{bmatrix} = \left\{ \begin{smallmatrix} \# \\ \# \end{smallmatrix} \right\}$$

For all $\begin{smallmatrix} \# & a \\ \# & b \end{smallmatrix} \in \Theta$ we define,

$$\varphi_r^i \begin{bmatrix} \# & a \\ \# & b \end{bmatrix}, Y\,Y \end{bmatrix} = \left\{ \# c \,\middle|\, \begin{smallmatrix} \# & b \\ \# & c \end{smallmatrix} \in \Theta \right\} \cup \left\{ \# \# \,\middle|\, \begin{smallmatrix} \# & b \\ \# & \# \end{smallmatrix} \in \Theta \right\}, \quad \varphi_c^d \begin{bmatrix} \Lambda, \begin{smallmatrix} a \\ b \end{smallmatrix} \end{bmatrix} = \left\{ \begin{smallmatrix} \# \\ \# \end{smallmatrix} \right\}$$

For all $\begin{smallmatrix} a & b \\ c & d \end{smallmatrix} \in \Theta$ we define,

$$\varphi_r^i \begin{bmatrix} a & b \\ c & d \end{bmatrix}, Y\,Y \end{bmatrix} = \left\{ e\,f \,\middle|\, \begin{smallmatrix} c & d \\ e & f \end{smallmatrix} \in \Theta \right\} \cup \left\{ \# \# \,\middle|\, \begin{smallmatrix} c & d \\ \# & \# \end{smallmatrix} \in \Theta \right\}$$

For all $\begin{smallmatrix} a & \# \\ b & \# \end{smallmatrix} \in \Theta$ we define,

$$\varphi_r^i \begin{bmatrix} a & \# \\ b & \# \end{bmatrix}, Y\,Y \end{bmatrix} = \left\{ c\,\# \,\middle|\, \begin{smallmatrix} b & \# \\ c & \# \end{smallmatrix} \in \Theta \right\} \cup \left\{ \# \# \,\middle|\, \begin{smallmatrix} b & \# \\ \# & \# \end{smallmatrix} \in \Theta \right\}, \quad \varphi_c^d \begin{bmatrix} a \\ b \end{bmatrix}, \Lambda \end{bmatrix} = \left\{ \begin{smallmatrix} \# \\ \# \end{smallmatrix} \right\}$$

For all $\begin{smallmatrix} \# & a \\ \# & \# \end{smallmatrix} \in \Theta$ we define,

$$\varphi_c^d \begin{bmatrix} \Lambda, \begin{smallmatrix} a \\ \# \end{smallmatrix} \end{bmatrix} = \left\{ \begin{smallmatrix} \# \\ \# \end{smallmatrix} \right\}$$

For all $\begin{smallmatrix} a & \# \\ \# & \# \end{smallmatrix} \in \Theta$ we define,

$$\varphi_c^d \begin{bmatrix} \begin{smallmatrix} a \\ \# \end{smallmatrix}, \Lambda \end{bmatrix} = \left\{ \begin{smallmatrix} \# \\ \# \end{smallmatrix} \right\}$$

For all $\begin{smallmatrix} a & b \\ \# & \# \end{smallmatrix} \in \Theta$ we define,

$$\varphi_r^d \begin{bmatrix} a\,b, \Lambda \end{bmatrix} = \left\{ \# \# \right\}$$

Additionally we also define, $\varphi_c^d \begin{bmatrix} \# \\ \# \end{bmatrix}, \Lambda \end{bmatrix} = \left\{ \begin{smallmatrix} Y \\ Y \end{smallmatrix} \right\}$, $\varphi_r^d \begin{bmatrix} \# \#, \Lambda \end{bmatrix} = \left\{ Y\,Y \right\}$.

The working is as follows: First the tile of the form $\begin{smallmatrix} \# & \# \\ \# & a \end{smallmatrix}$ is considered and by column concatenating the tile with $\begin{smallmatrix} Y \\ Y \end{smallmatrix}$, the array $\begin{smallmatrix} \# & \# & Y \\ \# & a & Y \end{smallmatrix}$ in the axiom set M is obtained. Then based on the tile $\begin{smallmatrix} \# & \# \\ a & b \end{smallmatrix}$, we consider parallel contextual column insertion rules which help in increasing the column size which is the horizontal growth. The horizontal growth can be stopped by using the parallel contextual column insertion rules which is based on the tile $\begin{smallmatrix} \# & \# \\ a & \# \end{smallmatrix}$. For increasing the row size, we use for the vertical growth the parallel contextual row insertion rules based on the tiles $\begin{smallmatrix} \# & a \\ \# & b \end{smallmatrix}, \begin{smallmatrix} a & b \\ c & d \end{smallmatrix}$ and $\begin{smallmatrix} a & \# \\ b & \# \end{smallmatrix}$. The vertical growth can be stopped by using the

parallel contextual row insertion rules based on the tiles $\dfrac{\#\ a}{\#\ \#}, \dfrac{a\ b}{\#\ \#}$ and $\dfrac{a\ \#}{\#\ \#}$.
Then we can subsequently use parallel contextual column deletion rules and parallel contextual row deletion rules in any order to remove a column and a row full of Ys. Then we make use of the parallel contextual column deletion rules based on the tiles $\dfrac{\#\ \#}{\#\ a}, \dfrac{\#\ a}{\#\ b}, \dfrac{\#\ a}{\#\ \#}, \dfrac{\#\ \#}{a\ \#}, \dfrac{a\ \#}{b\ \#}$ and $\dfrac{a\ \#}{\#\ \#}$ to delete the columns of #s on the extreme ends of the resulting array obtained from the previous step. Finally we make use of the parallel contextual row deletion rules based on the tiles $\dfrac{\#\ \#}{a\ b}$ and $\dfrac{a\ b}{\#\ \#}$ to delete the rows of #s on the extreme ends of the resulting array obtained from the previous step and arrive at an array which belongs to $L(G)$.

Clearly, G can generate any language in LOC and hence $LOC \subseteq PCAIDG$.

Now to prove the proper inclusion, we consider the language $L = \{(X)_m^3 | m \geq 1\}$. This language, L is not in LOC as can be seen in [6]. But this language can be generated by the PCAIDG, $G = (V, T, M, C, R, \varphi_c^i, \varphi_r^i, \varphi_c^d, \varphi_r^d)$, where $V = \{X\}$, $T = \{X\}$, $M = \begin{Bmatrix} X\ X\ X \\ X\ X\ X \end{Bmatrix}$, $C = \emptyset$, $R = \{X\ X\}$, $\varphi_c^i = \emptyset$, $\varphi_r^i [X\ X, X\ X] = X\ X$, $\varphi_c^d = \emptyset$, $\varphi_r^d = \emptyset$. Hence LOC is properly contained in $PCAIDG$.

Now we compare $PCAIDG$ with the family of recognizable picture languages [6,7] and find an interesting result.

Theorem 3. $REC \subsetneq PCAIDG$.

Proof. $REC \subseteq PCAIDG$ follows from Theorems 1 and 2, since every recognizable language is a projection of a local language.

Now the proper inclusion can be proved easily by giving an example of a picture language which cannot be in REC but in PCAIDG.

Now we compare $PCAIDG$ with the family of Siromoney matrix languages.

Note 1. We can represent $\dfrac{\#\ \#\ \#\ \#}{a\ a\ a\ a}$ as $\dfrac{\#}{a^4}$. In same way we can also represent $\dfrac{\#\ \#\ \#\ \#}{a\ b\ c\ d}$ with $\alpha = abcd$ as $\dfrac{\#}{\alpha}$.

Definition 8. *A Context-sensitive matrix grammar (CSMG) is defined by a 7-tuple $G = (V_h, V_v, \Sigma_I, \Sigma, S, HR, VR)$, where: V_h is a finite set of horizontal nonterminals; V_v is a finite set of vertical nonterminals; $\Sigma_I \subseteq V_v$ is a finite set of intermediates; Σ is a finite set of terminals; $S \in V_h$ is a starting symbol; HR is a finite set of horizontal context sensitive rules; VR is a finite set of vertical right-linear rules.*

There are two phases of derivation of the Siromoney Context-sensitive Matrix Grammars. In the first phase, a horizontal string of intermediate symbols is generated by means of context-sensitive grammar rules in R_h. During the second phase treating each intermediate as a start symbol, vertical generation of the actual picture is done in parallel, by applying R_v. Parallel application ensures that the terminating rules are all applied simultaneously in every column and that the column grows only in downward direction. The language generated by a CSMG is called a CSML. For more information, we can refer [19]. We denote the family of Siromoney context-sensitive matrix languages by $\mathfrak{L}(CSML)$.

Theorem 4. $\mathfrak{L}(CSML) \subsetneq PCAIDG.$

Proof. $\mathfrak{L}(CSML) \subseteq PCAIDG$ can be proved by the following construction.

Consider any CSMG, $G_m = (V_h, V_v, \Sigma_I, \Sigma, S, HR, VR)$. We construct a parallel contextual array insertion deletion grammar $G = (V, T, M, C, R, \varphi_c^i, \varphi_r^i, \varphi_c^d, \varphi_r^d)$ generating L such that $L = L(G_m)$. $V = V_h \cup V_v \cup \Sigma \cup \{\#\}$, $T = \Sigma$, $M = \left\{ \begin{matrix} \# & \# & \# \\ \# & S & \# \end{matrix} \middle| S \in V_h \text{ is the start symbol} \right\}$,

$$C = \left\{ \frac{\#}{\alpha} \middle| S \to \alpha \in HR, \alpha \in (V_h \cup \Sigma_I)^+ \right\} \cup \left\{ \frac{\#}{S} \middle| S \to \alpha \in HR \right\} \cup \left\{ \frac{\#}{\gamma} \middle| \beta \to \right.$$

$$\left. \gamma \in HR, |\beta| \leq |\gamma| \right\} \cup \left\{ \frac{\#}{\beta} \middle| \beta \to \gamma \in HR, |\beta| \leq |\gamma| \right\},$$

$$R = \left\{ \begin{matrix} \# & b \\ \# & B' \end{matrix} \middle| B \to bB' \in VR, B' \in V_v \right\} \cup \left\{ \begin{matrix} \# & b \\ \# & \# \end{matrix} \middle| B \to b \in VR \right\} \cup \left\{ \begin{matrix} b & c \\ B' & C' \end{matrix} \middle| B \to \right.$$

$$\left. bB', C \to cC' \in VR, B' \neq C, B \neq C' \right\} \cup \left\{ \begin{matrix} b & c \\ \# & \# \end{matrix} \middle| B \to b, C \to c \in VR \right\} \cup$$

$$\left\{ \begin{matrix} b & \# \\ B' & \# \end{matrix} \middle| B \to bB' \in VR, B' \in V_v \right\} \cup \left\{ \begin{matrix} b & \# \\ \# & \# \end{matrix} \middle| B \to b \in VR \right\} \cup \left\{ \# B \middle| B \to bB' \in \right.$$

$$\left. VR, B' \in V_v \right\} \cup \left\{ \# B \middle| B \to b \in VR \right\} \cup \left\{ B C \middle| B \to bB', C \to cC' \in VR, B' \neq \right.$$

$$\left. C, B \neq C' \right\} \cup \left\{ B C \middle| B \to b, C \to c \in VR \right\} \cup \left\{ B \# \middle| B \to bB' \in VR, B' \in \right.$$

$$\left. V_v \right\} \cup \left\{ B \# \middle| B \to b \in VR \right\},$$

$$\varphi_c^i \begin{bmatrix} \# & \# \\ \#, & S \end{bmatrix} = \left\{ \frac{\#}{\alpha} \middle| S \to \alpha \in HR, \alpha \in (V_h \cup \Sigma_I)^+ \right\},$$

$$\varphi_c^d \begin{bmatrix} \# & \# \\ \alpha, & \# \end{bmatrix} = \left\{ \frac{\#}{S} \middle| S \to \alpha \in HR \right\},$$

$$\varphi_c^i \begin{bmatrix} \# & \# \\ \#, & \beta \end{bmatrix} = \left\{ \frac{\#}{\gamma} \middle| \beta \to \gamma \in HR, |\beta| \leq |\gamma| \right\},$$

$$\varphi_c^d \begin{bmatrix} \# & \# \\ \gamma, & \# \end{bmatrix} = \left\{ \frac{\#}{\beta} \middle| \beta \to \gamma \in HR, |\beta| \leq |\gamma| \right\},$$

For all $A \in (V_h \cup \Sigma_I)$,

$$\varphi_c^i \begin{bmatrix} \# & \# \\ A, & \beta \end{bmatrix} = \left\{ \frac{\#}{\gamma} \middle| \beta \to \gamma \in HR, |\beta| \leq |\gamma| \right\},$$

$$\varphi_c^d \begin{bmatrix} \# & \# \\ \gamma, & A \end{bmatrix} = \left\{ \frac{\#}{\beta} \middle| \beta \to \gamma \in HR, |\beta| \leq |\gamma| \right\},$$

For all $B, C \in \Sigma_I$,

$$\varphi_r^i \left[\# \#, \# B\right] = \left\{\begin{matrix} \# & b \\ \# & B' \end{matrix} \middle| B \to bB' \in VR, B' \in V_v \right\},$$

$$\varphi_r^i \left[\# \#, \# B\right] = \left\{\begin{matrix} \# & b \\ \# & \# \end{matrix} \middle| B \to b \in VR \right\},$$

$$\varphi_r^i \left[\# \#, B\ C\right] = \left\{\begin{matrix} b & c \\ B' & C' \end{matrix} \middle| B \to bB', C \to cC' \in VR, B' \neq C, B \neq C' \right\},$$

$$\varphi_r^i \left[\# \#, B\ C\right] = \left\{\begin{matrix} b & c \\ \# & \# \end{matrix} \middle| B \to b, C \to c \in VR \right\},$$

$$\varphi_r^i \left[\# \#, B\ \#\right] = \left\{\begin{matrix} b & \# \\ B' & \# \end{matrix} \middle| B \to bB' \in VR, B' \in V_v \right\},$$

$$\varphi_r^i \left[\# \#, B\ \#\right] = \left\{\begin{matrix} b & \# \\ \# & \# \end{matrix} \middle| B \to b \in VR \right\},$$

$$\varphi_r^d \left[\begin{matrix} \# & b \\ \# & B'' \end{matrix}, \lambda\ \lambda\right] = \left\{\# B \middle| B \to bB' \in VR, B' \in V_v \right\},$$

$$\varphi_r^d \left[\begin{matrix} \# & b \\ \# & \# \end{matrix}, \lambda\ \lambda\right] = \left\{\# B \middle| B \to b \in VR \right\},$$

$$\varphi_r^d \left[\begin{matrix} b & c \\ B' & C'' \end{matrix}, \lambda\ \lambda\right] = \left\{B\ C \middle| B \to bB', C \to cC' \in VR, B' \neq C, B \neq C' \right\},$$

$$\varphi_r^d \left[\begin{matrix} b & c \\ \# & \# \end{matrix}, \lambda\ \lambda\right] = \left\{B\ C \middle| B \to b, C \to c \in VR \right\},$$

$$\varphi_r^d \left[\begin{matrix} b & \# \\ B' & \# \end{matrix}, \lambda\ \lambda\right] = \left\{B\ \# \middle| B \to bB' \in VR, B' \in V_v \right\},$$

$$\varphi_r^d \left[\begin{matrix} b & \# \\ \# & \# \end{matrix}, \lambda\ \lambda\right] = \left\{B\ \# \middle| B \to b \in VR \right\},$$

For all $D, E \in V_v$ and $b, c \in \Sigma$

$$\varphi_r^i \left[\# b, \# D\right] = \left\{\begin{matrix} \# & d \\ \# & D' \end{matrix} \middle| D \to dD' \in VR, D' \in V_v \right\},$$

$$\varphi_r^i \left[\# b, \# D\right] = \left\{\begin{matrix} \# & d \\ \# & \# \end{matrix} \middle| D \to d \in VR \right\},$$

$$\varphi_r^i \left[b\ c, D\ E\right] = \left\{\begin{matrix} d & e \\ D' & E' \end{matrix} \middle| D \to dD', E \to eE' \in VR, D' \neq E, D \neq E' \right\},$$

$$\varphi_r^i \left[b\ c, D\ E\right] = \left\{\begin{matrix} d & e \\ \# & \# \end{matrix} \middle| D \to d, E \to e \in VR \right\},$$

$$\varphi_r^i \left[b\ \#, D\ \#\right] = \left\{\begin{matrix} d & \# \\ D' & \# \end{matrix} \middle| D \to dD' \in VR, D' \in V_v \right\},$$

$$\varphi_r^i \left[b\ \#, D\ \#\right] = \left\{\begin{matrix} d & \# \\ \# & \# \end{matrix} \middle| D \to d \in VR \right\},$$

$$\varphi_r^d \left[\begin{matrix} \# & d \\ \# & D'' \end{matrix}, \lambda\ \lambda\right] = \left\{\# D \middle| D \to dD' \in VR, D' \in V_v \right\},$$

$$\varphi_r^d \left[\begin{matrix} \# & d \\ \# & \# \end{matrix}, \lambda\ \lambda\right] = \left\{\# D \middle| D \to d \in VR \right\},$$

$$\varphi_r^d \left[\begin{matrix} d & e \\ D' & E'' \end{matrix}, \lambda\ \lambda\right] = \left\{D\ E \middle| D \to dD', E \to eE' \in VR, D' \neq E, D \neq E' \right\},$$

$$\varphi_r^d \begin{bmatrix} d & e \\ \# & \# \end{bmatrix}, \lambda \, \lambda = \left\{ D \, E \middle| D \to d, E \to e \in VR \right\},$$

$$\varphi_r^d \begin{bmatrix} d & \# \\ D' & \# \end{bmatrix}, \lambda \, \lambda = \left\{ D \, \# \middle| D \to dD' \in VR, D' \in V_v \right\},$$

$$\varphi_r^d \begin{bmatrix} d & \# \\ \# & \# \end{bmatrix}, \lambda \, \lambda = \left\{ D \, \# \middle| D \to d \in VR \right\},$$

For all $a, b \in \Sigma$,

$$\varphi_c^d \begin{bmatrix} \lambda & \# \\ \lambda & a \end{bmatrix} = \left\{ \begin{matrix} \# \\ \# \end{matrix} \right\}, \; \varphi_c^d \begin{bmatrix} \lambda & a \\ \lambda & b \end{bmatrix} = \left\{ \begin{matrix} \# \\ \# \end{matrix} \right\}, \; \varphi_c^d \begin{bmatrix} \lambda & a \\ \lambda & \# \end{bmatrix} = \left\{ \begin{matrix} \# \\ \# \end{matrix} \right\},$$

$$\varphi_c^d \begin{bmatrix} \# & \lambda \\ a & \lambda \end{bmatrix} = \left\{ \begin{matrix} \# \\ \# \end{matrix} \right\}, \; \varphi_c^d \begin{bmatrix} a & \lambda \\ b & \lambda \end{bmatrix} = \left\{ \begin{matrix} \# \\ \# \end{matrix} \right\}, \; \varphi_c^d \begin{bmatrix} a & \lambda \\ \# & \lambda \end{bmatrix} = \left\{ \begin{matrix} \# \\ \# \end{matrix} \right\},$$

$$\varphi_r^d \begin{bmatrix} \lambda & \lambda, a & b \end{bmatrix} = \{\# \, \#\}, \; \varphi_r^d \begin{bmatrix} a & b, \lambda & \lambda \end{bmatrix} = \{\# \, \#\}.$$

The working is as follows: The axiom set consists of arrays of the form $\begin{matrix} \# & \# & \# \\ \# & S & \# \end{matrix}$ based on the starting symbol S of the CSMG. We consider the rules which are based on the horizontal production rules of the CSMG to perform the parallel contextual column insertion operation. Parallel contextual column insertion operation and deletion operation are performed alternatively to simulate the generation of horizontal strings of intermediates based on the CSMG. Now we consider the rules based on the vertical production rules of the CSMG to perform the parallel contextual row insertion operation. Parallel contextual row insertion operation and deletion operation are performed alternatively to simulate the vertical generation of the actual picture based on the CSMG. Then using the parallel contextual column deletion operation the #'s on the extreme ends of the column are deleted and finally using the parallel contextual row deletion operation the #'s on the extreme ends of the rows are deleted resulting in an array which belongs to $L(G)$.

We now prove the proper inclusion. Consider the language

$$L = \left\{ \begin{pmatrix} (\bullet)_n \\ (X)_n \\ (\bullet)_n \end{pmatrix}^n \begin{pmatrix} (X)_n \\ (X)_n \\ (\bullet)_n \end{pmatrix}^n \begin{pmatrix} (\bullet)_n \\ (\bullet)_n \\ (\bullet)_n \end{pmatrix}^n \right\}.$$ This language cannot be generated by any $CSMG$ as can be seen in [20]. But this language can be generated by a $PCAIDG$ as seen in Example 1. Hence we see that the family of languages generated by context-sensitive matrix grammar is properly included in $PCAIDG$.

4 Conclusion

This paper presents novel theoretical results which contribute to the research on picture languages. It deals with a new type of grammar PCAIDG for generating 2D-pictures i.e., arrays of characters. Comparison results of PCAIDG with LOC, REC and $\mathfrak{L}(CSML)$ are dealt with. It is worth investigating to compare the power of this new grammar with tile rewriting grammars, regional grammars, kolam grammars and many specific other models (see Matz [12], Crespi Reghizzi and Pradella [14], Prusa [15], Subramanian et al. [22], Fernau et al. [2,3], etc.). We are pursuing this study. A related study based on the idea of array insertion and deletion operations in the field of membrane computing has been done by the authors which is of interest to read [9].

Acknowledgement. The authors are thankful to Prof. Henning Fernau (Fachbereich 4-Abteilung Informatik, Universität Trier, D-54286 Trier, Germany) for his valuable input to this paper. A four page abstract of this paper (not refereed) has appeared in the technical report of Theorietag 2017 held at Bonn, Germany during September 18–22, 2017. (See: [PDF] Theorietag 2017-Uni.Trier, page 41–44).

References

1. Ehrenfeucht, A., Păun, Gh., Rozenberg, G.: Contextual grammars and formal languages. In: Rozenberg, G., Salomaa, A. (eds.) Handbook of Formal Languages, pp. 237–293. Springer, Heidelberg (1997). https://doi.org/10.1007/978-3-662-07675-0_6

2. Fernau, H., Freund, R., Schmid, M.L., Subramanian, K.G., Wielderhold, P.: Contextual array grammars and array P systems. Ann. Math. Artif. Intell. **75**, 5–26 (2015)

3. Fernau, H., Paramasivan, M., Schmid, M.L., Thomas, D.G.: Some picture processing based on finite automata and regular grammars. J. Comput. Syst. Sci. **95**, 232–258 (2018)

4. Freund, R.: Array grammars. Technical report No. 15/00. Universitat Rovirai Virgili (2000)

5. Freund, R., Păun, Gh., Rozenberg, G.: Contextual array grammars. In: Subramanian, K.G., Rangarajan, K., Mukund, M. (eds.) Formal Models, Languages and Application Series in Machine Perception and Artificial Intelligence, vol. 66, pp. 112–136. World Scientific (2007)

6. Giammarresi, D., Restivo, A.: Two-dimensional languages. In: Rozenberg, G., Salomaa, A. (eds.) Handbook of Formal Languages, vol. 3, pp. 215–267. Springer, Heidelberg (1997). https://doi.org/10.1007/978-3-642-59126-6_4

7. Giammarresi, D., Restivo, A.: Recognizable picture languages. Int. J. Pattern Recognit. Artif. Intell. **6**, 241–256 (1992)

8. Helen Chandra, P., Subramanian, K.G., Thomas, D.G.: Parallel contextual array grammars and languages. Electron. Not. Discrete Math. **12**, 106–117 (2003)

9. James Immanuel, S., Thomas, D.G., Thamburaj, R., Nagar, A.K.: Parallel contextual array insertion deletion P system. In: Brimkov, V.E., Barneva, R.P. (eds.) IWCIA 2017. LNCS, vol. 10256, pp. 170–183. Springer, Cham (2017). https://doi.org/10.1007/978-3-319-59108-7_14

10. Krithivasan, K., Balan, M.S., Rama, R.: Array contextual grammars. In: Martin-Vide,C., Păun, Gh. (eds.) Recent Topics in Mathematical and Computational Linguistics, pp. 154–168. The Publishing House of the Romanian Academy (2000)

11. Marcus, S.: Contextual grammars. Rev. Roum. Math. Pures et Appl. **14**(10), 1525–1534 (1969)

12. Matz, O.: Regular expressions and context-free grammars for picture languages. In: Reischuk, R., Morvan, M. (eds.) STACS 1997. LNCS, vol. 1200, pp. 283–294. Springer, Heidelberg (1997). https://doi.org/10.1007/BFb0023466

13. Păun, Gh.: Marcus Contextual Grammars. Kluwer, Dordrecht (1997)

14. Pradella, M., Cherubini, A., Reghizzi, C.: A unifying approach to picture grammars. Inf. Comput. **209**, 1246–1267 (2011)

15. Prusa, D.: Two dimensional languages. Ph.D. thesis. Charles University, Faculty of Mathematics and Physics, Czech Republic (2004)
16. Rama, R., Smitha, T.A.: Some results on array contextual grammars. Int. J. Pattern Recognit. Artif. Intell. **14**, 537–550 (2000)
17. Rosenfeld, A.: Isotonic grammars, parallel grammars and picture grammars. In: Michie, D., Meltzer, D. (eds.) Machine Intelligence VI, pp. 281–294. University of Edinburgh Press, Scotland (1971)
18. Rosenfeld, A.: Picture Languages: Formal Models for Picture Recognition. Academic Press, Cambridge (1979)
19. Siromoney, G., Siromoney, R., Krithivasan, K.: Abstract families of matrices and picture languages. Comput. Graph. Image Process. **1**, 234–307 (1972)
20. Siromoney, G., Siromoney, R., Krithivasan, K.: Picture languages with array rewriting rules. Inf. Control **22**, 447–470 (1973)
21. Subramanian, K.G., Van, D.L., Chandra, P.H., Quyen, N.D.: Array grammars with contextual operations. Fund. Info. **83**, 411–428 (2008)
22. Subramanian, K.G., Revathi, L., Siromoney, R.: Siromoney array grammars and applications. Int. J. Pattern Recognit. Artif. Intell. **3**, 333–351 (1989)

Chain Code P System for Generation of Approximation Patterns of Sierpiński Curve

A. Dharani[1], R. Stella Maragatham[1], Atulya K. Nagar[2],
and K. G. Subramanian[2(✉)]

[1] Department of Mathematics, Queen Mary's College, Chennai 600004, India
[2] Department of Mathematics and Computer Science, Faculty of Science,
Liverpool Hope University, Hope Park, Liverpool L16 9JD, UK
kgsmani1948@gmail.com

Abstract. A sequence of approximating geometric patterns that define in the limit, the Sierpiński space filling curve is considered and the problem of generation of the infinite set of these patterns is investigated. A P system model in the bio-inspired area of membrane computing is constructed to generate the language of chain code kind of words that describe the approximating geometric patterns of Sierpiński curve.

Keywords: Space-filling curve · Sierpiński curve
Membrane computing · Chain codes

1 Introduction

Space-filling curves, also called square-filling curves, have attracted the attention of several researchers in the past, after Peano [17] constructed in 1890, the first space-filling curve, followed by Hilbert's space-filling curve [10] in 1891, with Hilbert providing a geometrical generating procedure. This topic of space-filling curves continues to be of interest both in theoretical investigations [11,21,23] and in practical applications [4]. Sagan [19] provides a comprehensive account of many aspects of several space-filling curves, especially, those of Peano, Hilbert and Sierpiński, while Bader's monograph [3] on space-filling curves with applications in scientific computing is a more recent one. Basically, a space-filling curve is a curve passing through every point of a two-dimensional region with positive area.

In the field of two-dimensional formal language theory, different kinds of theoretical models [8] with grammatical formalism have been introduced with motivation from different problems arising in the broad areas of image analysis, computer vision, pattern recognition and others. Chain code grammars [13] constitute one such grammar formalism for describing chain code pictures composed of horizontal and vertical unit lines. A chain code picture in two-dimensional plane, in its basic form, is encoded by a word over the symbols l, r, u, d standing

© Springer Nature Switzerland AG 2018
R. P. Barneva et al. (Eds.): IWCIA 2018, LNCS 11255, pp. 43–52, 2018.
https://doi.org/10.1007/978-3-030-05288-1_4

for unit moves to the left (l), right (r), up (u) and down (d) neighbours of a point $p = (x, y)$ in the chain code picture, where x, y are integers. There have been many studies [6,7] on theoretical aspects and applications of chain code picture grammars and languages. Generation of geometrical approximation patterns of Peano and Hilbert space-filling curves in terms of chain code grammars and other kinds of syntactic models has been investigated [21,23].

On the other hand, in the area of membrane computing [15,16] with its origin in certain biological features and their functioning, a novel computing model, generally called P system was introduced by Păun [14] and this model and its many variants have been used in providing solutions for problems in different application areas [16,24,26]. A Chain code P system involving a sequential mode of rewriting with context-free grammar type rules and the terminal alphabet $\{l, r, u, d\}$ with the interpretation as mentioned earlier, was proposed in [25] while in [5], rewriting in parallel mode was employed in the chain code P system and thereby a parallel chain code P system was proposed. In these models the problem of generation of the approximation patterns of the Peano and Hilbert space-filling curves are considered.

Here we consider Sierpiński space-filling curve which was introduced by Sierpiński [22] in 1912. We take the view [19, p. 50] of this curve as a map from the closed unit interval [0, 1] to an isosceles right triangle. We construct a Parallel chain code P system generating chain code words over $\{l, r, u, d\}$ representing the polygonal approximation patterns of the Sierpiński space-filling curve.

2 Basic Notions

For notions related to formal language theory we refer to [18,20], for chain code grammars to [13] and for P systems to [14].

If V is a finite alphabet, a word or a string α over V is a sequence of symbols taken from V. The set of all words over V, including the empty word λ with no symbols, is denoted by V^*. The length of the word α is denoted by $|\alpha|$.

2.1 Chain Code Pictures

A chain code picture in the two-dimensional plane is basically composed of horizontal and vertical unit lines and the ends of a unit line are points with integer coordinates. Starting from an end of a unit line in a chain code picture and tracing through all the unit lines of the picture and reaching an end of a unit line in the picture, we can obtain a word over the symbols $\{l, r, u, d\}$, called the chain code word of the picture, with each of the symbols being interpreted as tracing a unit line in the picture in the appropriate direction: left, right, up or down. A chain code picture language is a set of chain code words, with each word corresponding to a chain code picture. For formal definitions relating to chain code picture we refer to [7,13]. Figure 1 shows a chain code picture in the form of the letter I and the chain code word $rrrrlluuuurrllll$ describes this chain code picture starting from the leftmost position of the lower horizontal line and ending in the leftmost position of the upper horizontal line. There can be several chain code words describing the same chain code picture depending on the start and end points and also the moves of tracing the picture.

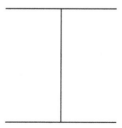

Fig. 1. A chain code picture which is in the form of letter I for the code word *rrrrlluuuurrllll*

2.2   Chain Code P Systems

We now recall the chain code P system [5] with a parallel mode of rewriting the string objects in the membranes.

A context-free parallel chain code P system Π of degree $m, m \geq 1$, is given by $\Pi = (N, \Sigma, \mu, L_1, \cdots, L_m, R_1, \cdots, R_m, i_0)$ where N is a finite set of nonterminals, Σ is a finite set of chain-code symbols, μ is a membrane structure with each membrane labelled in a one-to-one way with $1, 2, \cdots, m$. Initially, each membrane or region can have a finite set L_i, $1 \leq i \leq m$, of strings over $N \cup \Sigma$. Each region has a finite set (which can also be empty) R_i, $1 \leq i \leq m$, of context-free rules of the form $X \to \gamma(tar)$, where $X \in N$, $\gamma \in (N \cup \Sigma)^*$ with each rule having an attached target *here, out, in* The target indicates the region where the result of the rewriting should be placed in the next step: *here* means that the result remains in the same region where the rule was applied, *out* means that the string is to be sent to the immediately outer region and *in* means that the string is sent to one of the directly inner membranes, if any exists. Generally, the target *here* is understood and not mentioned. The output membrane has label i_0.

In a step of computation of Π, in every region each string is rewritten by at most one nondeterministically chosen and applicable rule at a time; if no such rule exists, the string remains unchanged. A computation halts with no rule is applicable in the regions. The strings generated over Σ and collected in the output membrane constitute the chain code picture language of the system Π. The set of all chain code picture languages generated by context-free parallel chain code P systems with m membranes is denoted by $PCCP_m(CF)$.

We illustrate constructing a context-free parallel chain code P system Π_I generating the chain code picture language $L_I = \{r^{2n}l^nu^{2n}r^nl^{2n}\}$ with each word in L_I corresponding to an encoding of a chain code picture in the form of letter I (Fig. 1) of increasing sizes.

Let

$$\Pi_I = (\{A, B, C\}, \{l, r, u, d\}, [_1 [_2]_2]_1, \{ABC\}, \emptyset, R_1, R_2, 2)$$

where the sets of rules are

$$R_1 = \{A \rightarrow r^2 Al, B \rightarrow u^2 B, C \rightarrow rCl^2, A \rightarrow r^2 Al(in),$$

$$B \rightarrow u^2 B(in), C \rightarrow rCl^2(in)\}, R_2 = \emptyset.$$

Since region 1 only has an initial word ABC, a computation can start with this initial word. Note that applicable rules with the same target could be applied. If the rules $A \rightarrow r^2 Al, B \rightarrow u^2 B, C \rightarrow rCl^2$ are applied $n-1$ times, then the word generated is $r^{2(n-1)} l^{n-1} u^{2n} r^{n-1} l^{2(n-1)}$. If now the rules $A \rightarrow r^2 Al(in), B \rightarrow u^2 B(in), C \rightarrow rCl^2(in)$ are applied, the string obtained is $r^{2n} l^n u^{2n} r^n l^{2n}$ which is sent to the output region 2 and is collected in the language generated. Note that on interpreting the symbols l, r, u, d in the word $r^{2n} l^n u^{2n} r^n l^{2n}$ as mentioned earlier we can obtain the picture in the form of the letter I of a size depending on n.

3   Approximating Polygon Patterns in Isosceles Right Triangle for the Sierpiński Curve

We consider approximating polygon patterns [19, p. 52] of the Sierpiński's space filling curve [22], based on the view of the curve as a map from a closed unit interval onto a isosceles right triangle. The first few members of the sequence of continuous polygons, ultimately converging to the Sierpiński's curve, are shown in Figs. 2, 3, 4, 5, 6, 7, 8 and 9. The polygons are drawn to pass through adjacent subtriangles of the isosceles triangle. For more mathematical discussion on this aspect of Sierpiński's curve, we refer to [19, Chap. 4.2].

We consider the basic chain code symbols l, r, u, d with interpretation as described earlier in Sect. 2.1 and additional chain code kind of symbols n_1, n_2, s_1, s_2 respectively corresponding to unit moves from a point in the 2D plane along the *north-east, north-west, south-east, south-west* directions. Based on these eight symbols, on tracing the polygon starting from the open left end, the corresponding chain code words of the sequence of approximating polygon patterns of the Sierpiński curve is given by

$$S_1 = r, \ S_2 = n_1 r s_1, \ S_3 = r n_1 u r d s_1 r$$

$$S_4 = n_1 r s_1 n_1 n_2 u n_1 r s_1 d s_2 s_1 n_1 r s_1$$

$$S_5 = r n_1 u r d s_1 r n_1 u n_2 l u r n_1 u r d s_1 r d l s_2 d s_1 r n_1 u r d s_1 r$$

and so on. In fact for $n > 3$,

$$S_{n+1} = h_1(S_n) r h_2(S_n)$$

where h_1, h_2, are given by

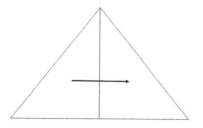

Fig. 2. First Polygon of Sierpiński Curve in isosceles right triangle

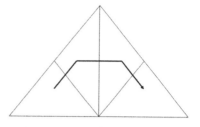

Fig. 3. Second Polygon of Sierpiński Curve in isosceles right triangle

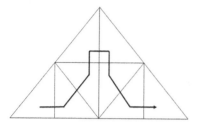

Fig. 4. Third Polygon of Sierpiński Curve in isosceles right triangle

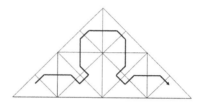

Fig. 5. Fourth Polygon of Sierpiński Curve in isosceles right triangle

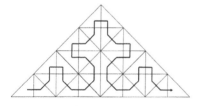

Fig. 6. Fifth Polygon of Sierpiński Curve in isosceles right triangle

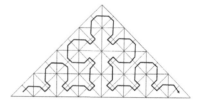

Fig. 7. Sixth Polygon of Sierpiński Curve in isosceles right triangle

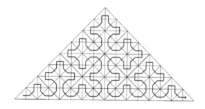

Fig. 8. Seventh Polygon of Sierpiński Curve in isosceles right triangle

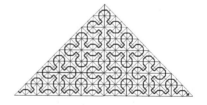

Fig. 9. Eighth Polygon of Sierpiński Curve in isosceles right triangle

$$h_1(n_1) = r, h_1(r) = n_1, h_1(n_2) = d, h_1(d) = n_2,$$

$$h_1(s_1) = u, h_1(u) = s_1, h_1(s_2) = l, h_1(l) = s_2$$

$$h_2(n_1) = d, h_2(d) = n_1, h_2(n_2) = l, h_2(l) = n_2,$$

$$h_2(s_1) = r, h_2(r) = s_1, h_2(s_2) = u, h_2(u) = s_2$$

We construct a context-free parallel chain code system Π_S generating the language of words corresponding to the approximating polygon patterns of the Sierpiński's space filling curve in a right isosceles triangle. But the set Σ of terminal symbols is taken as $\{l, r, u, d, n_1, n_2, s_1, s_2\}$ with the interpretation for the symbols as mentioned earlier.

Let $\Pi_S = (N, \Sigma, [_1 [_2]_2]_1, L_1, L_2, R_1, R_2, 2)$ where $N = \{A, B, C, D, E, F, X, Y\}$, $L_1 = \{A\}$, $L_2 = \{r, n_1 r s_1\}$, $R_2 = \emptyset$. The set of rules in region 1 is

$$R_1 = \{1 : A \rightarrow BrD, 2 : B \rightarrow An_1C, 3 : D \rightarrow Es_1A,$$

$$4 : C \rightarrow FuB, 5 : E \rightarrow DdX,$$

$$6 : F \rightarrow Cn_2Y, 7 : X \rightarrow Ys_2E, 8 : Y \rightarrow XlF, \}$$

$$\cup \{9 : A \rightarrow rn_1urds_1r(in), 10 : B \rightarrow n_1rs_1n_1n_2un_1(in),$$

$$11 : D \rightarrow s_1ds_2s_1n_1rs_1(in), 12 : C \rightarrow un_2lurn_1u(in),$$

$$13 : E \rightarrow ds_1rdls_2d(in), 14 : F \rightarrow n_2un_1n_2s_2ln_2(in),$$

$$15 : X \rightarrow s_2ln_2s_2s_1ds_2(in), 16 : Y \rightarrow ls_2dlun_2l(in)\}.$$

Theorem 1. *The P system Π_S mentioned above generates in membrane 2 the language of the words S_n, where S_n is the n-th approximating polygon pattern of the Sierpiński Curve in a right isoceles triangle.*

Proof. We give an outline of the proof. In a computation of the P system Π_S, starting from the initial word A in region, if the rule 9 is applied, the word rn_1urds_1r is obtained and is sent to the output region 2 while in region 2, there are no rules but the initial words r and n_1rs_1 are already in the output region. These three words $S_1 = r$, $S_2 = n_1rs_1$, $S_3 = rn_1urds_1r$ correspond to the Figs. 2, 3 and 4 respectively. If in region 1, rule 1 is applied on the initial word A followed by rules 10 and 11 applied in parallel, then the word $S_4 = n_1rs_1n_1n_2un_1rs_1ds_2s_1n_1rs_1$ is generated and is sent to region 2. Thus starting from the initial word A, the applicable rules among 1 to 8 can be used in parallel as many times as needed and the applicable rules among 9 to 16 can be used to terminate the derivation yielding the elements S_n for some $n \geq 3$ and sent to the output region 2, thus generating the language L_S. $\qquad\square$

We note that the nonterminals A to Y correspond to the sub-polygonal lines shown in Fig. 10, and these are suitably connected to give rise to the approximation polygon patterns of the Sierpiński curve.

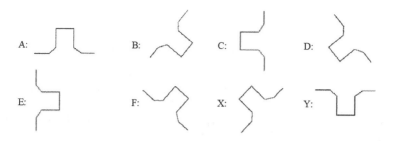

Fig. 10. Polygonal lines corresponding to the indicated nonterminal

4 Approximating Polygon Patterns in a Square for the Sierpiński Curve

We now consider approximating polygon patterns [19, p. 51] of the Sierpiński's space filling curve [22] in a square. In this case the curve is considered as a map from a closed unit interval onto a square, which is in fact the original construction [19, p. 50]. Again for mathematical aspects of this curve, we refer to [19, p. 50]. The first few members of the sequence of these approximation polygon patterns are shown in Fig. 11, 12 and 13. As in the case of isoceles triangle considered in Sect. 3, here again the polygons pass through adjacent subtriangles of the square.

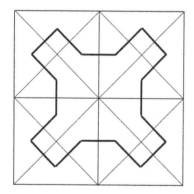

Fig. 11. First Polygon of Sierpiński Curve in a square

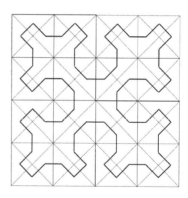

Fig. 12. Second Polygon of Sierpiński Curve in a square

Also the chain code symbols $l, r, u, d, n_1, n_2, s_1, s_2$ with interpretation as described earlier, can be used in encoding as words, the approximation polygon patterns of the Sierpiński's space filling curve [22] in a square. On tracing the polygon stating from the lowermost triangle on the left edge of the square, the sequence of chain code words S^n corresponding to the approximating polygon patterns of the Sierpiński curve in a square is given by

$$S^1 = n_1 s_1 s_2 n_2, \ S^2 = n_1 u n_2 n_1 s_1 r n_1 s_1 s_2 d s_1 s_2 n_2 l s_2 n_2,$$

$$S^3 = n_1un_2n_1s_1rn_1un_2ls_2n_2n_1un_2n_1s_1rn_1s_1s_2ds_1rn_1un_2n_1s_1rn_1s_1$$

$$s_2ds_1s_2n_2ls_2ds_1rn_1s_1s_2ds_1s_2n_2ls_2n_2n_1un_2ls_2ds_1s_2n_2ls_2n_2$$

and so on.

We construct a context-free parallel chain code system Π^S to generate the language of words corresponding to the approximating polygon patterns of the Sierpiński's space filling curve in a square. The set Σ of terminal symbols is $\{l, r, u, d, n_1, n_2, s_1, s_2\}$ with the interpretation for the symbols as mentioned earlier. Let $\Pi^S = (N, \Sigma, [_1[_2]_2]_1, L'_1, L'_2, R'_1, R'_2, 2)$ where $N = \{A, B, C, D\}$, $L'_1 = \{As_1Bn_2\}$, $L'_2 = \{n_1s_1s_2n_2\}$, $R'_2 = \emptyset$. The set of rules in region 1 is

$$R'_1 = \{1 : A \to AuCn_1DrA, 2 : B \to BdDs_2ClB,$$

$$3 : C \to ClBn_2AuC, 4 : D \to DrAs_1BdD\}$$

$$\cup\{5 : A \to n_1un_2n_1s_1rn_1(in), 6 : B \to s_2ds_1s_2n_2ls_2(in),$$

$$7 : C \to n_2ls_2n_2n_1un_2(in), 8 : D \to s_1rn_1s_1s_2ds_1(in)\}.$$

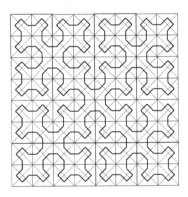

Fig. 13. Third Polygon of Sierpiński Curve in a square

Theorem 2. *The P system Π^S mentioned above generates in membrane 2 the language of words S^n describing the approximating polygon patterns of the Sierpiński curve in a square.*

The proof of this Theorem is similar to the Proof of Theorem 1. The word $n_1s_1s_2n_2$ which corresponds to the polygon in Fig. 11, is already in the output region as an initial word. Since the initial word in region 1 is As_1Bn_2, on applying in parallel, the rules 5 and 6, the word generated is $n_1un_2n_1s_1rn_1s_1s_2ds_1s_2n_2ls_2n_2$ which is sent to the output region 2, since the target of the rules 5 and 6 is *in*. Thus starting from the initial word As_1Bn_2, the applicable rules among 1 to 4 can be used in parallel as many times as needed and the applicable rules among 5 to 8 can be used to terminate the derivation yielding the elements S^n for some $n \geq 3$ and sent to the output region 2, thus generating the language of words S^n describing the approximating polygon patterns of the Sierpiński curve in a square.

5   Conclusion and Future Work

The problem of generation of the approximation patterns of Sierpiński curve in the two-dimensional (2D) plane has been considered here. Sierpiński curve in three-dimensional (3D) space has also been considered [3]. Generation of these 3D approximation patterns of Sierpiński curve in the framework of P systems can be studied. Besides theoretical studies of Space-filling curves, a number of applications [1–3, 9, 12] of space-filling curves, in particular of Sierpiński curves (see, for example, [4]) have been investigated. It will be of interest to study the role of P systems in the context of these applications.

Acknowledgement. The authors thank the reviewers for their useful comments which helped for a better presentation of the paper.

References

1. Aftosmis, M.J., Berger, M.J., Murman, S.M.: Applications of space-filling curves to Cartesian methods for CFD. In: 42nd Aerospace Sciences Meeting and Exhibit, Reno, Nevada (2004)
2. Ali, M.A., Ladhake, S.A.: Overview of space-filling curves and their applications in scheduling. Int. J. Adv. Eng. Technol. **1**(4), 148–154 (2011)
3. Bader, M.: Space-filling Curves - An Introduction with Applications in Scientific Computing. Texts in Computational Science and Engineering. Springer, Heidelberg (2013). https://doi.org/10.1007/978-3-642-31046-1
4. Bader, M., Schraufstetter, S., Vigh, C.A., Behrens, J.: Memory efficient adaptive mesh generation and implementation of multigrid algorithms using Sierpiński curves. Int. J. Comput. Sci. Eng. **4**(1), 12–21 (2008)
5. Ceterchi, R., Subramanian, K.G., Venkat, I.: P systems with parallel rewriting for chain code picture languages. In: Beckmann, A., Mitrana, V., Soskova, M. (eds.) CiE 2015. LNCS, vol. 9136, pp. 145–155. Springer, Cham (2015). https://doi.org/10.1007/978-3-319-20028-6_15
6. Dassow, J., Habel, A., Taubenberger, S.: Chain-code pictures and collages generated by hyperedge replacement. In: Cuny, J., Ehrig, H., Engels, G., Rozenberg, G. (eds.) Graph Grammars 1994. LNCS, vol. 1073, pp. 412–427. Springer, Heidelberg (1996). https://doi.org/10.1007/3-540-61228-9_102
7. Drewes, F.: Some remarks on the generative power of collage grammars and chain-code grammars. In: Ehrig, H., Engels, G., Kreowski, H.-J., Rozenberg, G. (eds.) TAGT 1998. LNCS, vol. 1764, pp. 1–14. Springer, Heidelberg (2000). https://doi.org/10.1007/978-3-540-46464-8_1
8. Giammarresi, D., Restivo, A.: Two-dimensional languages. In: Rozenberg, G., Salomaa, A. (eds.) Handbook of Formal Languages, vol. 3, pp. 215–267. Springer, Heidelberg (1997). https://doi.org/10.1007/978-3-642-59126-6_4
9. He, Y., Li, L., Zhai, H., Dang, X., Liang, C.-H., Liu, Q.H.: Sierpinski space-filling curves and their application in high-speed circuits for ultrawideband SSN suppression. IEEE Antennas Wirel. Propag. Lett. **9**, 568–571 (2010)
10. Hilbert, D.: Über die stetige Abbildung einer Linie auf ein Flächenstück. Math. Annln. **38**, 459–460 (1891)
11. Kitaev, S., Mansour, T., Seebold, P.: The Peano curve and counting occurrences of some patterns. J. Autom. Lang. Combin. **9**(4), 439–455 (2004)

12. Lawder, J.: The application of space-filling curves to the storage and retrieval of multi-dimensional data. Ph.D thesis. University of London (1999)
13. Maurer, H.A., Rozenberg, G., Welzl, E.: Using string languages to describe picture languages. Inform. Control **54**, 155–185 (1982)
14. Păun, Gh.: Computing with membranes. J. Comput. Syst. Sci. **61**, 108–143 (2000)
15. Păun, Gh.: Membrane Computing: An Introduction. Springer, Heidelbrg (2000). https://doi.org/10.1007/978-3-642-56196-2
16. Păun, Gh., Rozenberg, G., Salomaa, A.: The Oxford Handbook of Membrane Computing. Oxford University Press, New York (2010)
17. Peano, G.: Sur une courbe qui remplit toute une aire plane. Math. Annln. **36**, 157–160 (1890)
18. Rozenberg, G., Salomaa, A. (eds.): Handbook of Formal Languages (3 Volumes). Springer, Berlin (1997). https://doi.org/10.1007/978-3-642-59126-6
19. Sagan, H.: Space-Filling Curves. Springer, New York (1994). https://doi.org/10.1007/978-1-4612-0871-6
20. Salomaa, A.: Formal Languages. Academic Press, London (1973)
21. Seebold, P.: Tag system for the Hilbert curve. Discrete Math. Theoret. Comput. Sci. **9**, 213–226 (2007)
22. Sierpiński, W.: Sur une nouvelle courbe continnue qui remplit toute une aire plane. Bull. Acad. Sci. de Cracovie (Sci. math et nat.) Série A, 462–478 (1912)
23. Siromoney, R., Subramanian, K.G.: Space-filling curves and infinite graphs. In: Ehrig, H., Nagl, M., Rozenberg, G. (eds.) Graph Grammars 1982. LNCS, vol. 153, pp. 380–391. Springer, Heidelberg (1983). https://doi.org/10.1007/BFb0000120
24. Subramanian, K.G.: P systems and picture languages. In: Durand-Lose, J., Margenstern, M. (eds.) MCU 2007. LNCS, vol. 4664, pp. 99–109. Springer, Heidelberg (2007). https://doi.org/10.1007/978-3-540-74593-8_9
25. Subramanian, K.G., Venkat, I., Pan, L.: P systems generating chain code picture languages. In: Proceedings of Asian Conference on Membrane Computing, pp. 115–123 (2012)
26. Zhang, G., Pérez-Jiménez, M.J., Gheorghe, M.: Real-life Applications with Membrane Computing. ECC, vol. 25. Springer, Cham (2017). https://doi.org/10.1007/978-3-319-55989-6

Digitized Rotations of Closest Neighborhood on the Triangular Grid

Aydın Avkan, Benedek Nagy, and Müge Saadetoğlu[(✉)]

Faculty of Arts and Sciences, Department of Mathematics,
Eastern Mediterranean University, North Cyprus via Mersin 10,
Famagusta, Turkey
{aydin.avkan, muge.saadetoglu}@emu.edu.tr,
nbenedek.inf@gmail.com

Abstract. Rigid motions on the plane play an important role in image processing and in image manipulation. They have many properties including the bijectivity and the isometry. On the other hand, digitized rigid motions may fail to satisfy this injectivity or surjectivity properties. Pluta et al. investigated digitized rigid motions locally on the square grid and the hexagonal grid by using neighborhood motion maps. In this paper we show digitized rigid rotations of a pixel and its closest neighbors on the triangular grid. In particular, different rotation centers are considered with respect to the corresponding main pixel, e.g. edge midpoints and corner points. Angles of all bijective and non-bijective rotations are proven for rotations described above.

Keywords: Digital rotations · Discrete motions · Non-traditional grid Neighborhood maps

1 Introduction

Grids play an important role in digital geometry and in digital image processing. There are 3 regular tessellations of the plane which are the square, the hexagonal and the triangular grids (Fig. 1). The square grid and its n-dimensional extensions are well known since their coordinate systems are the Cartesian coordinate systems. There is good literature on the research on the hexagonal grid as well. The hexagonal grid has more symmetry axes and every pixel has six neighbors. As a third type, we have the triangular grid (which is the dual of the hexagonal grid) which is also a valid alternative of the above mentioned two regular grids in more and more applications. Like the hexagonal grid, the triangular grid also has a triangular symmetry, which is better fit for the human eye than the square grid. One of the basic transformations of digital images is their rotation. While in the Euclidean plane, rotations are isometric and bijective, this generally does not hold for the digital pictures. Rotations in a grid usually do not map the grid into itself, thus digitized rotations are equipped with a kind of rounding/digitizing operator. Rotations that map the grid into itself have been described in [5, 6] for the triangular grid. In general, bijectivity of a rotation is important as this notion determines the information preserving and loss in image processing. Non-bijectivity usually causes information loss in the processed image. In [9, 10] Nouvel and Rémila

© Springer Nature Switzerland AG 2018
R. P. Barneva et al. (Eds.): IWCIA 2018, LNCS 11255, pp. 53–67, 2018.
https://doi.org/10.1007/978-3-030-05288-1_5

characterized bijective digitized rotations on the square grid, by specifically studying the non-bijective ones. In [11] Pluta et al. extended this study to characterize the bijective rigid motions on the square grid by focusing on the local description (neighborhood motion map) of the 4 and the 8-neighborhoods, hence extending the characterization of bijective digitized rotations already examined in [8]. Also in [11] two different algorithms are proposed to test whether a given subset of the square grid is transformed bijectively by a digitized rigid motion. Later on, in [12], the same authors studied the differences between the digitized rigid motion defined on both the square and the hexagonal grids. Their approach was an extension to the hexagonal grid of the previous study of the digitized rigid motions of the square grid in the framework of neighborhood motion maps. In particular, they give a comparison of the loss of information (under the digitized rigid motion) between the two grids.

Working on the triangular grid is a relatively new and uninvestigated field in digital geometry, even though various combinatorial image processing algorithms are investigated recently [1, 3, 4, 7]. There are still some interesting questions that need to be answered. Motion map is one of these unanalyzed concepts.

In this paper we examine the neighborhood motion maps of the closest neighbors on the triangular grid. We consider the digitized rigid motions by taking the translation vector as the null vector. In the earlier works on the topic [11, 12], the center of rotation was always the midpoint of a pixel. However, in our work the center of rotations will be at various points of the given (main) pixel. Specifically, we consider the midpoint, the corner points and the edge midpoints as rotation centers for the corresponding even or odd pixel. All rotations will be taken in the positive (anti-clockwise) direction.

2   Preliminaries

In this section we recall some basic concepts from the literature mentioned earlier. $\mathbb{R}$ denotes the set of real numbers while $\mathbb{Z}$ is the set of integers.

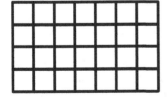 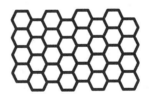 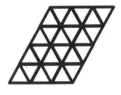

Fig. 1. The Square grid (left), the hexagonal grid (middle) and the triangular grid (right).

2.1   Basic Notations

Definition 1 (Rigid Motions on $\mathbb{R}^2$). Rigid motions on $\mathbb{R}^2$ are bijective distance and angle preserving maps (isometries). They consist of translations, rotations and their compositions. $\breve{U}: \mathbb{R}^2 \to \mathbb{R}^2$ where $x \to Rx + t$ will be the generalized form of the rigid motion, where the rotation matrix is R and t is the translation vector (t_1, t_2).

In our paper we do not use translation, thus $t = (0, 0)$.

Let us consider rigid motions on $\mathbb{Z}^2$. If we apply the rigid motion to a point with integer coordinates, the resulting image may not have integer coordinates. Therefore we need to define digitized rigid motions which map $\mathbb{Z}^2$ to $\mathbb{Z}^2$.

Definition 2 (Digitized Rigid Motion). Digitized rigid motion U is the composition of two functions; the rigid motion $\widetilde{U_{\mathbb{Z}^2}}$ restricted to the domain $\mathbb{Z}^2$ and the digitization operator $D : \mathbb{R}^2 \to \mathbb{Z}^2$. Therefore, the digitized rigid motions are defined by : $\mathbb{Z}^2 \to \mathbb{Z}^2$, where $\widetilde{U_{\mathbb{Z}^2}}$.

2.2 The Triangular Grid

The triangular grid is built up by pixels with 2 different orientations. With respect to these orientations we introduce pixels as even "Δ" or as odd "∇" triangles. In some cases the triangular grid gives more accurate results compared to the square grid, since it has a larger neighborhood relation and better symmetric properties.

Definition 3 (Triangular Grid). A triangular grid is a grid formed by a tessellation of $\mathbb{R}^2$ by regular triangles of side length $\sqrt{3}$ and of height 1.5 units.

Definition 4 (Neighborhood). Triangular grid has 3 types of neighbor relations. Each pixel has three 1-neighbors (closest neighbors), nine 2-neighbors (closest ones counted as well) and twelve 3-neighbors (the closest and 2 neighbors counted as well) (Fig. 2).

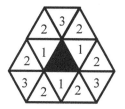

Fig. 2. Neighborhood relation.

2.3 Digitized Cell on the Triangular Grid

While in the square grid, simple rounding operation can be used for digitization, it is not straightforward to define the digitization on the triangular grid. We use digitized cell to map the image of the point after rotation to the center of the belonging pixel. If the midpoint of a given pixel falls inside of any pixel then the image point should belong to the corresponding pixel (Fig. 3, left).

We now consider the next case where the midpoint of the original pixel does not fall inside, but just gets mapped on the edge of a pixel instead. We need to define the digitized cell to show on which pixel midpoint this image point should get mapped to. If the point lies on any diagonal line (grid line with negative slope), then it should be mapped to the corresponding odd triangle, if it lies on any horizontal grid line or anti-diagonal line (grid line with positive slope), then it is going to be mapped to the corresponding even triangle. If the center point of any pixel is mapped on the left corner of an even pixel after the rotation (which lies between the diagonal and the horizontal grid lines corresponding to this pixel), then we map it to that even pixel (Fig. 3, right).

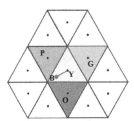 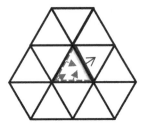

Fig. 3. The triangle Y denotes the main pixel whereas the triangles P, G and O are the closest neighbors of the former. The point B gets mapped to the midpoint of the corresponding pixel after the digitization operator (left). Edges indicated by broken lines belong to the corresponding even triangle, while the solid edge belongs to the corresponding odd one. Left corner of even triangle belongs to the even triangle itself (right).

In this paper, we check the bijectivity corresponding to digitized rigid motions (rotations) with some critical angles ($0° \leq \theta \leq 360°$). Here we consider 3 possible choices for the center of rotation: midpoint of the pixel, the corner points of the pixel, and finally, the midpoint of its edges, where the pixels are the triangles of the grid. Note that exactly these three types of rotation centers have rotation angles that map the grid exactly to itself [5, 6].

3   Bijectivity of the Neighborhood Motion Maps Corresponding to Rotations

The non-injectivity and/or the non-surjectivity of the digitized rigid motion may appear with the existence of 2 and/or 0 preimages respectively (Fig. 4). To observe these local alterations of 1-neighbors, we consider the neighborhood motion map concept on the grid defined as set of vectors, one for each rigid motion of a neighbor. In Fig. 4, the points p, q, r and s are the center points of the corresponding pixels before the rotation. The point p is the center of the main pixel and the other 3 points are the centers of the closest neighbors, respectively. Point c is the rotation center and the rotation angle is 40° in positive direction (anti-clockwise). The points p', q', r' and s' are the rotated images of the points p, q, r and s, respectively. As one can observe this digitized rotation is non-bijective. The images of the points p and q lie in the same, in fact the main, pixel.

Further in this section, the center of rotation will have the coordinates (0,0) and bijectivity and non-bijectivity will be proven by computing the image points.

For each of the propositions, even and odd orientations of the original pixels are analyzed separately. We will use the name main pixel for the pixel that we analyze with its neighbors.

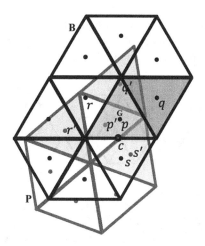

Fig. 4. The grid part denoted by P is a part of the rotated form of the grid denoted by B, 40° around the point c. The green cell, G (with midpoint p) is non-injective since it contains double points (pixels with centers p' and q') after the rotation. (Color figure online)

This section is organized in the following way; in Sect. 3.1 we consider the digitized rigid rotations of the closest neighbors when the rotation center is a corner point of the main pixel. Similarly, in Sects. 3.2 and 3.3, rotation centers are taken to be the center and the edge mid-points of the main pixel respectively.

3.1   Rotations Around a Corner of the Triangle

The grid is mapped to itself by the angle of rotation $\theta \in \{n60° : n \in \mathbb{Z}\}$ when the center of rotation is a corner point [6].

Proposition 1. If the center of rotation is the left corner of an even pixel, then by considering the closest neighbors, the digitized rigid motions are given in Fig. 5.

The changes of the image of the mapped neighborhood occur at the angles

$\sin^{-1}(0.75) - 30°, 30°, 30°, \cos^{-1}(0.75), 30° + \sin^{-1}(0.75), 90°,$
$60° + \cos^{-1}(0.75), 90° + \sin^{-1}(0.75), 150°, 150°, 120° + \cos^{-1}(0.75),$
$150° + \sin^{-1}(0.75), 210°, 210°, 180° + \cos^{-1}(0.75), 210° + \sin^{-1}(0.75), 270°,$
$240° + \cos^{-1}(0.75), 270° + \sin^{-1}(0.75), 330°, 330°, 300° + \cos^{-1}(0.75).$

Their approximated values are shown in Fig. 5.

Proof. The angles are calculated by using polar coordinates, where $x = r \cos \theta$ and $y = r \sin \theta$. In Fig. 6, the point c is the rotation center. The points p and p' are the neighbor pixel center and its position after the rotation, respectively. The angle α denotes the angle between the solid arrow (which connects the point p' to the origin) and the positive x-axis, and the angle $\theta_1 = \alpha - 30°$. The angle α is calculated in the following way; $y = 1.5$ units and the radius (the length of both of the arrows cp and cp') is 2 units. Angle θ_1 is computed as shown in Fig. 6. $1.5 = 2 \sin \alpha \Rightarrow$ $\alpha = \sin^{-1}(0.75)$, $\theta_1 = \sin^{-1}(0.75) - 30°$, where $30°$ is the angle between the x-axis and the dotted arrow, which connects the point p to the origin c.

The other angles are computed in a similar manner.

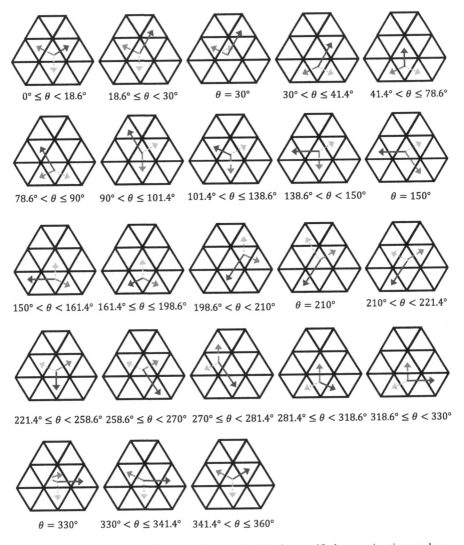

$0° \leq \theta < 18.6°$ $18.6° \leq \theta < 30°$ $\theta = 30°$ $30° < \theta \leq 41.4°$ $41.4° < \theta \leq 78.6°$

$78.6° < \theta \leq 90°$ $90° < \theta \leq 101.4°$ $101.4° < \theta \leq 138.6°$ $138.6° < \theta < 150°$ $\theta = 150°$

$150° < \theta < 161.4°$ $161.4° \leq \theta \leq 198.6°$ $198.6° < \theta < 210°$ $\theta = 210°$ $210° < \theta < 221.4°$

$221.4° \leq \theta < 258.6°$ $258.6° \leq \theta < 270°$ $270° \leq \theta < 281.4°$ $281.4° \leq \theta < 318.6°$ $318.6° \leq \theta < 330°$

$\theta = 330°$ $330° < \theta \leq 341.4°$ $341.4° < \theta \leq 360°$

Fig. 5. Neighborhood motion maps after rotation by the specified approximation angles.

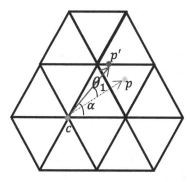

Fig. 6. Center of rotation (blue point, c), neighbor pixel center point (light pink, p), rotated form of the center point (pink point p'). (Color figure online)

Proposition 2. If the center of rotation is the left corner of an even pixel, then the digitized rigid motion is non-injective if and only if $\theta \in \{30° + n360° : n \in \mathbb{Z}\}$ or $\theta \in \{330° + n360° : n \in \mathbb{Z}\}$.

Proof. Non-bijectivity occurs when 2 different pixels lie in the same pixel after the rotation. Based on Proposition 1 (Fig. 5) the only non-bijective maps are at 30° and 330° in the range $[0°, 360°]$.

For example, Fig. 7 shows the non-injective case of the rotation by showing the pixel to which two pixels are mapped. Point c is the center of rotation with angle 30°. The points p and q are the center of the main pixel and the center of one its neighbor, respectively. The points p' and q' are the rotated images of the points p and q in the given order. By the digitized cell, the points p' and q' lie in the same pixel since p' is on the anti-diagonal and q' is on the horizontal line.

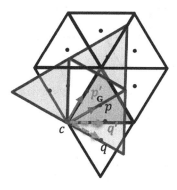

Fig. 7. Solid arrows shows how the center point p of the green pixel moves to p' and broken arrows shows how the center q moves to q'. Both points lie in the green pixel (G) after rotation. (Color figure online)

Now we consider other corners of the main pixel as rotation centers and/or also odd main pixels.

Proposition 3. At every 60° turn, the center of rotation is changed to another corner and the digitized rigid motions for this center can be observed from Proposition 1, Fig. 5. Figure 8 shows the changes of rotation centers with respect to the angles 0°, 60°, 120°, 180°, 240° and 300°.

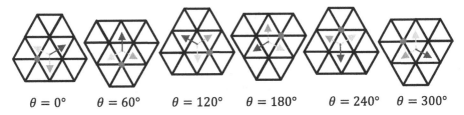

$\theta = 0°$ $\theta = 60°$ $\theta = 120°$ $\theta = 180°$ $\theta = 240°$ $\theta = 300°$

Fig. 8. Changes of rotation centers with respect to the angles.

Remark 1. The images with respect to different corner positions of the center of rotation can be observed by the images of Fig. 5 in the same order with various starting images.

Instead of the formal description of the previous statements we give an example to show how they can be understood. The motion maps from the right corner of an odd pixel can be observed directly from Fig. 5 (Line 3, second image). Figure 9 shows the first 2 images of this rotation by the specified approximation angles. The first image is exactly 180° rotated form of the first image of Fig. 5. The order of the images and angles of the digitized rotations from the right corner of the odd pixel follows the order of Fig. 5 with the starting image the interval containing 180°.

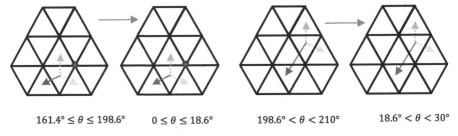

161.4° ≤ θ ≤ 198.6°   0 ≤ θ ≤ 18.6°   198.6° < θ < 210°   18.6° < θ < 30°

Fig. 9. The first image of rotation from the right corner of the odd pixel (2 images on the left), the second image of rotation from the right corner of the odd pixel. (2 images on the right).

The images and the angles of all rotations from any corner point can be obtained in a similar way.

- 0° is the starting point of rotation from the left corner of the even pixel (Proposition 1, Fig. 5).
- Image of the interval which contains 60° is the first image of rotation from the bottom corner of the odd-pixel.

- Image of the interval which contains 120° is the first image of rotation from the right corner of the even pixel.
- Image of the interval which contains 180° is the first image of rotation from the right corner of the odd pixel.
- Image of the interval which contains 240° is the first image of rotation from the upper corner of the even pixel.
- Image of the interval which contains 300° is the first image of rotation from the left corner of the odd pixel.

3.2 Rotations Around the Center of the Triangle

The grid is mapped to itself by the angle of rotation $\theta \in \{n120° : n \in \mathbb{Z}\}$ when the center of rotation is the center of the pixels [5]. The proofs of the next propositions are excluded.

Proposition 4. If the center of rotation is the midpoint of an even pixel, then by considering the closest neighbors, the digitized rigid motions are given in Fig. 10.

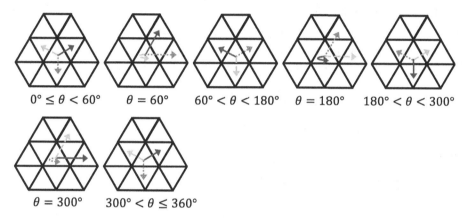

Fig. 10. Neighborhood motion maps after rotation by the specified angles.

Proposition 5. If the center of rotation is the midpoint of an even pixel, then the digitized rigid motion is non-injective if and only if $\theta \in \{60° + n360° : n \in \mathbb{Z}\}$, $\theta \in \{180° + n360° : n \in \mathbb{Z}\}$ or $\theta \in \{300° + n360° : n \in \mathbb{Z}\}$.

Proposition 6. If the center of rotation is the midpoint of an odd pixel, then by considering the closest neighbors, the digitized rigid motions are given in Fig. 11.

Remark 2. If the center of rotation is the midpoint of the odd pixel then the digitized rigid motion is always injective and thus bijective.

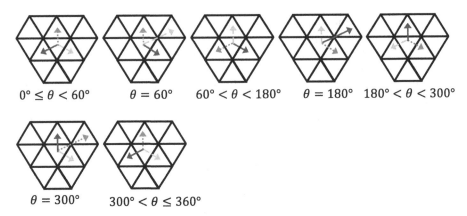

$$0° \leq \theta < 60° \qquad \theta = 60° \qquad 60° < \theta < 180° \qquad \theta = 180° \quad 180° < \theta < 300°$$

$$\theta = 300° \qquad 300° < \theta \leq 360°$$

Fig. 11. Neighborhood motion maps after rotation by the specified angles.

3.3 Rotations Around the Midpoint of an Edge of the Triangle

The grid is mapped to itself by the angle of rotation $\theta \in \{180°n : n \in \mathbb{Z}\}$ when the center of rotation is the midpoint of an edge.

Proposition 7. If the center of rotation is the midpoint of the lower edge of an even pixel, then by considering closest neighbors, the digitized rigid motions are given in Fig. 12. The changes of the motion map occur for the angles

$$\cos^{-1}\left(\tfrac{-6\sqrt{3}-2\sqrt{19}}{8\sqrt{7}}\right) - \cos^{-1}\left(-\sqrt{\tfrac{3}{7}}\right), \ \cos^{-1}\left(\tfrac{6\sqrt{3}-2\sqrt{19}}{8\sqrt{7}}\right) - \cos^{-1}\left(\sqrt{\tfrac{3}{7}}\right),$$

$$\cos^{-1}\left(\tfrac{-6\sqrt{3}+2\sqrt{19}}{8\sqrt{7}}\right) - \cos^{-1}\left(\sqrt{\tfrac{3}{7}}\right), \ 180° - \cos^{-1}\left(-\sqrt{\tfrac{3}{7}}\right),$$

$$360° - \cos^{-1}\left(\tfrac{-6\sqrt{3}-2\sqrt{19}}{8\sqrt{7}}\right) - \cos^{-1}\left(-\sqrt{\tfrac{3}{7}}\right), \ 90°, \ 90°,$$

$$\cos^{-1}\left(\tfrac{-6\sqrt{3}-2\sqrt{19}}{8\sqrt{7}}\right) - \cos^{-1}\left(\sqrt{\tfrac{3}{7}}\right), \ 180° - \cos^{-1}\left(\sqrt{\tfrac{3}{7}}\right),$$

$$360° - \cos^{-1}\left(\tfrac{-6\sqrt{3}+2\sqrt{19}}{8\sqrt{7}}\right) - \cos^{-1}\left(-\sqrt{\tfrac{3}{7}}\right),$$

$$360° - \cos^{-1}\left(\tfrac{6\sqrt{3}-2\sqrt{19}}{8\sqrt{7}}\right) - \cos^{-1}\left(-\sqrt{\tfrac{3}{7}}\right),$$

$$360° - \cos^{-1}\left(\tfrac{-6\sqrt{3}-2\sqrt{19}}{8\sqrt{7}}\right) - \cos^{-1}\left(\sqrt{\tfrac{3}{7}}\right),$$

$$360° - \cos^{-1}\left(\tfrac{6\sqrt{3}+2\sqrt{19}}{8\sqrt{7}}\right) - \cos^{-1}\left(-\sqrt{\tfrac{3}{7}}\right),$$

$$360° - \cos^{-1}\left(\tfrac{-6\sqrt{3}+2\sqrt{19}}{8\sqrt{7}}\right) - \cos^{-1}\left(\sqrt{\tfrac{3}{7}}\right),$$

$$360° - \cos^{-1}\left(\tfrac{6\sqrt{3}-2\sqrt{19}}{8\sqrt{7}}\right) - \cos^{-1}\left(\sqrt{\tfrac{3}{7}}\right), \ 360° - \cos^{-1}\left(-\sqrt{\tfrac{3}{7}}\right),$$

$$360° + \cos^{-1}\left(\tfrac{6\sqrt{3}+2\sqrt{19}}{8\sqrt{7}}\right) - \cos^{-1}\left(-\sqrt{\tfrac{3}{7}}\right), \ 270°, \ 270°,$$

$$360° - \cos^{-1}\left(\tfrac{6\sqrt{3}+2\sqrt{19}}{8\sqrt{7}}\right) - \cos^{-1}\left(\sqrt{\tfrac{3}{7}}\right), \ 360° - \cos^{-1}\left(\sqrt{\tfrac{3}{7}}\right),$$

$$360° - \cos^{-1}\left(\tfrac{-6\sqrt{3}+2\sqrt{19}}{8\sqrt{7}}\right) + \cos^{-1}\left(\sqrt{\tfrac{3}{7}}\right), \ 360° - \cos^{-1}\left(\tfrac{6\sqrt{3}-2\sqrt{19}}{8\sqrt{7}}\right) + \cos^{-1}\left(\sqrt{\tfrac{3}{7}}\right).$$

Their approximate values are shown in Fig. 12.

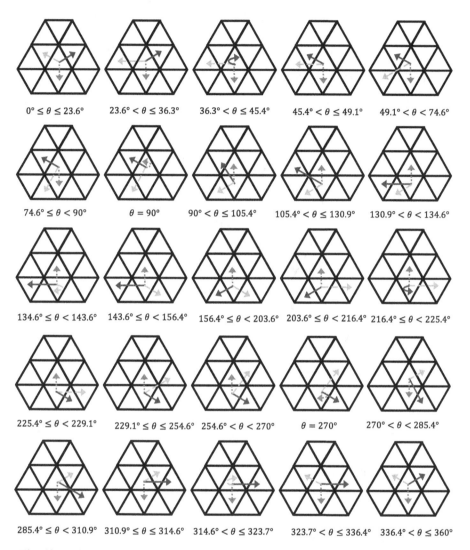

Fig. 12. Neighborhood motion maps after rotation by the specified approximation angles.

Proof. The angles are calculated by using polar coordinates, where $x = r \cos \theta$ and $y = r \sin \theta$. Figure 13 shows that the point c is the midpoint of the bottom edge of the main pixel, which is the rotation center as well. The point p is the center of the neighbor pixel. The line, L, is the line that passes through the right edge of the main pixel and the circle, C, is the circle whose radius is equal to the distance between c and p. The angles α and β denote the angles between the horizontal line (holding the point c) and the arrows which connect the points p and p' to the center of rotation, c, respectively.

The equation of the line L is $y = -\sqrt{3}x + 1.5$ and the equation of the circle C is $x^2 + y^2 = \frac{7}{4}$. The point p' is the intersection point of L and C, Then the x-coordinate of this point is $\frac{3\sqrt{3}-\sqrt{19}}{8}$. Since $x = r \cos \beta$ and $r = \frac{\sqrt{7}}{2}$, then $\beta = \cos^{-1}\left(\frac{6\sqrt{3}-2\sqrt{19}}{8\sqrt{7}}\right)$, thus the angle of rotation is equal to $\cos^{-1}\left(\frac{6\sqrt{3}-2\sqrt{19}}{8\sqrt{7}}\right) - \cos^{-1}\left(\sqrt{\frac{3}{7}}\right)$ where $\cos^{-1}\left(\sqrt{\frac{3}{7}}\right) = \alpha$. Other angles are computed similarly.

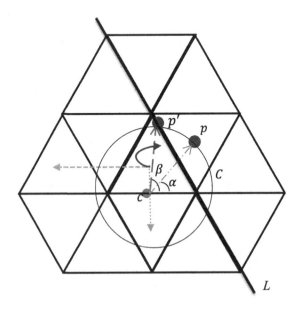

Fig. 13. Blue dot c indicates the center of rotation where the pink dots p and p' indicate the center of the right neighbor pixel and its image after rotation, respectively. (Color figure online)

Proposition 8. If the center of rotation is the midpoint of the lower edge of an even pixel, then the digitized rigid motion is non-injective for the following intervals of the rotation angle, where $n \in \mathbb{Z}$.

- $\left(\cos^{-1}\left(\frac{6\sqrt{3}-2\sqrt{19}}{8\sqrt{7}}\right) - \cos^{-1}\left(\sqrt{\frac{3}{7}}\right) + n360°,\right.$
  $\left. \cos^{-1}\left(\frac{-6\sqrt{3}+2\sqrt{19}}{8\sqrt{7}}\right) - \cos^{-1}\left(\sqrt{\frac{3}{7}}\right) + n360°\right]$
- $[90° + n360°, 90° + n360°]$ (they contain exactly one angle for each n)
- $\left[360° - \cos^{-1}\left(\frac{-6\sqrt{3}+2\sqrt{19}}{8\sqrt{7}}\right) - \cos^{-1}\left(-\sqrt{\frac{3}{7}}\right) + n360°,\right.$
  $\left. 360° - \cos^{-1}\left(\frac{6\sqrt{3}-2\sqrt{19}}{8\sqrt{7}}\right) - \cos^{-1}\left(-\sqrt{\frac{3}{7}}\right) + n360°\right)$
- $\left[360° - \cos^{-1}\left(\frac{-6\sqrt{3}+2\sqrt{19}}{8\sqrt{7}}\right) - \cos^{-1}\left(\sqrt{\frac{3}{7}}\right) + n360°,\right.$
  $\left. 360° - \cos^{-1}\left(\frac{6\sqrt{3}-2\sqrt{19}}{8\sqrt{7}}\right) - \cos^{-1}\left(\sqrt{\frac{3}{7}}\right) + n360°\right)$

- $[270° + n360°, 270° + n360°]$ (they contain exactly one angle for each n)

- $\left[360° - \cos^{-1}\left(\frac{-6\sqrt{3}+2\sqrt{19}}{8\sqrt{7}}\right) + \cos^{-1}\left(\sqrt{\frac{3}{7}}\right) + n360°,\right.$
$\left. 360° - \cos^{-1}\left(\frac{6\sqrt{3}-2\sqrt{19}}{8\sqrt{7}}\right) + \cos^{-1}\left(\sqrt{\frac{3}{7}}\right) + n360°\right).$

Proof. It is a consequence of the result of Proposition 7, Fig. 12.

Proposition 9. Digitized rigid motion maps for rotation center at the other edge midpoints are obtained from Fig. 12 as described below.

– The first 3 neighborhood motion maps of rotations centered at the left edge midpoint of an even triangle is shown in Fig. 14. (240° rotated forms of Fig. 12).

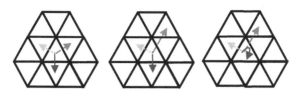

Fig. 14. The first 3 neighborhood motion maps of rotations centered at the left edge midpoint of an even triangle.

– The first 3 neighborhood motion maps of rotations centered at the right edge midpoint of an even triangle is shown in Fig. 15. (120° rotated forms of the images of Fig. 12).

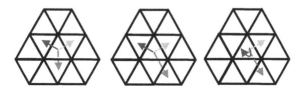

Fig. 15. The first 3 neighborhood motion maps of rotations centered at the right edge midpoint of an even triangle.

Remark 3. The images of Fig. 16 (for rotation from the midpoints of odd triangle edges) can be observed by 180° rotation from the corresponding edge of the even triangle.

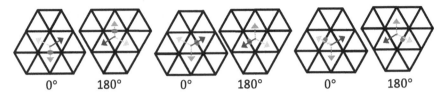

Fig. 16. Bottom edge midpoint of an even pixel is mapped to the upper edge midpoint of an odd pixel at 180°(first and second subfigures), right edge midpoint of an even pixel is mapped to the left edge midpoint of an odd pixel at 180° (third and fourth subfigures) and left edge midpoint of an even pixel is mapped to the right edge midpoint of an odd pixel at 180° (fifth and sixth subfigures).

4 Conclusion and Future Work Plans

In this paper we characterized bijective digitized rotations of the closest neighbors on the triangular grid. To do this different rotation centers on a given main pixel are considered. Specifically, we proved bijectivity angles for digitized rotations around the corners, the edge midpoints and the center of the given (main) pixel.

Our main perspective is to extend this work to characterize bijective digitized rotations of larger neighborhoods (including the 2-neighbors and the 3-neighbors). We also plan to investigate the bijectivity of the local neighborhoods of the triangular grid, when the rotation center is not nearby, but some distance away. Another way to continue the research is to combine rotations with other operations, e.g., translations [2].

References

1. Abdalla, M., Nagy, B.: Dilation and erosion on the triangular tessellation: an independent approach. IEEE Access **6**, 23108–23119 (2018)
2. Abuhmaidan, K., Nagy, B.: Non-bijective translations on the triangular plane. In: 2018 IEEE 16th World Symposium on Applied Machine Intelligence and Informatics (SAMI 2018), Kosice, Slovakia, pp. 183–188 (2018)
3. Balint, G.T., Nagy, B.: Finiteness of chain-code picture languages on the triangular grid. In: ISPA 2015: Int. Symp. on Image and Signal Processing and Analysis, IEEE, pp. 310–315 (2015)
4. Kardos, P., Palágyi, K.: On topology preservation of mixed operators in triangular, square, and hexagonal grids. Discrete Appl. Math. **216**, 441–448 (2017)
5. Nagy, B.: Isometric transformations of the dual of the hexagonal lattice, ISPA 2009: 6th International Symposium on Image and Signal Processing and Analysis, Salzburg, Austria, pp. 432–437 (2009)
6. Nagy, B.: Transformations of the triangular grid, GRAFGEO: Third Hungarian Conference on Computer Graphics and Geometry, Budapest, Hungary, pp. 155–162 (2005)
7. Nagy, B., Moisi, E.V.: Memetic algorithms for reconstruction of binary images on triangular grids with 3 and 6 projections. Appl. Soft Comput. **52**, 549–565 (2017)
8. Nouvel, B., Rémila, E.: Characterization of bijective discretized rotations. In: Klette, R., Žunić, J. (eds.) IWCIA 2004. LNCS, vol. 3322, pp. 248–259. Springer, Heidelberg (2004). https://doi.org/10.1007/978-3-540-30503-3_19

9. Nouvel, B., Rémila, E.: Configurations induced by discrete rotations: Periodicity and quasi-periodicity properties. Discrete Appl. Math. **147**, 323–343 (2005)

10. Nouvel, B., Rémila, É.: On colorations induced by discrete rotations. In: Nyström, I., Sanniti di Baja, G., Svensson, S. (eds.) DGCI 2003. LNCS, vol. 2886, pp. 174–183. Springer, Heidelberg (2003). https://doi.org/10.1007/978-3-540-39966-7_16

11. Pluta, K., Romon, P., Kenmochi, Y., Passat, N.: Bijective digitized rigid motions on subsets of the plane. J. Math. Imaging Vis. **59**, 84–105 (2017)

12. Pluta, K., Romon, P., Kenmochi, Y., Passat, N.: Honeycomb geometry: rigid motions on the hexagonal grid. In: Kropatsch, W., Artner, N., Janusch, I. (eds.) DGCI 2017. LNCS, vol. 10502, pp. 33–45. Springer, Cham (2017). https://doi.org/10.1007/978-3-319-66272-5_4

Binary Tomography on Triangular Grid Involving Hexagonal Grid Approach

Benedek Nagy[1] and Tibor Lukić[2(✉)]

[1] Faculty of Arts and Sciences, Eastern Mediterranean University, North Cyprus, Mersin-10, Famagusta, Turkey
nbenedek.inf@gmail.com
[2] Faculty of Technical Sciences, University of Novi Sad, Novi Sad, Serbia
tibor@uns.ac.rs

Abstract. In this paper, we consider the binary tomography reconstruction problem of images on the triangular grid. The reconstruction process is based on three natural directions of projections, defined by the lane directions of the triangular grid (they are analogous to row and column directions on the square grid). The recently proposed shifted projection approach is applied, which allows that the number of delta and nabla shape triangular pixels in each lane to be exactly determined. The structure of the set of the same type pixels coincides with the structure of the hexagonal grid. The proposed new reconstruction process solve separately the task for the delta and nabla shape pixels on two hexagonal grids. Experimental results on a number of test images is presented and analyzed. The new method shows advantage in both aspects, quality of the reconstructions and running times.

Keywords: Discrete tomography · Triangular grid · Hexagonal grid
Shifted projection approach · Independent approach

1 Introduction

In digital image processing the images consist of a finite number of pixels. The most usual grid is the square grid that contains square pixels and thus the images are usually considered in rectangular frames. The most image processing algorithms use this grid; however, in 2D, i.e., in the plane, the triangular and hexagonal grids are valid alternatives [1,13–15] The development of theory on the hexagonal grid and the respective applications have started nearly a half century ago, right after similar investigations on the square (rectangular) grid have started, see e.g., [4,5,7,9,16]. In this paper, binary tomography (BT) problems on the triangular grid is considered. The BT is a restricted subfield of general tomography and deals with the reconstructions of binary images. In many real cases, the object being studied may consists of a material with homogeneous structure. Therefore, the absence or the presence of such material can be represented by 0 and 1, respectively. As a field of BT application, we first mention the human radiology. One of the most important uses in radiology is the reconstruction of images representing blood vessels or organs (angiograms), obtained by X-ray tomography methods,

R. P. Barneva et al. (Eds.): IWCIA 2018, LNCS 11255, pp. 68–81, 2018.
https://doi.org/10.1007/978-3-030-05288-1_6

[28]. The homogeneous structure is achieved by injecting a special contrast agent into the part of the body being examined. In the field of industry, it is often necessary to examine the quality of the interior of an object with homogeneous structure, without damaging it. In such cases, for example in damage assessment of a metal turbine blade, BT can be a useful tool as a non-destructive testing approach, for more details see [11].

Recently, various binary tomography reconstruction methods were proposed on the triangular grid. We mention the stochastic [18,23] and deterministic [19] methods. In the dense projection approach (DPA) [26], increased projection emission/radiation is used requiring increased memory space. As a consequence, greater running time is needed for the reconstruction process to obtain better results. Therefore, it is of high importance to develop methods which can give at least the same quality result with less radiation. In our recent paper [27], we proposed a shifted projection approach which provides the same quality of reconstruction as the DPA method, but does not require increase of the projection data. In this paper, we make a step further and propose a more efficient method on the basis of shifted projection approach. The new approach is based on the duality between triangular and hexagonal grids. We suggest transforming the reconstruction problem, originally given on triangular grid, into two new problems on two hexagonal grids, with a halved dimension compared to the original problem. These two new smaller hexagonal problems are also mutually independent and parallel processing is possible. Hexagonal problems are solved by gradient based deterministic algorithms. The reduced dimension also reduces the number of switching components, which make hexagonal subproblems easier for processing by optimization algorithm.

This paper is organized as follows. Section 2 gives a brief description of the triangular grid and the shifted projection approach. In Sect. 3, the hexagonal grid and the corresponding deterministic binary tomography reconstruction method are shortly presented. Section 4 contains the description of the proposed combined triangular-hexagonal grid method. In Sect. 5, an experimental evaluation of the proposed method is given. Finally, Sect. 6 concludes the paper.

2 The Triangular Grid

The often used Cartesian coordinate system made the square grid the most wide spread and most used regular tessellation of the plane. The rows and the columns of a picture are addressed by two independent integer coordinates. Usually, the considered shapes are embedded in rectangles on the square grid. The triangular grid can also be described elegantly by three coordinates, as it can be seen in Fig. 1. Although the coordinates are not independent, this description mirrors the symmetry of the grid. The triangular grid is not a point lattice, due to the fact that there are two types of triangles (pixels). The pixels having coordinate sum 0 are called even pixels, their shape is Δ (delta) in this paper. The ones having coordinate sum 1 are called odd pixels and has shape ∇ (nabla). The triplets to address the pixels of the grid are exactly those integer triplets that having sum zero or one. More properties of the coordinate system and the grid can be seen, e.g., in [24], including the way how neighbor pixels can easily be addressed. Each pixel (triangle) has three closest neighbors. These can be found by changing one of the coordinate values by 1 (each of them has opposite shape than the original pixel). For

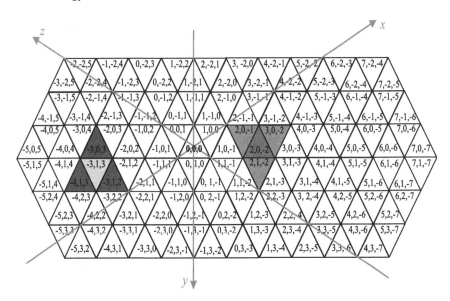

Fig. 1. The symmetric coordinate system for the triangular grid, with an even and an odd pixel and their closest neighbors.

each pixel there are six same type pixels that can be reached by increasing a coordinate value and decreasing another by 1. A pixel and its six neighbors generated this way will play an important role later on. The sets of pixels for which one of the coordinate values is fixed are called lanes (e.g., $y = -2$ for the horizontal lane on the top of Fig. 1). Lanes give the natural directions of the grid, they play similar role as columns and rows in the square grid. Naturally, the images are embedded in hexagons on the triangular grid [25]. In this paper, binary images with regular hexagonal shapes are considered.

As we have already mentioned, we are using only projections that are in the directions of the underlying grid. On the square grid these directions are the usual vertical and horizontal directions (column and row sums, respectively). On the triangular grid the projections go by lanes. Binary tomography has been defined and analyzed both for the square grid with these two projections (see, e.g., [8,29] for founding papers) and for the triangular grid by lanes (see [18,19,22]).

In this paper, we are reconstructing images with regular hexagonal shape on the triangular grid. In the next subsection the base of the shifted projection approach is recalled from [27].

2.1 The Shifted Projection Approach

The shifted projection approach means that the projection ray goes through pixels (triangles) parallel with lane, but not along the middle of lane, as it is usually suggested, see [18,19]. The projection ray is shifted/moved from the middle, see illustration in Fig. 2. For simplicity, we assume that the length of triangle sides is one. The value of α is the ray length through delta shape pixels, while $1 - \alpha$ is the length through nabla

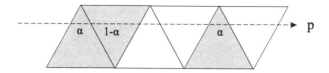

Fig. 2. Shifted projection ray penetrating trough a triangular grid lane.

shape pixels. α is selected from interval $(0,1)$, where $\alpha \neq 0.5$. This "shifted" choice of α provides additional information about the nabla and delta pixels belonging to the object. Namely, it determines the exact number of the shaded pixels in each grid lane. In a case when α is an irrational number from the predefined interval, it can easily be proven that the number of nabla and delta type pixels per lane are uniquely determined by the given projection value p, see Fig. 2 and [27] for more details. Thus, the proposed shift projection approach on the triangular grid provides additional information about the pixels belonging to the object: the number of nabla and delta type pixels per lane.

In practice, one may not need to use irrational number for α. In our recent paper [27] is shown that $\alpha = \frac{22}{31}$ is also good enough choice for the test images of 26 lanes per hexagonal side, what we use in our experiments.

3   The Hexagonal Grid

It is well known that the hexagonal grid defines the closest packing of same size disks in the plane, that is, this grid has a much lower rotational dependency than the square grid has. The hexagonal grid has various other advantages over the traditional square grid by its geometry discussed by various authors in the literature [6, 12]. Now we recall that the hexagonal grid also has a nice and symmetric description introduced by Her (see, e.g., [10]) by three coordinate values, as it can be seen in Fig. 3. The three coordinate axes have angles $2\pi/3$. Observe that in the hexagonal grid all the pixels (they are also called hexels due to their shape, see e.g., [21]) have coordinate sum 0, and exactly those integer triplets are used to address hexels which have this property. As the three coordinate values are dependent on each other any two of them would be enough to address the hexels (as it was used, e.g., in [16]). However, it is recommended to use all the three values to capture the symmetry of the grid and have a more elegant and simple way of description. With the symmetric coordinate system the neighborhood criteria of hexels can formally be written as follows. Two distinct hexels (x_1,y_1,z_1) and (x_2,y_2,z_2) are neighbors if and only if $|x_1 - x_2| \leq 1, |y_1 - y_2| \leq 1, |z_1 - z_2| \leq 1$, or, equivalently, $|x_1 - x_2| + |y_1 - y_2| + |z_1 - z_2| = 2$. Actually, due to the zero-sum restriction of triplets addressing hexels, it is equivalent to the following condition: exactly one of the coordinate values is increased by 1 and exactly one of them decreased by 1 comparing (x_1,y_1,z_1) and (x_2,y_2,z_2). Observe the 6 neighbors of the hexel $(0,0,0)$ in Fig. 3; they are $(0,1,-1),(1,0,-1),(1,-1,0),(0,-1,1),(-1,0,1)$ and $(-1,1,0)$. Remember that we have also 6 same type triangle pixels of any pixel of the triangular grid described by exactly these vectors. This mean that, effectively, the triangular grid can be seen as a union of two "independent" hexagonal grids, one with the delta and

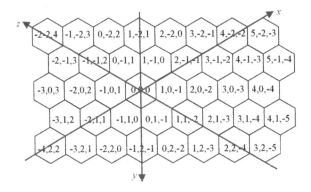

Fig. 3. The symmetric coordinate system for the hexagonal grid [10].

the other with the nabla shape pixels. Coming back to the hexagonal grid, the next important thing is to consider somewhat similar set of pixels as the rows and columns of the rectangular grid. We recall the notion of lanes from [24] similarly as it was already mentioned for the triangular grid. The lanes are sets of pixels for which one of the coordinate values is fixed (e.g., $y = -2$ for the horizontal lane can be seen on the top of Fig. 3). Lanes give the natural directions of the grid, observe that they are orthogonal to a chosen coordinate axis. Two lanes are parallel if they are orthogonal to the same axis. The intersection of two non-parallel lanes contains exactly one hexel; the coordinate triplet of that pixel is determined by the lanes.

3.1 Reconstruction Method on Hexagonal Grid

We consider three projection directions orthogonal to the coordinate axes. In this way the sum of the 1's by lanes are counted. Lanes orthogonal to coordinate axes are reached by fixing the corresponding coordinate value (see Fig. 3).

The following linear system of equations represents the binary tomography (BT) image reconstruction problem:

$$Au = b, \quad A \in \mathbb{R}^{m \times n}, \ u \in \{0,1\}^n, \ b \in \mathbb{R}^m.$$

The matrix A is a so-called projection matrix, whose each row corresponds to one projection ray. The corresponding components of vector b contain the detected m projection value. The binary-vector u represents the unknown image to be reconstructed. Each row entry $a_{i,.}$ of A represents the length of the intersection of the hexel and the projection ray passing through it. We assume that the ray always passing trough the center of hexels and the length of hexel side is one. It is easy to check, that in the considered directions (orthogonal to coordinate axes) these values are $\sqrt{3}$. The projection value measured by a projection ray is calculated as a sum of products of the pixel's intensity and the corresponding length of the projection ray through that pixel ($\sqrt{3}$). Projections are taken from three different directions, orthogonal to the three coordinate axes. For each direction, every possible lane, parallel to the considered direction, is taken.

For the reconstruction on hexagonal grid, we use the method proposed in [20]. Below is a brief description of this method.

We reformulate the BT problem into an energy-minimization problem given by

$$\min_{u \in \{0,1\}^n} E(u) := \frac{1}{2} \left(\|Au - b\|_2^2 + \lambda \sum_i \sum_{j \in \Upsilon(i)} (u_i - u_j)^2 \right), \tag{1}$$

The first term in (1) is called the *data fitting* term and measures the accordance of a solution with a projection data. The second term is the so-called *smooth regularization* term and its role is to enforce the coherency of the solution. Its application is based on the prior knowledge that the original image is composed from compact regions of pixels with homogeneous intensities. This holds for every real image with a relatively good resolution, however it does not hold for random images. The parameter $\lambda > 0$ is the balancing parameter between data fitting and smoothing terms.

By $\Upsilon(i)$ in (1) we denote the set of indices of three neighboring hexels of u_i. In three of the considered directions: for a hexel (x, y, z) the following hexels are used as neighbors: $(x + 1, y, z - 1)$, $(x, y + 1, z - 1)$ and $(x - 1, y + 1, z)$. In this way, each difference of two closest neighborhood hexels, in entire gird, is used exactly once in the regularization term of (1).

The problem (1) can be considered in a relaxed form

$$\min_{u \in [0,1]^n} E_R(u; \mu) := E(u) + \mu \langle u, \tau - u \rangle, \quad \mu > 0, \tag{2}$$

where $\tau = [1, 1, \ldots, 1]^T$. Parameter μ regulates the influence of the added concave regularization term $\langle u, \tau - u \rangle$, which enforces the binary solution. The problem (2), for fixed $\mu > 0$, can be treated by a convex constrained optimization method. We utilize the Spectral Projected Gradient (SPG), iterative and gradient based, optimization algorithm [2] for this task, already used in similar problems [17]. For detailed description and analysis of the reconstruction process (2), we refer the reader to [20].

4   Proposed Combined Triangular-Hexagonal Grid Method

The main idea, suggested in this paper, predicts transforming the reconstruction problem, originally given on triangular grid, into two "smaller" problems on hexagonal grid. After finding solutions on hexagonal grid, we transfer obtained solutions back to the triangular grid and get the final solution. This approach is mainly based on the duality between triangular and hexagonal grids.

The task is to reconstruct triangular grid based binary images, with regular hexagonal shapes, from the given projective data. Three "natural" projective directions are used, orthogonal to x, y and z coordinate axes (1). We accept the shifted projection approach, described in our earlier paper [27], which allows to determine the number of nabla and delta type pixels per each projection lane. Using this information, we form two separate hexagonal grids. One of the hexagonal grid is associated only with nabla triangles, while the other is associated only with delta triangles. More precisely, coordinate values of the hexagonal girds are determined in the following way. Let (x, y, z) is

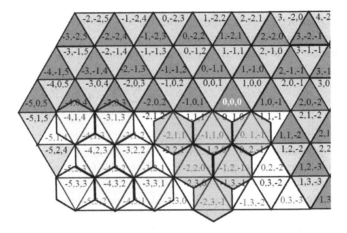

Fig. 4. The triangular grid parts of its corresponding hexagonal grids H_∇ (in bright gray) and H_Δ (in darker gray).

a coordinate triplet of the given triangular grid T. Coordinate triplets $(x_\nabla, y_\nabla, z_\nabla)$ and $(x_\Delta, y_\Delta, z_\Delta)$ of the corresponding hexagonal grids H_∇ and H_Δ, respectively, are determined by

$$\text{If } x + y + z = 0 \text{ then } (x_\Delta, y_\Delta, z_\Delta) = (x, y, z) \text{ and}$$

$$\text{If } x + y + z = 1 \text{ then } (x_\nabla, y_\nabla, z_\nabla) = (x - 1, y, z).$$

It is easy to see, that new hexagonal grids, H_∇ and H_Δ, have half of the pixels than the given triangular grid, see Fig. 4. The applied shifted projection approach on triangular gird determines the number of ∇ and Δ pixels. The gird H_∇ is associated with nabla pixels in triangular grid, which number (those with an intensity of 1) is known in each lane. Therefore, we can calculate the projection values for all lanes of the hexagonal grid H_∇. By this way, we obtained a reconstruction problem on the hexagonal grid H_∇, determined by three "natural" projection directions, orthogonal to the coordinate axes. In a similar way, but now using information about the number of Δ pixels per lanes, we obtained the second reconstruction problem, based on the hexagonal grid H_Δ. Hence, we have transformed the given reconstruction problem on the triangular grid into two reconstruction (sub-)problems on hexagonal grids - whose dimensions are twice smaller as the original problem. As a next step, we solve these two reconstruction problems by a deterministic and gradient based method, described in details in [20]. These two problems are mutually independent, therefore parallel processing is possible, which additionally speeds up the process. After finding solutions on hexagonal grids H_∇ and H_Δ, their pixel intensity values are transferred back to the given triangular grid and the final solution is determined. More precisely, this "inverse process" can be described in the following way:

$$\text{If } x + y + z = 0 \text{ then } T(x, y, z) = H_\Delta(x, y, z) \text{ and}$$

$$\text{If } x + y + z = 1 \text{ then } T(x, y, z) = H_\nabla(x - 1, y, z),$$

where (x, y, z) is a coordinate triplet belongs to the triangular grid T. By $T(x, y, z)$, $H_\Delta(x, y, z)$ and $H_\nabla(x, y, z)$ intensities of pixels at the point (x, y, z) are denoted.

As we see above, the suggested new approach instead on originally given triangular grid, solves two smaller problems on hexagonal grids. These two subproblems, with halved dimensions, are simpler for handling by minimization methods, because the switching components and the number of compliant solutions are also reduced. On the other hand, smaller dimensions implies reduction of running time too. In addition, the hexagonal subproblems are mutually independent, allowing parallel computing, which further reduces the running time. In the following, we denote the new method by CB-T associating that it combines triangular and hexagonal grids.

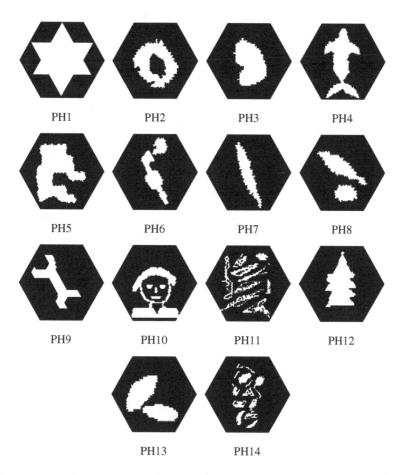

Fig. 5. Original images used in the experiments. All images have the same size: 26 by 26 by 26 (regular hexagons), i.e., 4056 pixels/triangles.

5 Experimental Results

This section presents experimental evaluation of the performance of the proposed CB-T reconstruction method. There are only few tomography methods designed for triangular gird, see [18,19,26,27]. The performance of the CB-T method is compared with two reconstruction methods with, which provided best results, so far. These two methods are the SPG optimization algorithm [2,3] based, "standard", one projection ray per lane approach (SPG-T) and the method based on the shifted projection approach (SH-T). The SPG-T method is proposed, analyzed and completely described in [19], while the SH-T method is introduced in [27]. All three methods are implemented in MATLAB environment.

In evaluation process, we use the set of 14 binary test images of size 26 by 26 by 26 (regular hexagons with side length of 26), each contains 4056 pixel triangles. Note that this resolution is close to the resolution of 64×64 image in square grid. The original test images are presented in Fig. 5.

The projection data is collected using three projection directions. These directions are by lanes, i.e., they are perpendicular to the coordinate axes. We evaluate the performance of the proposed CB-T method by reconstructing the test images from the given projection data. The obtained results are compared with reconstruction results provided by SPG-T and SH-T methods on the same set of images and using projections from the same three directions. We analyze the quality of the reconstructions and the required running times.

The quality of the reconstructions is indicated by three quality/error measures. The absolute number of misclassified pixels in reconstructions are indicated by PE (pixel error), and it is simply calculated by $PE = \|u^r - u^{orig}\|_1$, where u^r and u^{orig} represents the reconstruction and its original image, respectively. In fact, it is the Hamming distance of the original and the reconstructed images. The designation $\nabla\Delta$ presents the sum of the deviation of the number of odd and even pixels in reconstructed image from the correct number in each lane, calculated by

$$\nabla\Delta = \sum_{i=1}^{nr.lanes} |sr_i - sorig_i| + |lr_i - lorig_i|,$$

where sr_i and lr_i are the number of odd and even pixels, respectively, in i-th lane of the reconstructed image, while $sorig_i$ and $lorig_i$ are their counterparts regarding the original image. The projection error, denoted by PRE, measures the accordance of the reconstruction with the given projection data. We defined it by $PRE = \|Au^r - b\|_2$.

Three reconstruction examples are shown in Fig. 6. For each test image, below the reconstructed image, we can see the corresponding difference image, indicating the positions of misclassified pixels. The pixel error PE and the relative number of misclassified pixels (in brackets), are also shown. In all three cases, the new CB-T method provided results with lowest errors. Table 1 summarize the obtained error for all 14 test images. From the total of 14 reconstructions, in 11 cases the proposed CB-T method shows minimal pixel errors, comparing PE values. The projection errors PRE show that the projection data are better fitted for CB-T in 10 cases. Values of $\nabla\Delta$ are also significantly decreased for CB-T method and they have minimal values in all cases.

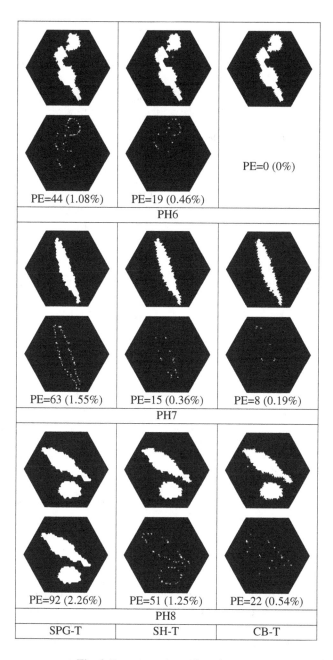

Fig. 6. Reconstructions of test images.

Table 1. Pixel (*PE*), nabla-delta ($\nabla\Delta$) and projection errors (*PRE*) for SPG-T, SH-T and CB-T methods.

	SPG-T	SH-T	CB-T	SPG-T	SH-T	CB-T
	PH1			PH2		
PE	0/0%	0/0%	0/0%	90/2.21%	45/1.10%	67/1.65%
$\nabla\Delta$	0	0	0	48	16	4
PRE	0	0	0	3.08	2.04	2.76
	PH3			PH4		
PE	32/0.78%	0/0%	0/0%	67/1.65%	0/0%	0/0%
$\nabla\Delta$	18	0	0	49	0	0
PRE	2.73	0	0	3.04	0	0
	PH5			PH6		
PE	42/1.03%	0/0%	0/0%	55/1.35%	19/0.46%	0/0%
$\nabla\Delta$	30	0	0	48	10	0
PRE	2.44	0	0	3.12	2.02	0
	PH7			PH8		
PE	63/1.55%	15/0.36%	8/0%	92/2.26%	51/1.25%	22/0.54%
$\nabla\Delta$	47	8	0	50	25	8
PRE	3.20	2.13	1.53	3.31	2.86	2.65
	PH9			PH10		
PE	5/0.12%	0/0%	0/0%	293/7.22%	286/7.05%	306/7.54%
$\nabla\Delta$	6	0	0	38	26	14
PRE	1.65	0	0	2.87	2.81	4.25
	PH11			PH12		
PE	963/23.74%	921/22.70%	985/24.28%	5/0.12%	0/0%	0/0%
$\nabla\Delta$	85	53	12	7	0	0
PRE	3.57	3.84	4.08	1.50	0	0
	PH13			PH14		
PE	48/1.18%	11/0.27%	0/0%	556/13.70%	541/13.33%	520/12.82%
$\nabla\Delta$	37	9	0	64	30	13
PRE	3.00	2.44	0	3.08	4.11	3.86

In Table 2 elapsed running times are presented for all test images. In Sect. 4 we already concluded that the proposed CB-T method consists of two subproblems, when each has halved dimensions compared to SPG-T and SH-T. In addition to that, these two subproblems are mutually independent, which allows parallel computation. These fact make the obtained results in Table 2 expected, where CB-T achieved significantly less running times in all cases. Based on the obtained experimental results, this reduction is on average approximately 80% per image.

Table 2. Elapsed running times in minutes for SPG-T, SH-T and CB-T methods.

SPG-T	SH-T	CB-T	SPG-T	SH-T	CB-T
PH1			PH2		
17.45	17.25	3.50	27.13	28.11	5.35
PH3			PH4		
20.34	21.03	4.09	18.78	19.23	3.91
PH5			PH6		
23.30	24.10	4.79	25.78	25.81	5.09
PH7			PH8		
33.2	35.1	7.22	30.89	31.12	6.11
PH9			PH10		
34.11	33.34	7.33	31.89	31.95	6.30
PH11			PH12		
32.53	32.89	6.57	21.67	22.45	4.55
PH13			PH14		
19.78	19.93	4.07	32.47	33.27	6.23

6 Conclusions

In this paper we have proposed a new binary tomography reconstruction method for images on the triangular grid. The new method predicts to transfer the problem given on the triangular grid to two subproblems defined on hexagonal grids. These two hexagonal subproblems processing separately the nabla and delta type pixels of the triangular grid. Important advantage is that subproblems have halved dimensions compared to the given problem on the triangular grid. Also, they can be solved simultaneously, i.e., parallel computing is possible. Experimental results shows its good performance regarding the quality of reconstructions in comparison with already suggested reconstruction methods. Also, great progress has been made in terms of required running times. Based on experiments, the new method, on average, reduced the running time for 80% in comparison with other relevant reconstruction algorithms.

Acknowledgement. Tibor Lukić acknowledges the Ministry of Education and Sciences of the R. of Serbia for support via projects OI-174008 and III-44006. He also acknowledges support received from the Hungarian Academy of Sciences through the DOMUS project.

References

1. Abdalla, M., Nagy, B.: Dilation and erosion on the triangular tessellation: an independent approach. IEEE Access **6**, 23108–23119 (2018)
2. Birgin, E.G., Martínez, J.M., Raydan, M.: Algorithm 813: SPG - software for convex-constrained optimization. ACM Trans. Math. Softw. **27**, 340–349 (2001)

3. Birgin, E., Martínez, J.: A box-constrained optimization algorithm with negative curvature directions and spectral projected gradients. In: Alefeld, G., Chen, X. (eds.) Topics in Numerical Analysis. COMPUTING, vol. 15, pp. 49–60. Springer, Vienna (2001). https://doi.org/10.1007/978-3-7091-6217-0_5

4. Borgefors, G.: Distance transformations on hexagonal grids. Pattern Recogn. Lett. **9**(2), 97–105 (1989)

5. Brimkov, V.E., Barneva, R.P.: "Honeycomb" vs square and cubic models. Electron. Notes Theoret. Comput. Sci. **46**, 321–338 (2001)

6. Brimkov, V.E., Barneva, R.P.: Analytical honeycomb geometry for raster and volume graphics. Comput. J. **48**(2), 180–199 (2005)

7. Deutsch, E.S.: Thinning algorithms on rectangular, hexagonal and triangular arrays. Commun. ACM **15**(3), 827–837 (1972)

8. Gale, D.: A theorem on flows in networks. Pacific J. Math. **7**(2), 1073–1082 (1957)

9. Golay, M.: Hexagonal parallel pattern transformations. IEEE Trans. Comput. **18**, 733–740 (1969)

10. Her, I.: Geometric transformations on the hexagonal grid. IEEE Trans. Image Process. **4**, 1213–1222 (1995)

11. Herman, G.T., Kuba, A.: Advances in Discrete Tomography and Its Applications. Birkhäuser, Basel (2007)

12. Kardos, P., Palagyi, K.: Hexagonal parallel thinning algorithms based on sufficient conditions for topology preservation. In: Proceedings of the International Symposium CompIMAGE, pp. 63–68 (2012)

13. Kardos, P., Palagyi, K.: On topology preservation in triangular. In: Proceedings of the International Symposium on Image and Signal Processing and Analysis (ISPA), pp. 789–794 (2013)

14. Kardos, P., Palagyi, K.: On topology preservation of mixed operators in triangular, square, and hexagonal grids. Discrete Appl. Math. **216**, 441–448 (2017)

15. Klette, R., Rosenfeld, A.: Digital Geometry. Geometric Methods for Digital Picture Analysis. Morgan Kaufmann Publishers/Elsevier Science B.V., San Francisco/Amsterdam (2004)

16. Luczak, E., Rosenfeld, A.: Distance on a hexagonal grid. IEEE Trans. Comput. **C–25**(5), 532–533 (1976)

17. Lukić, T., Balázs, P.: Binary tomography reconstruction based on shape orientation. Pattern Recogn. Lett. **79**, 18–24 (2016)

18. Lukić, T., Nagy, B.: Energy-minimization based discrete tomography reconstruction method for images on triangular grid. In: Barneva, R.P., Brimkov, V.E., Aggarwal, J.K. (eds.) IWCIA 2012. LNCS, vol. 7655, pp. 274–284. Springer, Heidelberg (2012). https://doi.org/10.1007/978-3-642-34732-0_21

19. Lukić, T., Nagy, B.: Deterministic discrete tomography reconstruction by energy minimization method on the triangular grid. Pattern Recogn. Lett. **49**, 11–16 (2014)

20. Lukić, T., Nagy, B.: Regularized Binary Tomography on The Hexagonal Grid (2018, Submitted)

21. Matej, S., Herman, G.T., Vardi, A.: Binary tomography on the hexagonal grid using Gibbs priors. Int. J. Imaging Syst. Technol. **9**, 126–131 (1998)

22. Moisi, E., Nagy, B.: Discrete tomography on the triangular grid: a memetic approach. In: Proceedings of 7th International Symposium on Image and Signal Processing and Analysis (ISPA 2011), pp. 579–584, Dubrovnik, Croatia (2011)

23. Moisi, E., Nagy, B., Cretu, V.: Reconstruction of binary images represented on equilateral triangular grid using evolutionary algorithms. In: Balas, V., Fodor, J., Várkonyi-Kóczy, A., Dombi, J., Jain, L. (eds.) Soft Computing Applications. AISC, vol. 195, pp. 561–571. Springer, Heidelberg (2013). https://doi.org/10.1007/978-3-642-33941-7_49

24. Nagy, B.: Shortest paths in triangular grids with neighbourhood sequences. J. Comput. Inf. Technol. **11**, 111–122 (2003)
25. Nagy, B., Barczi, K.: Isoperimetrically optimal polygons in the triangular grid with jordan-type neighbourhood on the boundary. Int. J. Comput. Math. **90**, 1629–1652 (2013)
26. Nagy, B., Lukić, T.: Dense projection tomography on the triangular tiling. Fundamenta Informaticae **145**, 125–141 (2016)
27. Nagy, B., Lukić, T.: New projection approach for binary tomography on triangular grid (2018, Submitted)
28. Prause, G., Onnasch, D.: Binary reconstruction of the heart chambers from biplane angiographic image sequences. IEEE Trans. Med. Imag. **15**, 532–46 (1997)
29. Ryser, H.J.: Combinatorial properties of matrices of zeros and ones. Can. J. Math. **9**, 371–377 (1957)

Sphere Construction on the FCC Grid Interpreted as Layered Hexagonal Grids in 3D

Girish Koshti[1], Ranita Biswas[1(✉)], Gaëlle Largeteau-Skapin[2], Rita Zrour[2], Eric Andres[2], and Partha Bhowmick[3]

[1] Department of Computer Science and Engineering,
Indian Institute of Technology Roorkee, Roorkee, India
gkoshti01@gmail.com, biswas.ranita@gmail.com
[2] University of Poitiers, Laboratory XLIM, ASALI, UMR CNRS 7252, BP 30179,
86962 Futuroscope Chasseneuil, France
{gaelle.largeteau.skapin,rita.zrour,eric.andres}@univ-poitiers.fr
[3] Department of Computer Science and Engineering,
Indian Institute of Technology Kharagpur, Kharagpur, India
bhowmick@gmail.com

Abstract. In this paper, we propose an algorithm to build discrete spherical shell having integer center and real-valued inner and outer radii on the face-centered cubic (FCC) grid. We address the problem by mapping it to a 2D scenario and building the shell layer by layer on hexagonal grids with additive manufacturing in mind. The layered hexagonal grids get shifted according to need as we move from one layer to another and forms the FCC grid in 3D. However, we restrict our computation strictly to 2D in order to utilize symmetry and simplicity.

Keywords: Discrete sphere · Hexagonal grid
Face-centered cubic grid · Digital geometry · Additive manufacturing

1 Introduction

Additive manufacturing has become widespread and offers many possibilities for system design and operational planning [7,8,10,13,14,19]. Additive manufacturing includes many branches like 3D printing, rapid prototyping and direct digital manufacturing. Designing algorithms for efficient additive manufacturing of primitive geometric objects is of significant importance. A typical method consists of layer based manufacturing techniques that maximizes properties such as self alignment, rigid connection to neighbors, complete tessellation of $\mathbb{R}^3$, etc. [9]. Spherical material powder particles form a close sphere packing in 3D which allows us to obtain the highly desirable properties. The corresponding grid is the FCC grid in 3D. The shape of the cells in an FCC grid is rhombic dodecahedron, which is a space filling polyhedron.

© Springer Nature Switzerland AG 2018
R. P. Barneva et al. (Eds.): IWCIA 2018, LNCS 11255, pp. 82–96, 2018.
https://doi.org/10.1007/978-3-030-05288-1_7

In this paper, we propose an algorithm to build discrete spherical shells of integer center and real-valued inner and outer radii. The close packing of spherical voxels which gives us the FCC grid in 3D corresponds to layers of hexagonal grids with a shift from one layer to the next [17]. We address the problem of building discrete spherical shells by mapping it to a 2D scenario and building the shell layer by layer on hexagonal grids. For each layer, we generate a set of Andres circles [3] in the hexagonal grid. The definition of Andres hyperspheres [3], or digital hyperspheres in general, constitutes one of the most basic digital primitive that has been widely studied in the research community. Andres hyperspheres have been considered mainly in the square grid. However, recently, researchers have proposed digital circle definitions on other types of grids such as hexagonal grid [12].

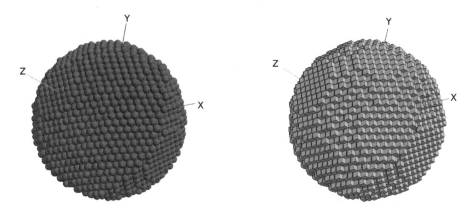

Fig. 1. A discrete sphere computed by our algorithm using layered hexagonal grids. We visualize using spherical voxels (left) and rhombic dodecahedron space filling voxels (right).

1.1 Our Contribution

Our main contribution in this work is to propose an algorithm to build discrete spherical shells of integer center and real-valued inner and outer radii on the FCC grid by addressing the problem and mapping it to a 2D scenario; the shells are built layer by layer in shifted hexagonal grids. All the computation are strictly done in 2D, layer by layer, by taking advantage of inherent symmetries in the hexagonal grids. The layered hexagonal grids get shifted as we move from one layer to another according to the 3D FCC grid they are representing. Such an algorithm is compatible with powder type additive manufacturing techniques. Experiments showed promising results and a linear time computation which is expected for rapid prototyping. A constructed discrete sphere using our proposed algorithm is shown in Fig. 1, visualized using spherical voxels on the left and space filling rhombic dodecahedra on the right.

The organization of the paper is as follows. In Sect. 2, we present some preliminaries and discussions about Andres circle and hexagonal grid. Section 3 explains the sphere construction layer by layer in hexagonal grids and Andres circle on hexagonal grid and explains the symmetries and separability properties. Section 4 discusses the sphere layering algorithms as well as results and visualizations. We conclude and present perspectives in Sect. 5.

2   Preliminaries

In this section, we discuss the FCC grid obtained from the close packing of spherical voxels in 3D. We then give a general characterization of the hexagonal grid in 2D and describe a 2-coordinate system to represent all the grid cells on this grid by integer pairs. We explain the conversion to and from the Cartesian coordinate system and this proposed 2-coordinate system; the concepts of distance calculation, neighborhood, adjacency, connectivity, and separability in this grid. These leads us to the characterization of the FCC grid by layers of shifted hexagonal grids. We formulate the horizontal and vertical shifts during grid layering to obtain close sphere packing. The definition of Andres circle on conventional square grid [3] is also recalled at the end of this section.

2.1   FCC Grid—Layered Hexagonal Grids in 3D

Close (and dense) packing of spherical voxels corresponds to two type of 3D grids, the FCC grid and the hexagonal close packing grid (also called diamond grid) [18]. In this paper, we are considering the FCC grid that can be seen as layers forming hexagonal grids. In the FCC grid, each layer of hexagons is shifted. Without shift it corresponds to the honeycomb grid in 3D which is also very popular in 3D printing. The shape of a cell in an FCC grid is the rhombic dodecahedron, which is a space filling polyhedron.

Hexagonal Grid. Each layer in an FCC sphere packing corresponds to a 2D hexagonal grid. Various coordinate systems for hexagonal grids have been proposed so far. The elementary coordinate system for the hexagonal grid uses 3-coordinate values to address every vertex of the grid [11,16]. However, the three values are not independent and are characterized by their sum, which is equal to 0 or 1. The points having 0-sum coordinate values are called even, the points with 1-sum are called odd.

In this paper, we chose to use a 2-coordinate system for the hexagonal grid as proposed in [2,15]. In this approach, the hexagonal x-axis is given by the Cartesian vector $(1,0)$ and the second coordinate, the hexagonal y-axis, is defined by the Cartesian vector $\left(\frac{1}{2}, \frac{\sqrt{3}}{2}\right)$. Figure 2 gives a visualization of such a grid. The hexagonal cells (centered on the grid point) are *pointy top* hexagons (two sides of the hexagons are parallel to the ordinate axis of the classical Euclidean coordinate system). It should be easy to transpose this work for other hexagon orientations or hexagon sizes. The hexagons are regular with a side length of $\frac{1}{\sqrt{3}}$. This means that the distance between the centroids of two neighboring hexagons is 1.

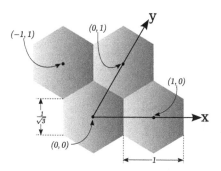

Fig. 2. Hexagonal grid coordinate system and size of individual hexagons.

The coordinate transforms from the Cartesian grid to the hexagonal grid and vice versa are given by the following mapping functions ([15]):

$$\mathcal{F}_{\bigcirc} : (\hat{x}, \hat{y}) \mapsto (x, y) = \left(\hat{x} - \frac{\hat{y}}{\sqrt{3}}, \frac{2\hat{y}}{\sqrt{3}} \right)$$

$$\mathcal{F}_{\square} : (x, y) \mapsto (\hat{x}, \hat{y}) = \left(x + \frac{y}{2}, \frac{y\sqrt{3}}{2} \right)$$

While considering the close packing of spherical voxels in a layer by layer fashion, from one layer to the next layer, we not only move vertically, but we also need to shift the next hexagonal grid layer as to make the spherical voxels of the next layer to fit correctly to the concavities produced in the last layer of spheres. Furthermore, as a consequence, even if the height of an individual layer is one, with spherical voxels of diameter one, vertical distance between two consecutive layers is less than an unit.

Proposition 1 (Horizontal Shift). *Horizontal translation between two consecutive hexagonal grid layer is given by $(-\frac{1}{3}, -\frac{1}{3})$ in the proposed hexagonal grid coordinate system.*

Proof. It is a direct consequence of the 3D sphere packing. While stacking the hexagonal grid layers, the center of the grid moves from a hexagon centroid to the hexagon edge end-points and then coming back to the centroid of some other hexagon and this process repeats.   □

The required vertical translation needed to move from one layer to its next layer can be calculated using the unit cell shape (rhombic dodecahedron) of an FCC grid.

Proposition 2 (Vertical Shift). *Vertical translation between each consecutive hexagonal grid layer is given by $\frac{\sqrt{6}}{3}$.*

Proof. Again, this is a direct consequence of sphere packing [6] as shown in Fig. 3.   □

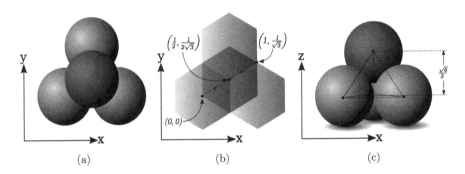

Fig. 3. Horizontal and vertical shifts calculation of layered hexagonal grids; the gray voxels are on the lower layer i.e. layer 0 and the red voxel is on the next upper layer i.e. layer 1. (a) Top view of stacking of spherical voxels. (b) Corresponding hexagonal cells of the spheres from (a) and horizontal shift of the layers. (c) Side view of the stacking of spherical voxels and vertical shift of the layers. (Color figure online)

2.2   Andres Spheres, Circles and Annuli

Andres spheres of radius r (without loss of generality, the center of the sphere has been assumed as the origin, if not mentioned otherwise) on a 3D regular square grid is given by [1,3]

$$\mathbb{S}(r) = \left\{ (i,j,k) \in \mathbb{Z}^3 : \left(r - \tfrac{1}{2}\right)^2 \leqslant i^2 + j^2 + k^2 < \left(r + \tfrac{1}{2}\right)^2 \right\}. \qquad (1)$$

The equation can be generalized in higher dimensions keeping the lower and upper bounds same, and can also be generalized to the concept of offset-circle and hypersphere by replacing $\frac{1}{2}$ by variable τ offset [5]. A generalization of the Andres hypersphere is focus based digital objects [4]. Some important properties and an algorithm for construction of the Andres circle and hypersphere can be seen in [3]. The Euclidean distance of each voxel of $\mathbb{S}(r)$ from the corresponding sphere is bounded from above by $\frac{1}{2}$. This makes an Andres sphere maintain the property of tiling space without any gap when the radius is increased in unit steps. The spheres generated by this method are not irreducible but have the property of $(n-1)$-separability in nD-space.

  This definition can be generalized to shells defined by an inner radius r and an outer radius R as

$$\mathbb{S}(r, R) = \left\{ (i,j,k) \in \mathbb{Z}^3 : r^2 \leqslant i^2 + j^2 + k^2 < R^2 \right\}. \qquad (2)$$

One of the fundamental properties is that for a given z_o, a digital 2D slice of an Andres sphere or shell forms an annulus as

$$\mathbb{C}(r, R) = \left\{(i, j) \in \mathbb{Z}^2 : r^2 - z_o^2 \leqslant i^2 + j^2 < R^2 - z_o^2\right\}. \qquad (3)$$

With $r = r' - \frac{1}{2}$ and $R = r' + \frac{1}{2}$, for some $r' \in \mathbb{Z}^2$, we have an Andres circle [1,3]. The whole idea of our layered approach is to generate those digital Andres circles in the hexagonal grid, layer by layer. However, to define Andres circles in the hexagonal grid, we have to use a distance defined in this grid.

Proposition 3. *The Euclidean distance between two centroids with coordinates (x_1, y_1) and (x_2, y_2) on the hexagonal grid is given by*

$$d_{\bigcirc}\left((x_1, y_1), (x_2, y_2)\right) = \sqrt{(x_1 - x_2)^2 + (y_1 - y_2)^2 + (x_1 - x_2)(y_1 - y_2)} \qquad (4)$$

Proof. This stems from the Euclidean distance $d_{\square}$ definition between the two points $\mathcal{F}_{\square}(x_1, y_1)$ and $\mathcal{F}_{\square}(x_2, y_2)$.

$$d_{\bigcirc}\left((x_1, y_1), (x_2, y_2)\right) = d_{\square}(\mathcal{F}_{\square}((x_1, y_1)), \mathcal{F}_{\square}(x_2, y_2))$$

$$= d_{\square}\left(\left(x_1 + \tfrac{y_1}{2}, \tfrac{y_1\sqrt{3}}{2}\right), \left(x_2 + \tfrac{y_2}{2}, \tfrac{y_2\sqrt{3}}{2}\right)\right)$$

$$= \sqrt{\left(x_1 + \tfrac{y_1}{2} - x_2 - \tfrac{y_2}{2}\right)^2 + \left(\tfrac{y_1\sqrt{3}}{2} - \tfrac{y_2\sqrt{3}}{2}\right)^2}$$

$$= \sqrt{(x_1 - x_2)^2 + (y_1 - y_2)^2 + (x_1 - x_2)(y_1 - y_2)}$$

$\square$

3 Sphere Construction Using Layered Hexagonal Grid

With the definition of the Andres circle on the conventional square grid and the coordinate system we have for hexagonal grid, in this section, we first give the characterization of Andres circle on the hexagonal grid. Then, we use this characterization to define a spherical shell which can be thought of as an amalgamation of multiple layers of 2D digital annulus. We present here how to define the layers to obtain the shell. And, then we also detail the symmetries in each layer, which are eventually used in our proposed algorithm in Sect. 4, to optimize the construction of the shell. Since each of these layers are Andres annuli, we can deduce separability properties of the whole shell depending on its thickness.

3.1 Andres Circle on Hexagonal Grid

The separability and tiling property of an Andres circle directly relates to the upper and lower limits of $\frac{1}{2}$ as we take from the actual radius. This single thickness model ensures that no pixel from the inside of the Andres circle is edge-connected with any pixel from the outside, and hence conforming separability of space.

Similar to the square grid, any two edge-connected neighbors, or simply neighbors as there is no vertex adjacency in the hexagonal grid, are single distance apart from each other in our 2-coordinate system. Hence, keeping the same upper and lower bounds to produce the Andres circle in the hexagonal grid gives us a separating and tileable object. However, we need to use the appropriate distance measure as described in Sect. 2. The Andres circle of radius r centered at the origin on the hexagonal grid is given by

$$\mathbb{C}(r) = \left\{ (i,j) | (r - \tfrac{1}{2})^2 \leqslant i^2 + j^2 + ij < (r + \tfrac{1}{2})^2 \right\}, \tag{5}$$

where (i,j) is a grid point on the hexagonal grid defined by the 2-coordinate system.

We can generalize this to discrete annulus where two radii and an arbitrary center are given as input. The discrete annulus of inner radius r and outer radius R centered at $c(c_x, c_y)$ on the hexagonal grid is given by

$$\mathbb{C}(r, R, c) = \left\{ (i,j) | r^2 \leqslant (i - c_x)^2 + (j - c_y)^2 + (i - c_x)(j - c_y) < R^2 \right\}. \tag{6}$$

It is quite evident that taking $r = R - 1$ in the Eq. 6 gives us the Andres circle of radius $r - \tfrac{1}{2}$ and taking $r = 0$ gives us a discrete disk of radius R. The center position can be moved to any other point without losing the characteristics of the discrete circle or annulus.

3.2   Layered Annulus Characterization

As discussed in Sect. 2, the FCC grid can be described as layered hexagonal grids with proper horizontal and vertical shifts given to the grid points. While generating a discrete spherical shell in a layered grid like this using a set of discrete annuli, the center and radius of the annulus to be constructed at each layer should be calculated conforming the shifting of the grid. Hereafter, we denote the i-th layer as $\mathcal{L}_i$ while the base of the hemisphere or the zeroth circle of latitude of the sphere is on $\mathcal{L}_0$.

Lemma 1 (Center Recurrence). *The center position of the annulus on $\mathcal{L}_i$ for $i > 0$ is given by*
$$c_i = c_0 + \left(\tfrac{1}{3}, \tfrac{1}{3} \right) * (i \mod 3),$$
where $c_0 \in \mathbb{Z}^2$ corresponds to the center used in $\mathcal{L}_0$, i.e. the input center.

Proof. As per the vertical shift between layers, the Cartesian center position of the annulus on $\mathcal{L}_i$ for $i \geqslant 0$ is given by

$$\hat{c}_i = \hat{c}_0 + \left(0, 0, \tfrac{\sqrt{6}}{3} i \right),$$

where $\hat{c}_0$ is the Cartesian equivalent of the input center. Now as the grids also get horizontally shifted by $(-\tfrac{1}{3}, -\tfrac{1}{3})$ at each layer, the center of the annulus gets coordinate translation by $(\tfrac{1}{3}, \tfrac{1}{3})$ and from $(0,0)$ in $\mathcal{L}_0$, moves to $(\tfrac{1}{3}, \tfrac{1}{3})$ in $\mathcal{L}_1$, to $(\tfrac{2}{3}, \tfrac{2}{3})$ in $\mathcal{L}_2$ and then we have a grid point again that we can simply consider as $(0,0)$ in the new layer.   □

Lemma 2 (Radius Recurrence). *The radius (lower or upper) of the annulus on $\mathcal{L}_i$ for $i > 0$ is given by*

$$\rho_i = \sqrt{\rho_0^2 - \frac{2i^2}{3}},$$

for $\rho \in \{r, R\}$, where ρ_0 corresponds to the respective radius used in $\mathcal{L}_0$, i.e. the input inner or outer radius.

Proof. As given in Proposition 2, the height or Cartesian z-coordinate of the annulus in $\mathcal{L}_i$ is $\frac{\sqrt{6}}{3}$ added to the z-coordinate of $\mathcal{L}_{i-1}$. Hence, the radius of the annulus can be directly computed by the change in z-coordinate.   □

Lemma 3 (Layer Count). *The number of layers in a single hemisphere of outer radius R is given by $h_R = \left\lceil \frac{3R}{\sqrt{6}} \right\rceil$.*

Proof. It follows directly from the fact that the vertical translation between each layer is given by $\frac{\sqrt{6}}{3}$. See Proposition 2.   □

Theorem 1 (Spherical Shell). *The spherical shell of inner radius r and outer radius R on the layered hexagonal grid is given by*

$$\mathbb{S}(r, R) = \bigcup_{i=-h_R}^{h_R} \mathbb{C}(r_i, R_i, c_i).$$

Proof. The theorem is a direct consequence of the construction of an Andres shell in 3D as presented in Eq. (3).   □

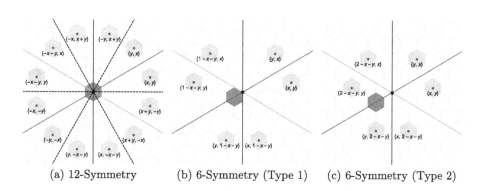

(a) 12-Symmetry   (b) 6-Symmetry (Type 1)   (c) 6-Symmetry (Type 2)

Fig. 4. 12 and 6 symmetries as occurring in our layered hexagonal grids. (Color figure online)

3.3 Symmetries

The symmetry group of regular hexagon is the dihedral group D_6, i.e. a group of order 12. However, when the center of symmetry is at a vertex of a grid cell, rather than the grid cell center, we get only 6-symmetry. The three different symmetries occurring in our layered hexagonal grids are discussed below.

Lemma 4 (12-Symmetry). *Any cell (x, y) on the hexagonal grid has a maximum of 12 symmetric images considering an integer point (i.e. cell center) as the center of symmetry.*

Proof. The dihedral group of a regular hexagon leads to 6 axes of symmetry in this case. Hence, maximum 12-symmetric points for a grid cell (x, y) as shown in Fig. 4(a), considering the symmetry center as the origin. The 6 symmetric axes are given as $x = y, x - 0, 2x = -y, x = -y, x = -2y, y = 0$ starting from the red line and moving counter-clockwise. ⊔⊓

Lemma 5 (6-Symmetry (Type 1)). *Any cell (x, y) on the hexagonal grid has a maximum of 6 symmetric images considering an integer point $+(\frac{1}{3}, \frac{1}{3})$ (i.e. right-upper vertex of a cell) as the center of symmetry.*

Proof. The dihedral group of a regular triangle leads to 3 axes of symmetry in this case. Hence, maximum 6-symmetric points for a grid cell (x, y) as shown in Fig. 4(b), considering the symmetry center as the right-upper vertex of the origin cell. The 3 symmetric axes are given as $x = y, 2x - 1 = -y, x - 1 = -2y$ starting from the red line and moving counter-clockwise. □

Lemma 6 (6-Symmetry (Type 2)). *Any cell (x, y) on the hexagonal grid has a maximum of 6 symmetric images considering an integer point $+(\frac{2}{3}, \frac{2}{3})$ (i.e. top vertex of a cell) as the center of symmetry.*

Proof. The dihedral group of a regular triangle leads to 3 axes of symmetry in this case. Hence, maximum 6-symmetric points for a grid cell (x, y) as shown in Fig. 4(c), considering the symmetry center as the top vertex of the $(1, 0)$ cell. The 3 symmetric axes are given as $x = y, 2x - 2 = -y, x - 2 = -2y$ starting from the red line and moving counter-clockwise. □

Theorem 2 (Symmetry). *The symmetry group of $\mathcal{L}_i$ for $i \geqslant 0$ is given by*

$$\mathcal{G}_i(x, y) = \{(x, y), (y, x), (-y, x + y), (-x, x + y), (-x - y, x), (-x - y, y),$$
$$(-x, -y), (-y, -x), (y, -x - y), (x, -x - y), (x + y, -x), (x + y, -y)\}, \text{ for } \iota = 0$$
$$= \{(x, y), (y, x), (\iota - x - y, x), (\iota - x - y, y), (x, \iota - x - y), (y, \iota - x - y)\}, \text{ for } \iota \neq 0,$$

where $\iota \equiv i (\mathrm{mod}\, 3)$.

Proof. Directly follows from Lemmas 4, 5, and 6. □

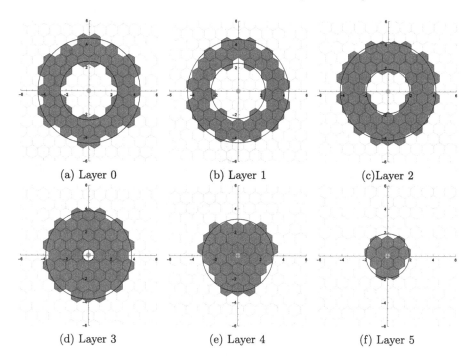

(a) Layer 0   (b) Layer 1   (c)Layer 2

(d) Layer 3   (e) Layer 4   (f) Layer 5

Fig. 5. Six different layers of the hemispherical shell corresponding to $\mathbb{S}(2.5, 4.5)$.

4 Sphere Layering Algorithm

In this section, we present the discrete sphere construction algorithm (Algorithm 1) on the FCC grid by using the layered hexagonal grid concept. Our algorithm takes an integer center c and real inner and outer radii, respectively r and R, as input and gives the sequence of coordinates in the layered hexagonal grid to form the hemispherical shell corresponding to $\mathbb{S}(r, R, c)$ (Fig. 5). This output sequence is suitable for additive manufacturing in a layer by layer fashion with the discrete annuli on each layer generated using an inside to outside circular motion. The algorithm can be easily augmented to generate the whole spherical shell by constructing the two hemispheres in parallel or in sequence and then fitting them together to avoid powder inside the sphere.

The main algorithm is a direct consequence of the lemmas and theorems presented in Sect. 3. As presented in Algorithm 1, we first compute the number of layers to be generated in a single hemispherical shell by using Lemma 3, and use that to set the upper bound for our loop counter. Each iteration of this loop constructs one layer calling the Procedure AnnulusHex and using the loop counter i to denote the layer number. At each increment of the layer count, we modify the inner radius r, outer radius R, and center coordinate c for the annulus to be constructed next. We use the center and radius recurrences as explained in Lemmas 1 and 2. The completion of the loop gives us the perfect sequence of coordinates for generating the hemispherical shell corresponding to $\mathbb{S}(r, R, c)$ in the FCC grid. Notice that, the coordinates are given in our 2-coordinate system and are easily convertible to Cartesian coordinates as required by using the layer number and the conversion formulas as given in Sect. 2.

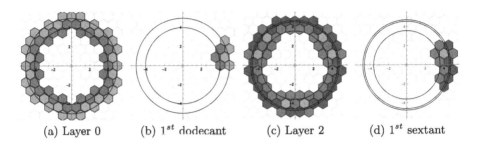

(a) Layer 0   (b) 1st dodecant   (c) Layer 2   (d) 1st sextant

Fig. 6. Two layers of the hemispherical shell $\mathbb{S}(3.5, 5.5)$ and their corresponding dodecant and sextant which where obtained by the circular motion building process with symmetry. The alternate Andres circles are colored using blue and yellow, and the cells that are computed twice are shown in green. (Color figure online)

Once the Procedure AnnulusHex is called with a center c and a pair of radii r and R, it generates the discrete annulus starting from the Andres circle having radius $r + \frac{1}{2}$ and continue giving unit increment to this radius until we reach the outer radius R. Each Andres circle is generated using a circular motion by the Procedure AndresCircleHex, which efficiently utilizes the symmetry properties as explored in Sect. 3. However, using unit incremental steps starting from $r + \frac{1}{2}$ does not guaranty to exactly reach the radius $R - \frac{1}{2}$ of the outermost Andres circle required to ensure completeness of our constructed annulus. To take care of this issue, after completing our loop, we add this specific Andres circle separately at the end of generated sequence.

In the Procedure AndresCircleHex, the symmetry group properties of each layer allows us to compute the points only on the first dodecant or first sextant as applicable and then use the symmetries to deduce the complete circle. If c is an integer point, we need to generate only the first dodecant and if it is not, then we need to generate the first sextant. Note that, from Lemmas 4, 5, and 6, our considered first dodecant is bounded by the translated version of the boundary lines $y = 0$ and $x = y$ according to the circle center, and the first sextant is bounded by the translated versions of boundary lines $x = -2y$ and $x = y$. For any center, we start with the point lying on the circle having y-coordinate equals to the nearest integer of the y-coordinate of the circle center and proceed towards $x = y$ line to generate the sequence of points for the first dodecant. Notice that, in this sequence, the only two possibilities of the next point of (p_x, p_y) is given by $(p_x - 1, p_y + 1)$ and $(p_x, p_y + 1)$. After completing the construction of the first dodecant, we either generate the symmetric points in sequence to get the complete Andres circle if the center is an integer point, or we proceed to generate the rest of the first sextant. In this second situation, we again come back to the starting point and generate the rest of the first sextant by proceeding towards $x = -2y$ line and preparing the obtained points in our sequence. Here, the two possibilities of the next point of (p_x, p_y) are (p_x, p_y-1) and (p_x+1, p_y-1). Once, we have the first sextant, we create the complete circle by using the 6-symmetry type 1 or type 2 as applicable.

Notice that, we utilize the following two lemmas to get the recurrence functions for calculating the distance of the next candidate points from the center of the circle using the calculated distance of the previous point.

Lemma 7. *The distance of the next candidate points $p_1(p_x - 1, p_y + 1)$ and $p_2(p_x, p_y + 1)$ of point $p(p_x, p_y)$ from the circle center $c(c_x, c_y)$ are given by the following recurrence.*

For p_1 :	For p_2 :
$d \leftarrow d + f_1$	$d \leftarrow d + f_2$
$f_1 \leftarrow f_1 + 2$	$f_1 \leftarrow f_1 + 1$
$f_2 \leftarrow f_2 + 1$	$f_2 \leftarrow f_2 + 2$

where, the values for the start point $p'(p'_x, p'_y)$ are computed as $d = d_\bigcirc(p', c)$, $f_1 = -(p'_x - c_x) + (p'_y - c_y) + 1$, $f_2 = (p'_x - c_x) + 2(p'_y - c_y) + 1$.

Proof. Without loss of generality, let us consider c as the origin. Hence, we get

$$d_\bigcirc(p_1, c) = (p_x - 1)^2 + (p_y + 1)^2 + (p_x - 1)(p_y + 1)$$
$$= p_x^2 + p_y^2 + p_x p_y - p_x + p_y + 1$$
$$= d_\bigcirc(p, c) + f_1$$

Computing the value of $d_\bigcirc((p_x - 2, p_y + 2), c)$ the recurrence on the factor f_1 can be obtained. And similarly, the recurrence for the other factor f_2 and the distance for p_2 can be computed. □

Lemma 8. *The distance of the next candidate points $p_1(p_x, p_y - 1)$ and $p_2(p_x + 1, p_y - 1)$ of point $p(p_x, p_y)$ from the circle center $c(c_x, c_y)$ are given by the following recurrence.*

For p_1 :	For p_2 :
$d \leftarrow d - f_1$	$d \leftarrow d - f_2$
$f_1 \leftarrow f_1 - 2$	$f_1 \leftarrow f_1 - 1$
$f_2 \leftarrow f_2 - 1$	$f_2 \leftarrow f_2 - 2$

where, the values for the start point $p'(p'_x, p'_y)$ are computed as $d = d_\bigcirc(p', c)$, $f_1 = (p'_x - c_x) + 2(p'_y - c_y) - 1$, $f_2 = -(p'_x - c_x) + (p'_y - c_y) - 1$.

Proof. Similar to Lemma 7. □

Algorithm 1. LAYERSPHEREHEX(r, R, c)

Input: int×int c, real r, real R
Output: $\mathbb{S}(c, r, R)$

1 int $h \leftarrow \left\lceil \frac{3R}{\sqrt{6}} \right\rceil, i \leftarrow 0, r_0 \leftarrow r, R_0 \leftarrow R, S \leftarrow \langle \rangle$ ▷ Lemma 3
2 **while** $i < h$ **do**
3   $\quad S \leftarrow S ^\frown \text{AnnulusHex}(c, r, R)$
4   $\quad i \leftarrow i + 1$
5   $\quad r \leftarrow \sqrt{r_0^2 - \frac{2i^2}{3}}, R \leftarrow \sqrt{R_0^2 - \frac{2i^2}{3}}, c \leftarrow c + \left(\frac{1}{3}, \frac{1}{3}\right) - (i \mid 3, i \mid 3)$ ▷ Lemma 1 & 2
6 **return** S

Procedure AnnulusHex(c, r, R)

Input: real r, real R, (int/3 × int/3) c,
Output: $\mathbb{C}(c, r, R)$

1 int $r \leftarrow r + \frac{1}{2}, \rho \leftarrow R - \frac{1}{2}, A \leftarrow \langle \rangle$
2 **while** $r < \rho$ **do**
3   $\quad A \leftarrow A ^\frown \text{AndresCircleHex}(c, r)$
4   $\quad r \leftarrow r + 1$
5 $A \leftarrow A ^\frown \text{AndresCircleHex}(c, \rho)$
6 **return** A

Procedure AndresCircleHex(c, r)

Input: (int/3 × int/3) $c \leftarrow (c_x, c_y)$, real r
Output: $\mathbb{C}(c, r)$

1 int $p_0 \leftarrow p \leftarrow (p_x, p_y) \leftarrow ([\lfloor c_x \rfloor + r], [c_y])$
2 int $d_0 \leftarrow d \leftarrow d_\bigcirc(p, c)^2, \underline{r} \leftarrow r - \frac{1}{2}, \bar{r} \leftarrow \underline{r} + 1, C \leftarrow \langle p \rangle$
3 int $f_{10} \leftarrow f_1 \leftarrow -(p_x - c_x) + (p_y - c_y) + 1$
4 int $f_{20} \leftarrow f_2 \leftarrow (p_x - c_x) + 2(p_y - c_y) + 1$
5 **while** $(p_x - c_x) > (p_y - c_y)$ **do**
6   $\quad p_1 \leftarrow (p_x - 1, p_y + 1), d_1 \leftarrow d + f_1$
7   $\quad$ **if** $\underline{r} \leqslant d_1 < \bar{r}$ **then** $C \leftarrow C ^\frown \langle p_1 \rangle$
8   $\quad p_2 \leftarrow (p_x, p_y + 1), d_2 \leftarrow d + f_2$
9   $\quad$ **if** $\underline{r} \leqslant d_2 < \bar{r}$ **then** $C \leftarrow C ^\frown \langle p_2 \rangle$
10 $\quad$ **if** $|r^2 - d_1| \leqslant |r^2 - d_2|$ **then** $p \leftarrow p_1, d \leftarrow d_1, f_1 \leftarrow f_1 + 2, f_2 \leftarrow f_2 + 1$
11 $\quad$ **else** $p \leftarrow p_2, d \leftarrow d_2, f_1 \leftarrow f_1 + 1, f_2 \leftarrow f_2 + 2$ ▷ Lemma 7
12 **if** $p_y = c_y$ **then** $C \leftarrow \text{Include12Symmetry}(C)$ ▷ Lemma 4
13 **else**
14 $\quad p \leftarrow p_0, d \leftarrow d_0, f_1 \leftarrow f_{20} - 2, f_2 \leftarrow f_{10} - 2$
15 $\quad$ **while** $(p_x - c_x) > -2(p_y - c_y)$ **do**
16 $\quad\quad p_1 \leftarrow (p_x, p_y - 1), d_1 \leftarrow d - f_1$
17 $\quad\quad$ **if** $\underline{r} \leqslant d_1 < \bar{r}$ **then** $C \leftarrow \langle p_1 \rangle ^\frown C$
18 $\quad\quad p_2 \leftarrow (p_x + 1, p_y - 1), d_2 \leftarrow d - f_2$
19 $\quad\quad$ **if** $\underline{r} \leqslant d_2 < \bar{r}$ **then** $C \leftarrow \langle p_2 \rangle ^\frown C$
20 $\quad\quad$ **if** $|r^2 - d_1| \leqslant |r^2 - d_2|$ **then** $p \leftarrow p_1, d \leftarrow d_1, f_1 \leftarrow f_1 - 2, f_2 \leftarrow f_2 - 1$
21 $\quad\quad$ **else** $p \leftarrow p_2, d \leftarrow d_2, f_1 \leftarrow f_1 - 1, f_2 \leftarrow f_2 - 2$ ▷ Lemma 8
22 $\quad$ **if** $p_y = \lfloor c_y \rfloor$ **then** $C \leftarrow \text{Include6SymmetryType1}(C)$ ▷ Lemma 5
23 $\quad$ **else** $C \leftarrow \text{Include6SymmetryType2}(C)$ ▷ Lemma 6
24 **return** C

Figure 6 presents two specific layers (layer 0 and layer 2) of $\mathbb{S}(3.5, 5.5)$. The alternate Andres circles are colored using blue and yellow, and the cells that are computed twice are shown in green. These twice computation of points happens for all those annulus where $R - r$ is not an integer and that makes the last two generated circles too close to each other creating overlaps. The black circles in the figure shows the real counterpart of the drawn Andres circles.

5   Conclusions

In this paper, we have proposed a generation algorithm for discrete spheres on the FCC grid using layered discrete annuli on hexagonal grids. The general idea is to propose digital primitive generation algorithms that are compatible with additive manufacturing techniques. We have characterized a discrete spherical shell as the union of multiple discrete annuli and have proposed an algorithm which generates the sequence of points of a discrete hemispherical shell by a layer by layer construction using these annuli. Individual annulus layer is constructed by generating smaller to bigger radii space-paving Andres circles, whereas each Andres circle is generated in a circular motion efficiently utilizing the symmetry groups appearing in the hexagonal grid layers.

References

1. Andres, E.: Discrete circles, rings and spheres. Comput. Graph. **18**(5), 695–706 (1994)
2. Andres, E.: Shear based bijective digital rotation in hexagonal grids. Pattern Recogn. Lett. (2018, submitted)
3. Andres, E., Jacob, M.: The discrete analytical hyperspheres. IEEE Trans. Visual. Comput. Graph. **3**, 75–86 (1997)
4. Andres, E., Biswas, R., Bhowmick, P.: Digital primitives defined by weighted focal set. In: 20th IAPR International Conference on Discrete Geometry for Computer Imagery, pp. 388–398 (2017)
5. Brimkov, V.E., Barneva, R.P., Brimkov, B.: Connected distance-based rasterization of objects in arbitrary dimension. Graph. Models **73**, 323–334 (2011)
6. Conway, J., Sloane, N., Bannai, E.: Sphere Packings, Lattices, and Groups (Sect. 6.3). Springer, New York (1999). https://doi.org/10.1007/978-1-4757-2249-9
7. Gao, W., et al.: The status, challenges, and future of additive manufacturing in engineering. Comput.-Aided Des. **69**, 65–89 (2015)
8. Hällgren, S., Pejryd, L., Ekengren, J.: (Re)design for additive manufacturing. Procedia CIRP **50**, 246–251 (2016)
9. Hiller, J., Lipson, H.: Design and analysis of digital materials for physical 3D voxel printing. Rapid Prototyping J. **15**, 137–149 (2009)
10. Hon, K.K.B.: Digital additive manufacturing: from rapid prototyping to rapid manufacturing. In: Hinduja, S., Fan, K.C. (eds.) 35th International MATADOR Conference, pp. 337–340. Springer, London (2007). https://doi.org/10.1007/978-1-84628-988-0_76
11. Nagy, B.: A symmetric coordinate frame for hexagonal networks. In: Theoretical Computer Science Information Society, pp. 193–196 (2004)

12. Nagy, B., Strand, R.: Approximating Euclidean circles by neighbourhood sequences in a hexagonal grid. Theor. Comput. Sci. **412**, 1364–1377 (2011)
13. Sá, A.M., Echavarria, K.R., Pietroni, N., Cignoni, P.: State of the art on functional fabrication. In: Eurographics Workshop on Graphics for Digital Fabrication (2016)
14. Salonitis, K., Zarban, S.A.: Redesign optimization for manufacturing using additive layer techniques. Procedia CIRP **36**, 193–198 (2015)
15. Snyder, W.E., Qi, H., Sander, W.A.: Coordinate system for hexagonal pixels. In: Medical Imaging: Image Processing, vol. 3661 (1999)
16. Stojmenović, I.: Honeycomb networks: topological properties and communication algorithms. IEEE Trans. Parallel Distrib. Syst. **8**(10), 1036–1042 (1997)
17. Strand, R.: Using the hexagonal grid for three-dimensional images: direct fourier method reconstruction and weighted distance transform. In: 18th International Conference on Pattern Recognition, vol. 2, pp. 1169–1172 (2006)
18. Strand, R., Nagy, B., Borgefors, G.: Digital distance functions on three-dimensional grids. Theor. Comput. Sci. **412**(15), 1350–1363 (2011)
19. Thompson, M.K., et al.: Design for additive manufacturing: trends, opportunities, considerations, and constraints. CIRP Ann. **65**(2), 737–760 (2016)

Quadrangular Mesh Generation Using Centroidal Voronoi Tessellation on Voxelized Surface

Ashutosh Soni and Partha Bhowmick[✉]

Department of Computer Science and Engineering, Indian Institute of Technology, Kharagpur, Kharagpur, India
ashu.soni.21690@gmail.com, pb@cse.iitkgp.ac.in

Abstract. We propose an efficient algorithm for isotropic tessellation on a voxelized surface. Owing to execution in the voxel space, the algorithm is easily compliant to parallel computation. We show how an input triangle mesh can readily be restructured to an isotropic quadrangular mesh after a post-processing on the tessellated surface. We also show how different regions of the quad mesh can be decimated to finer quads in an adaptive manner based on digital planarity. Necessary theoretical analysis and experimental results have been provided to adjudge its merit.

Keywords: Quad mesh · Triangle mesh · Voronoi tessellation
Centroidal Voronoi tessellation · Voxelized surface · Digital geometry

1 Introduction

Quadrangular (a.k.a. 'quad') meshes are made of 2-manifolds in the form of 3D quadrilaterals. They are used in a variety of geometric algorithms and applications, such as 2D and 3D object representation in CAD, finite element simulation, modeling, architecture and planning, and 3D printing.

A quad mesh can be classified as *regular*, *irregular*, or *semi-regular*, depending on 'valency' (i.e., degree of a vertex) [4]. Regular forms have each vertex with valency four and are widely used in texturing, mesh compression, etc. Because of the hard constraint on valency, shape of a quad often gets distorted, and hence the irregular form is used more often, as here unorthodox vertices (valency not equal to four) are allowed in an unlimited number to maintain the shapes of the quads. A semi-regular mesh is the one that allows a limited number of unorthodox vertices. In terms of quad size and shape, a mesh is also classified as *isotropic* or *anisotropic*. In an isotropic mesh, the quads are predominantly similar in size and shape, whereas it is not so for the anisotropic.

In this paper, we show how *centroidal Voronoi tessellation* (CVT) can be used for efficient construction of an isotropic and semi-regular quad mesh. The technique proposed by us is based on a novel idea of partitioning of a voxelized

© Springer Nature Switzerland AG 2018
R. P. Barneva et al. (Eds.): IWCIA 2018, LNCS 11255, pp. 97–111, 2018.
https://doi.org/10.1007/978-3-030-05288-1_8

mesh using functional components, minimization of a simple energy function, and quad decimation based on digital planarity. We briefly narrate in this section coverage by the existing works, followed by the contributions made by us.

1.1 State of the Art

CVT is a well-known concept in mesh processing, especially for restructuring a triangle mesh to a quad mesh [3,13]. In the literature, it is mostly found to be applied on triangle meshes (without any voxelization) under different metrics. The work in [21] shows that replacing the L_2 norm with an L_p norm for $p \geqslant 4$ can generate quadrangular Voronoi regions.

The idea of constrained CVT was introduced in [9] for surface re-meshing. Energy-based optimization for CVT construction was proposed in [22]. Techniques for construction of isotropic CVT on triangle mesh can be seen in [2,19,27,31], and those for anisotropic CVT in [10,20,28]. A GPU-based method for CVT computation has been presented in [25]. Intrinsic methods to generate CVT on curved surface have recently been proposed in [23,30]. All these methods operate in the real space and are based on discrete exponential map, energy minimization, etc.

For mesh subdivision, which is needed for smooth surface modeling, different techniques have been practiced since a long time [7,11,24,34]. Later advancements have been reported in [5,6,14–16,29,32]. None of these, however, has used voxelization, as proposed by us.

1.2 Our Motivation and Contribution

To the best of our knowledge, CVT computation based on geodesic distance on voxelized surface is not yet reported in the literature. Further, mesh subdivision using CVT on voxelized surface is worth studying in the context of surface re-meshing. The motivation of our work mainly rests on these two.

We have designed an efficient algorithm for construction of isotropic CVT on a voxelized surface. By 'isotropic tessellation', we mean the Voronoi regions are predominantly similar in size and shape. The proposed technique admits parallel computing and hence can easily be implemented on a GPU platform. Owing to the isotropic nature of CVT, an input triangle mesh can easily be restructured to an isotropic quadrangular mesh after a simple post-processing on the tessellated surface. We have also shown how different portions of the quad mesh can be decimated or subdivided to finer structures in an adaptive manner using the notion of digital planarity of the voxelized Voronoi regions. Some theoretical facts and experimental results have been added to demonstrate the novelty of our work.

2   Definitions and Terminologies

In this section, we discuss some basic concepts, mostly adopted from [17]. Further concepts, as and when needed, are put in the relevant sections.

A *voxel* is a 3-cell or unit cube determined by the integer grid and fully identified by its center, which is a point of $\mathbb{Z}^3$. A voxel consists of eight vertices (0-cells), twelve edges (1-cells), and six faces (2-cells). For $0 \leqslant k \leqslant l \leqslant 2$, two voxels are said to be k-*adjacent* if they share an l-cell. Note that this notion of 0-, 1-, and 2-adjacencies correspond respectively to the classical 26-, 18-, and 6-neighborhood notations used in [8].

A 3D digital object A is a finite set of 3-cells. For $k = 0, 1, 2$, a k-*path* in A is a sequence of 3-cells from A such that every two consecutive 3-cells are k-adjacent. A is called k-*connected* if there is a k-path connecting any two 3-cells of A. A k-*component* is a maximal k-connected subset of A.

Let B be a subset of A. If $A \smallsetminus B$ is not k-connected, then B is said to be k-*separating* in A. Let B be k-separating in A such that $A \smallsetminus B$ has exactly two k-components. A k-*simple cell* of B (w.r.t. A) is a 3-cell u such that $B \smallsetminus \{u\}$ is still k-separating in A. A k-separating digital object in A is k-*minimal* if it does not contain any k-simple cell. If B is not 2-separating in A, then B has *tunnels*; otherwise, it is *tunnel-free*.

We denote by $\mathcal{T}$ a triangle mesh, and by $\mathcal{V}$ the set of voxels obtained by voxelization of $\mathcal{T}$. We use the algorithm in [1] for mesh voxelization. The resultant voxel set is tunnel-free. For $k = 0, 1, 2$, we define the k-neighborhood of a voxel u in $\mathcal{V}$ as the set of all the voxels in $\mathcal{V}$ that are k-adjacent to u. We denote this set by $N_k(u)$, and we use $A_k(u)$ to denote $N_k(u) \cup \{u\}$. For a voxel $u \in \mathcal{V}$, we consider $A_0(u)$ to determine its functional plane, if any. The *functional plane(s)* of u is the principle plane(s), i.e., xy-, xz-, or yz-plane, if and only if $A_0(u)$ and its projection on that plane are in bijection with each other. For $k = 0, 1, 2$, a k-path from a voxel u to a voxel v in $\mathcal{V}$ is denoted by $\pi_k(u, v) := \langle u, v_1, v_2, \ldots, v_{t-1}, v \rangle$, and its length by $d_k(u, v) := t$. When the path is a/the shortest path, we call it a *geodesic path*. In our work, we consider 0-connected geodesic paths.

3 Proposed Work

The major steps of centroidal Voronoi tessellation (CVT) are shown in Fig. 1. In the following sections, we explain these in detail.

3.1 Surface Segmentation

With a voxelized surface $\mathcal{V}$ as input, we first perform a segmentation of $\mathcal{V}$ based on the idea of functional components. A *functional component* (FC) in $\mathcal{V}$ is the maximal 0-connected subset of $\mathcal{V}$ in which all the voxels have a common functional plane (FP). If a voxel u in $\mathcal{V}$ does not have an FP, then its FP is assigned as that of one of its surrounding voxels (the one in $A_2(u)$, $A_1(u)$, or $A_0(u)$, in that order). Based on the FPs of the voxels in $\mathcal{V}$, component labeling is done in GPU, using the technique of [33]. An example of surface segmentation is shown in Fig. 1c.

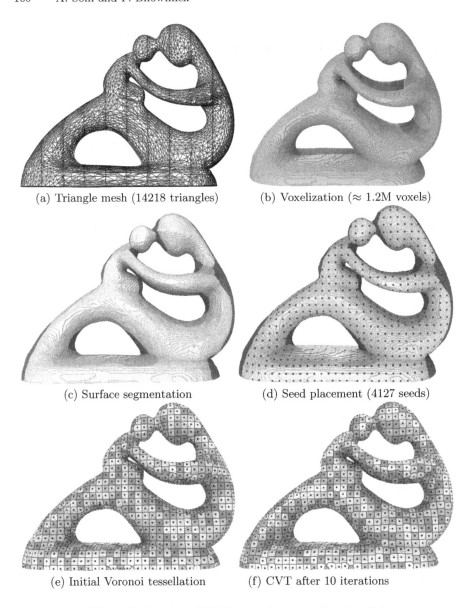

(a) Triangle mesh (14218 triangles)

(b) Voxelization ($\approx$ 1.2M voxels)

(c) Surface segmentation

(d) Seed placement (4127 seeds)

(e) Initial Voronoi tessellation

(f) CVT after 10 iterations

Fig. 1. Basic steps of CVT on `mother-and-child` model.

3.2   Voronoi Tessellation

To compute the Voronoi tessellation on a voxelized surface $\mathcal{V}$, we consider a set of sites/seeds, namely $\mathcal{S} = \{s_1, s_2, \ldots, s_n\}$, which is essentially a subset of $\mathcal{V}$. We consider the geodesic distance $d_0(u, v)$ between two voxels u and v as the metric in this tessellation. For a site s_i, its *Voronoi region* is defined as

$$\mathcal{R}(s_i) = \{u \in \mathcal{V} : d_0(u, s_i) \leqslant d_0(u, s_j) \; \forall s_j \in \mathcal{S}\}. \tag{1}$$

The resultant *Voronoi tessellation* is then given by

$$\mathcal{D}(\mathcal{V}, \mathcal{S}) = \bigcup_{s \in \mathcal{S}} \mathcal{R}(s). \tag{2}$$

Distribution of Seeds. Seed voxels are chosen from $\mathcal{V}$ in such a way that facilitates a Voronoi tessellation with regions of similar size and shape. This, in turn, results to generation of isotropic quadrangular mesh. Surface segmentation based on FCs helps in this process. Since each FC is in bijection with its projection (PFC) on its FP, we use this PFC for selection of seed voxels. We simply make a uniform selection of seed pixels from the PFC based on the size of a quad in the target quadrangular mesh. For this, let the desired size of a Voronoi region be $\rho \times \rho$. From the PFC we choose all those pixels as seeds which have either of their coordinates divisible by ρ. For example, if the PFC is on xy-plane, then a pixel $p(x, y)$ is chosen as a seed if and only if $x \bmod \rho = y \bmod \rho = 0$. We then project these seed pixels back to the corresponding FC to obtain the seed voxels which are in bijection with them.

Note that the seed points near the boundary of an FC may be either close or far with those near the boundary of its adjacent FC in terms of the geodesic distance. To see why, let C_1 and C_2 be two FCs adjacent to each other. Let, w.l.o.g., xy- and xz-planes be their respective FPs. Let $s_i(x_i, y_i, z_i) \in C_1$ and $s_j(x_j, y_j, z_j) \in C_2$ be two seed voxels such that

(i) $x_i = x_j$ and
(ii) (s_i, s_j) is the closest pair in $\{(s, s') : s \in C_1, s' \in C_2, x[s] = x[s'] = x_i\}$.

If $d_0(s_i, s_j) \leqslant \frac{3}{4}\rho$, then we replace s_i and s_j by the median voxel of $\pi_0(s_i, s_j)$. If $d_0(s_i, s_j) \geqslant \frac{3}{2}\rho$, then we add the median voxel of $\pi_0(s_i, s_j)$ as a new seed. This ensures that the geodesic distance between every two seeds in $\mathcal{S}$ ranges from $\frac{3}{4}\rho$ to $\frac{3}{2}\rho$. Such a policy follows the minimal and the maximal sampling-size property of Poisson disk sampling.

We now state few important characteristic properties of geodesic-based Voronoi tessellation on the voxelized surface. For this, we first define an *iso-contour* $K(u, \delta)$ as the set of voxels in $\mathcal{V}$ having a fixed geodesic distance δ from a given voxel $u \in \mathcal{V}$; i.e., $K(u, \delta) = \{v : (v \in \mathcal{V}) \wedge (d_0(u, v) = \delta)\}$. Clearly, an iso-contour can be obtained by breadth-first-search in $\mathcal{V}$ with u as the start vertex in the underlying graph (Fig. 2). We recall that a 0-DSS means the 0-path obtained by discretization of a straight line segment joining two pixels in 2D or two voxels in 3D, as applicable [17]. We also recall that *Chebyshev distance* between two n-dimensional points $p(p_1, p_2, \ldots, p_n)$ and $q(q_1, q_2, \ldots, q_n)$ is given by $d_\infty(p, q) = \max\{|p_i - q_i| : 1 \leqslant i \leqslant n\}$. Now we have the following lemma.

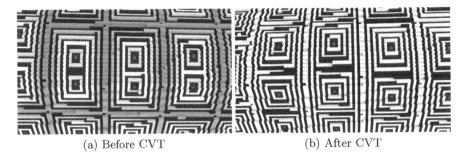

(a) Before CVT   (b) After CVT

Fig. 2. Iso-contours on a voxelized surface, shown alternately in white and blue, obtained w.r.t. the seed voxels shown in red. (Color figure online)

Lemma 1. *Let C be a functional component, F its functional plane, and u and v two voxels in C. Let C' be the projection of C on F, and u' and v' the respective projections of u and v on F. Let L be the 0-DSS connecting u' and v' on F. If L is contained in C', then its pre-image in C is a geodesic path $\pi_0(u, v)$ of length $d_\infty(u, v)$.*

Proof. Let, w.l.o.g., F be the xy-plane. Let $u = (x_u, y_u, z_u), u' = (x'_u, y'_u)$, etc. Since xy-plane serves here as the functional plane, we have:

(i) $x'_u = x_u, y'_u = y_u, x'_v = x_v, y'_v = y_v$;
(ii) $\max(|x_u - x_v|, |y_u - y_v|) \geqslant |z_u - z_v|$;
(iii) length of L (as a 0-path) is $\max(|x'_u - x'_v|, |y'_u - y'_v|)$.

Since L is 0-connected and there is a bijection between C and C' (Sect. 3.1), the pre-image of L is a 0-path in C and its length is $\max(|x_u - x_v|, |y_u - y_v|)$ by (i) and (iii), which, by (ii), equals $\max(|x_u - x_v|, |y_u - y_v|, |z_u - z_v|)$, i.e., length of the 0-DSS joining u and v in 3D. Since no geodesic path can be shorter than a 0-DSS, the pre-image is just a geodesic and its length equals the Chebyshev distance between u and v. □

We now introduce a special type of iso-contour referred to as *square iso-contour*. As before, we denote by C a functional component, by F its FP and by C' its projection on F, by u' the projection of a voxel $u \in C$ on F, and by L a 0-DSS on F. An iso-contour $K(u, \delta)$ in C is said to be a square iso-contour if its projection on F is a digital square. Here we use the term 'digital square' to mean a closed 1-path in 2D obtained by discretization of a rectilinear square with integer vertices. We have the following theorem for a square iso-contour.

Theorem 1. *Let $K(u, \delta)$ be an iso-contour belonging to a functional component, C. Let C' and $K'(u, \delta)$ be the respective projections of C and $K(u, \delta)$ on the functional plane, F. $K(u, \delta)$ is a square iso-contour if, for each voxel v in $K(u, \delta)$, there exists a pre-image of the 0-DSS $L(u', v')$ in C.*

Algorithm 1. COMPUTECVT($\mathcal{V}, \mathcal{S}, F$)

---

1 *Initialize*($\mathcal{V}, \mathcal{S}, L, D$)
2 *Compute VT*($\mathcal{V}, \mathcal{S}, L, D, F$)
3 $\mathcal{C} \leftarrow$ ComputeCentroid($\mathcal{V}, \mathcal{S}, L$)
4 float $\xi \leftarrow$ ComputeEVT($\mathcal{C}, \mathcal{S}$)
5 **do**
6 | float $\xi_0 \leftarrow \xi$
7 | *Compute VT*($\mathcal{V}, \mathcal{S}, L, D, F$)
8 | $\mathcal{C} \leftarrow$ ComputeCentroid($\mathcal{V}, \mathcal{S}, L$)
9 | $\xi \leftarrow$ ComputeEVT($\mathcal{C}, \mathcal{S}$)
10 | $\mathcal{S} \leftarrow \mathcal{C}$
11 **while** $|\xi_0 - \xi| \geqslant \varepsilon$;
12 **return** L

Proof. We use Lemma 1 for the proof. Since there exists a pre-image of $L(u', v')$ in C for each voxel v in $K(u, \delta)$, that pre-image is a geodesic path from u to v whose length equals the Chebyshev distance between u and v. The bijection between $K(u, \delta)$ and $K'(u, \delta)$ implies that for each voxel v in $K(u, \delta)$, there exists a geodesic path from u to v whose projection on F is a 0-DSS of length δ. Thus, $K'(u, \delta)$ is a digital square, which implies $K(u, \delta)$ is a square iso-contour. □

It is evident from Theorem 1 that if a functional component is sufficiently large in area compared to its perimeter such that it contains a large number of seeds that are uniformly distributed on it, then it will contain predominantly square iso-contours w.r.t. the seeds, and hence results to an almost isotropic tessellation. The result in Fig. 1(d–f) illustrates this fact.

3.3   Centroidal Voronoi Tessellation

Given a voxelized surface $\mathcal{V}$ and a set of n seeds $\mathcal{S} := \{s_1, s_2, \ldots, s_n\}$, we define *centroidal Voronoi tessellation energy* as

$$\xi(\mathcal{V}, \mathcal{S}, \mathcal{C}) = \frac{1}{n} \sum_{i=1}^{n} d_0(c_i, s_i). \tag{3}$$

Here, for each seed s_i, we denote by c_i the centroid of its Voronoi region, $\mathcal{R}(s_i)$. Computation of the centroid is discussed later in this section. Our objective is to minimize the value of the energy function by rearrangement of the seeds.

The steps for computing CVT are shown in Algorithm 1. Apart from $\mathcal{V}$ and $\mathcal{S}$, it takes as input an array F that contains the ID of FC corresponding to each voxel of $\mathcal{V}$. We use two other arrays, L and D, in the algorithm. For each voxel u in $\mathcal{V}$, $L(u)$ contains the label/ID of the seed s whose corresponding Voronoi region contains u, and $D(u)$ contains the geodesic distance of u from s. Their values are initialized in Line 1 using the procedure Initialize.

Procedure Initialize($\mathcal{V}, \mathcal{S}, L, D$)

---

1 **for** *each voxel $s \in \mathcal{S}$* **do** // one thread for each s
2     $D(s) \leftarrow 0$
3     $L(s) \leftarrow ID$ *of* s
4 **for** *each voxel $u \in \mathcal{V} \setminus \mathcal{S}$* **do** // one thread for each u
5     $D(u) \leftarrow \infty$
6     $L(u) \leftarrow 0$

Procedure ComputeCentroid($\mathcal{V}, \mathcal{S}, L$)

---

1 set $C \leftarrow \emptyset$
2 **for** *each voxel $s \in \mathcal{S}$* **do**
3     $s' \leftarrow \frac{1}{|\mathcal{R}(s)|} \sum\limits_{u \in \mathcal{R}(s)} u$
4     $s \leftarrow$ nearest voxel of s' in $\mathcal{R}(s)$
5     $C \leftarrow C \cup \{s\}$
6 **return** C

Procedure ComputeEVT($\mathcal{S}, \mathcal{C}$)

---

1 float $\xi \leftarrow 0$
2 **for** *each voxel $s \in \mathcal{S}$* **do** // one thread for each s
3     $\xi \leftarrow \xi + d_0(s, c)$ // c is the centroid of $\mathcal{R}(s)$
4 $\xi \leftarrow \frac{1}{n}\xi$
5 **return** ξ

Procedure ComputeVT($\mathcal{V}, \mathcal{S}, L, D, F$)

---

1 boolean *update* $\leftarrow$ TRUE
2 **while** *update* **do**
3   *update* $\leftarrow$ FALSE
4   **for** *each voxel $u \in \mathcal{V}$* **do** // one thread for each u
5   **for** *each voxel $v \in A_0(u)$* **do**
6   **if** $((F(L(u)) = F(L(v))) \wedge (D(u) > D(v) + 1))$ **then**
7              $D(u) \leftarrow D(v) + 1$
8              $L(u) \leftarrow L(v)$
9   *update* $\leftarrow$ TRUE
10   **else if** $((F(L(u)) \neq F(L(v)) \wedge (D(u) > D(v) + w))$ **then**
11              $D(u) \leftarrow D(v) + w$
12              $L(u) \leftarrow L(v)$
13   *update* $\leftarrow$ TRUE

The respective procedures ComputeVT and ComputeCentroid are iteratively called to modify the Voronoi tessellation and corresponding centroids, until con-

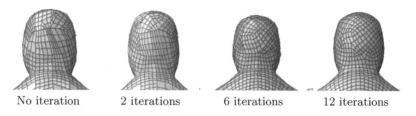

No iteration   2 iterations   6 iterations   12 iterations

Fig. 3. Quad meshes generated at different iterations by our algorithm.

vergence. The CVT energy is computed in Line 4 and Line 9 of Algorithm 1 by calling ComputeEVT, which outputs the average geodesic distance from all the centroids of the Voronoi regions to the corresponding seeds. Seeds are updated with centroids in Line 10. The convergence criterion in the **do-while** loop determines the terminating condition. If the absolute difference between the CVT energy in the current iteration with the CVT energy in the previous iteration is less then ε, then the algorithm terminates. The value of ε is typically set in the range from 1 to 5. An example of restructuring of quad mesh with the progress of our algorithm is shown in Fig. 3.

The procedure ComputeVT runs with a **while** loop, which terminates when the label of no voxel is updated. In every iteration, the labels and the distances of the voxels in $\mathcal{V}$ are updated. The updates occur for two possible cases: (i) the voxel u and its 0-adjacent voxel v have the same FC (Line 6) and (ii) u and v have different FC (Line 10). While updating the distance of u in the second case (Line 11), we use two sub-cases based on FCs of u and v, as follows. Let C_1 and C_2 be the FCs of u and v respectively. The *boundary* of C_1 w.r.t. C_2 is defined as $B_1 = \{p : (p \in C_1) \wedge (A_0(p) \not\subset C_1) \wedge (A_0(p) \subset C_1 \cup C_2)\}$. Similarly, we define $B_2 = \{p : (p \in C_2) \wedge (A_0(p) \not\subset C_2) \wedge (A_0(p) \subset C_1 \cup C_2)\}$. Hence, the boundary shared by C_1 and C_2 is taken as $B = B_1 \cup B_2$. Now, B_1 can have one or more than one FP, and so for B_2. That is, for $i = 1, 2$, we have either $|F(B_i)| = 1$ or $|F(B_i)| > 1$. Thus, we have the following two sub-cases:

1. $|F(B_1) \cup F(B_2)| = 2$: B possibly belongs to a high-curvature region. In this case, we assign $w = \rho/2$, where $\rho \times \rho$ is the desired size of a Voronoi region.
2. $|F(B_1) \cup F(B_2)| > 2$: B possibly belongs to a low-curvature region. We assign $w = 1$.

3.4 Parallel Computing and Time Complexity

There exist some Voronoi tessellation algorithms on GPU based on Euclidean norm [12,26]; however, they provide approximate solutions due to bounded-error problems and artifacts. Hence, we have designed and implemented a wavefront-based algorithm using shared memory (SM), which minimizes the number of kernel calls.

For functional segmentation, we use a CUDA kernel that activates a thread for each voxel in $\mathcal{V}$. It finds the functional plane for each voxel using the technique of [33] for functional-component labeling in GPU. For seed placement and

Voronoi tessellation, we use kernels based on SM. Let the size of an SM block be $\beta \times \beta \times \beta$. Let $\delta_{\max} = \max\{d_0(u, s) : u \in \mathcal{R}(s), s \in \mathcal{S}\}$. We have the following lemma on the number of kernel launches.

Lemma 2. *Number of kernel launches in* ComputeVT *is* $\lceil \delta_{\max}/\beta \rceil$.

Proof. First we explain the scenario without SM. Initially, no voxel in $\mathcal{V}$ is labeled excepting the seeds in $\mathcal{S}$, which have their distinct IDs. In the first kernel launch, each voxel u with $d_0(u, s) = 1$ for some seed s updates its label $L(u)$ to $L(s)$. In the $k (\geqslant 2)$th round of kernel launch, for each $u \in A_0(v)$ and $L(v) = L(s)$ for some seed s, the label $L(u)$ is updated to $L(s)$. Hence, the number of kernel launch is $\delta_{\max}$.

Now we go to the scenario with SM. There arise two cases as follows.

1. If $u \in \mathcal{R}(s)$ and s both lie in the same block of SM, then $L(u)$ will update to $L(s)$ in one kernel call.
2. If $u \in \mathcal{R}(s)$ and s lie in two different blocks, then the geodesic path $\pi(s, u)$ is partitioned into sub-paths: $\pi(s, v_1) \cup \pi(v_2, v_3) \cup \cdots \cup \pi(v_t, u)$, where, for $i = 1, 2, \ldots, t - 1$, each v_i is on the boundary of a block, and v_i and v_{i+1} are 0-adjacent. In first kernel launch, $\pi(s, v_1)$ is labeled with $L(s)$. In the second kernel call, $\pi(v_2, v_3)$ is labeled with $L(s)$. Thus, in t kernel calls, $\pi(s, u)$ is labeled with $L(s)$.

Thus, the number of kernel launches required for $\pi(u, s)$ is equal to the number of blocks $\pi(u, s)$ is covering, which gives the proof. $\qquad \square$

We use Lemma 2 to derive the time complexity of ComputeVT in the following theorem. For this, we use the notations: $b(= \beta^3) =$ block size, $n_b =$ number of blocks to accommodate the 3D array containing $\mathcal{V}$, $\mu =$ number of multiprocessors, $\kappa =$ number of cores per multiprocessor.

Theorem 2. *In a parallel computing framework, the time complexity of* ComputeVT *is given by*

$$O\left(\frac{n_b \cdot b \cdot \delta_{\max}}{\min(n_b, \mu) \cdot \min(b, \kappa)}\right).$$

Proof. Processing time per block is $O\left(\frac{b}{\min(b,\kappa)}\right)$. Number of blocks per multiprocessor is $O\left(\frac{n_b}{\min(n_b, \mu)}\right)$. For assignment of the label of a seed to the voxels in the portion of a geodesic in a block, we need $O(\beta)$ time. By Lemma 2, number of kernel launches is $O\left(\frac{\delta_{\max}}{\beta}\right)$. So, the time complexity of ComputeVT results to $O\left(\frac{n_b}{\min(n_b, \mu)} \cdot \frac{b}{\min(b, \kappa)} \cdot \beta \cdot \frac{\delta_{\max}}{\beta}\right) = O\left(\frac{n_b \cdot b \cdot \delta_{\max}}{\min(n_b, \mu) \cdot \min(b, \kappa)}\right).$ $\qquad \square$

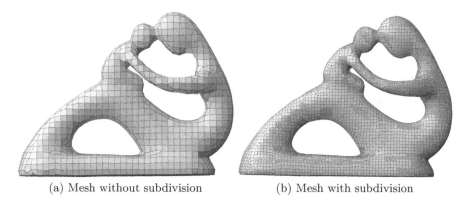

(a) Mesh without subdivision   (b) Mesh with subdivision

Fig. 4. An example of quad mesh constructed from the Voronoi tessellation shown in Fig. 1f.

3.5   Mesh Construction

Our mesh construction technique is different from the existing ones, which are mostly based on Delaunay triangulation; see, for example, [9, 23, 27, 30, 31] for triangle mesh and [3, 21] for quad mesh. We first extract vertex clusters from the Voronoi tessellation, compute a unique representative vertex for each cluster, and consider these representative vertices as vertices of the quad mesh. A *vertex cluster* K is defined as a subset of voxels in $\mathcal{V}$ such that each voxel $u \in K$ is 0-adjacent to at least three Voronoi regions and there exists some voxel v in $K \cap A_0(u)$. For every such cluster K, we consider its centroid as the representative. If there arise two representative voxels whose geodesic distance is less than $\frac{1}{4}\rho$, then we replace those two representatives by a median voxel in the corresponding geodesic path. These representative voxels are considered as the final vertices of the quadrangular mesh. An example of output generated by our technique is shown in Fig. 4a.

If a Voronoi region is lying in a non-planar area, then the corresponding quad is likely to deviate from the original surface by an undesirable amount. To resolve this, we adopt a strategy of subdivision of the Voronoi regions based on digital planarity. We use the technique of least-square fitting plane proposed in [18] for this purpose. An example of mesh subdivision generated by our algorithm is shown in Fig. 4b.

4   Experimental Results and Conclusion

We have written all our codes in C++ with CUDA library functions, and have run them on an Inspiron 15 7000 Gaming laptop. It has CUDA Driver Version 7.5, NVIDIA GeForce GTX 1050 Ti graphic card with 4GB GDDR5 graphics memory. GPU has 1290 clock rate, 768 cores. Its wrap size is 32 and maximum number of threads per block is 1024.

Table 1. Summary of results.

Object	#Tris	#Voxels	#Quads	ρ	GPU time (secs.)
mother-and-child	14,218	1.20M	19,438	21	13
bunny	69,451	1.10M	6,048	21	9
torus-knot	30,988	0.65M	11,824	21	11
duck	19,720	0.56M	14,152	15	5
mug	3,450	1.17M	25,116	21	12
machine-part	3,720	1.42M	23,041	17	19
hand	39,000	1.43M	8,041	40	19

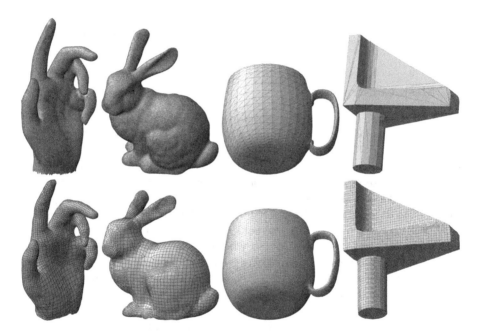

Fig. 5. Results of quadrangular mesh generation from triangle meshes (top: input, bottom: output).

Table 1 contains the data related to quad mesh generation for various kinds of models. It can be noticed that the model machine-part has taken a larger GPU time, as high-resolution voxel set is required to have enough seeds placed in between the 'sharp edges' present in a small locality. The objects like duck, torus-knot, and bunny have predominantly curved surfaces without sharp edges. Hence, a low-resolution voxelization is enough to keep the details of the original triangle mesh. The objects mug and machine-part are synthetic triangle meshes. Thus, they have more quads generated than the number of triangles in the original mesh. On the other hand, bunny, duck, and hand are scanned

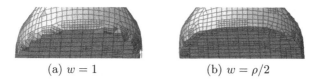

(a) $w = 1$ (b) $w = \rho/2$

Fig. 6. Impact of w on Voronoi vertices close to boundary of functional components.

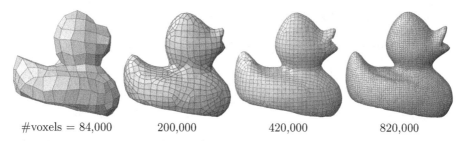

#voxels = 84,000   200,000   420,000   820,000

Fig. 7. Quad meshes generated with different resolutions of voxelization. Quad size ρ is fixed to 15.

models with curved surfaces, and hence their quads is less in number compared to triangles in the original mesh. The input and the output meshes for some of these objects are shown in Fig. 5.

An appropriate value of w (used in ComputeVT, Line 11) forces the Voronoi vertices corresponding to the seeds close to the boundary of an FP, to be placed on or near the boundary. It can be noticed from the results shown in Fig. 6. For a higher resolution of voxelization, quality of the quad mesh would be better. This is apparent from the results shown in Fig. 7.

The results presented here demonstrate the effectiveness of the proposed technique in quad mesh generation for objects of various types. The meshes generated by our algorithm are found to be isotropic and semi-regular, as evident from the results shown in this paper. For theoretical guarantee, we need to explore further on the tessellation created by our algorithm and the nature of distribution of seeds around the boundaries of functional components. Further, with different affine transforms like scaling and rotation, the invariance of result produced by our algorithm should also be comprehensively studied.

References

1. Bhunre, P.K., Bhowmick, P., Mukherjee, J.: On efficient computation of inter-simplex Chebyshev distance for voxelization of 2-manifold surface. Inf. Sci. (2018). https://doi.org/10.1016/j.ins.2018.03.006
2. Alliez, P., De Verdière, E.C., Devillers, O., Isenburg, M.: Isotropic surface remeshing. In: Shape Modeling International, pp. 49–58 (2003). https://doi.org/10.1109/SMI.2003.1199601

3. Baudouin, T.C., Remacle, J.-F., Marchandise, E., Lambrechts, J., Henrotte, F.: Lloyd's energy minimization in the L_p norm for quadrilateral surface mesh generation. Eng. Comput. **30**, 97–110 (2014). https://doi.org/10.1007/s00366-012-0290-x

4. Bommes, D., et al.: Quad-mesh generation and processing: a survey. Comput. Graph. Forum **32**, 51–76 (2013). https://doi.org/10.1111/cgf.12014

5. Boubekeur, T., Reuter, P., Schlick, C.:Visualization of point-based surfaces with locally reconstructed subdivision surfaces. In: Shape Modeling and Applications, pp. 23–32 (2005). https://doi.org/10.1109/SMI.2005.49

6. Cashman, T.J.: Beyond Catmull-Clark: a survey of advances in subdivision surface methods. Comput. Graph. Forum **31**, 42–61 (2012). https://doi.org/10.1111/j.1467-8659.2011.02083.x

7. Catmull, E., Clark, J.: Recursively generated B-spline surfaces on arbitrary topological meshes. Comput. Aided Des. **10**(6), 350–355 (1978)

8. Cohen-Or, D., Kaufman, A.: Fundamentals of surface voxelization. Graph. Models Image Process. **57**, 453–461 (1995). https://doi.org/10.1006/gmip.1995.1039

9. Du, Q., Gunzburger, M.D., Ju, L.: Constrained centroidal Voronoi tessellations for surfaces. SIAM J. Sci. Comput. **24**, 1488–1506 (2003). https://doi.org/10.1137/S1064827501391576

10. Du, Q., Wang, D.: Anisotropic centroidal Voronoi tessellations and their applications. SIAM J. Sci. Comput. **26**(3), 737–761 (2005). https://doi.org/10.1137/S1064827503428527

11. Dyn, N., Levin, D., Liu, D.: Interpolatory convexity-preserving subdivision schemes for curves and surfaces. Comput. Aided Des. **24**, 211–216 (1992). https://doi.org/10.1016/0010-4485(92)90057-H

12. Fischer, I., Gotsman, C.: Fast approximation of high-order Voronoi diagrams and distance transforms on the GPU. J. Graph. Tools **11**, 39–60 (2006). https://doi.org/10.1080/2151237X.2006.10129229

13. Hausner, A.: Simulating decorative mosaics. In: Computer Graphics & Interactive Techniques, pp. 573–580 (2001). https://doi.org/10.1145/383259.383327

14. Hu, K., Zhang, Y.J.: Centroidal Voronoi tessellation based polycube construction for adaptive all-hexahedral mesh generation. Comput. Methods Appl. Mech. Eng. **305**, 405–421 (2016). https://doi.org/10.1016/j.cma.2016.03.021

15. Ju, T., Carson, J., Liu, L., Warren, J., Bello, M., Kakadiaris, I.: Subdivision meshes for organizing spatial biomedical data. Methods **50**, 70–76 (2010). https://doi.org/10.1016/j.ymeth.2009.07.012

16. Karbacher, S., Seeger, S., Häusler, G.: A non-linear subdivision scheme for triangle meshes. In: Vision, Modeling and Visualization, pp. 163–170 (2000)

17. Klette, R., Rosenfeld, A.: Digital Geometry: Geometric Methods for Digital Picture Analysis (2004)

18. Klette, R., Stojmenović, I., Žunić, J.: A parametrization of digital planes by least-squares fits and generalizations. Graph. Models Image Process. 295–300 (1996). https://doi.org/10.1006/gmip.1996.0024

19. Leung, Y.-S., Wang, X., He, Y., Liu, Y.-J., Wang, C.C.: A unified framework for isotropic meshing based on narrow-band Euclidean distance transformation. Comput. Vis. Media **1**, 239–251 (2015). https://doi.org/10.1007/s41095-015-0022-4

20. Lévy, B., Bonneel, N.: Variational anisotropic surface meshing with Voronoi parallel linear enumeration. In: Jiao, X., Weill, J.C. (eds.) 21st International Meshing Roundtable, pp. 349–366. Springer, Heidelberg (2013). https://doi.org/10.1007/978-3-642-33573-0_21

21. Lévy, B., Liu, Y.: L_p centroidal Voronoi tessellation and its applications. ACM ToG, **29**, Article no. 119 (2010). https://doi.org/10.1145/1833349.1778856

22. Liu, Y., et al.: On centroidal Voronoi tessellation - energy smoothness and fast computation. ACM ToG **28**, Article no. 101 (2009). https://doi.org/10.1145/1559755.1559758

23. Liu, Y.-J., Xu, C.-X., Yi, R., Fan, D., He, Y.: Manifold differential evolution (MDE): a global optimization method for geodesic centroidal Voronoi tessellations on meshes. ACM ToG **35**, Article no. 243 (2016). https://doi.org/10.1145/2980179.2982424

24. Peters, J., Reif, U.: The simplest subdivision scheme for smoothing polyhedra. ACM ToG **16**, 420–431 (1997). https://doi.org/10.1145/263834.263851

25. Rong, G., Liu, Y., Wang, W., Yin, X., Gu, D., Guo, X.: GPU-assisted computation of centroidal Voronoi tessellation. IEEE TVCG **17**, 345–356 (2011). https://doi.org/10.1109/TVCG.2010.53

26. Rong, G., Tan, T.-S.: Jump flooding in GPU with applications to Voronoi diagram and distance transform. In: I3D 2006, pp. 109–116 (2006). https://doi.org/10.1145/1111411.1111431

27. Surazhsky, V., Alliez, P., Gotsman, C.: Isotropic remeshing of surfaces: a local parameterization approach. Ph.D thesis, INRIA (2003)

28. Valette, S., Chassery, J.-M.: Approximated centroidal Voronoi diagrams for uniform polygonal mesh coarsening. Comput. Graph. Forum **23**, 381–389 (2004). https://doi.org/10.1111/j.1467-8659.2004.00769.x

29. Velho, L., Zorin, D.: 4–8 subdivision. Comput. Aided Geom. Des. **18**, 397–427 (2001). https://doi.org/10.1016/S0167-8396(01)00039-5

30. Wang, X., et al.: Intrinsic computation of centroidal Voronoi tessellation (CVT) on meshes. Comput. Aided Des. **58**, 51–61 (2015). https://doi.org/10.1016/j.cad.2014.08.023

31. Yan, D.-M., Lévy, B., Liu, Y., Sun, F., Wang, W.: Isotropic remeshing with fast and exact computation of restricted Voronoi diagram. Comput. Graph. Forum **28**, 1445–1454 (2009). https://doi.org/10.1111/j.1467-8659.2009.01521.x

32. Yang, X.: Surface interpolation of meshes by geometric subdivision. Comput. Aided Des. **37**, 497–508 (2005). https://doi.org/10.1016/j.cad.2004.10.008

33. Yukihiro, K.: GPU-based cluster-labeling algorithm without the use of conventional iteration: application to the Swendsen-Wang multi-cluster spin flip algorithm. Comput. Phys. Commun. **194**(Sup. C), 54–58 (2015). https://doi.org/10.1016/j.cpc.2015.04.015

34. Zorin, D., Schröder, P., Sweldens, W.: Interpolating subdivision for meshes with arbitrary topology. In: Computer Graphics & Interactive Techniques, pp. 189–192 (1996). https://doi.org/10.1145/237170.237254

When Can l_p-norm Objective Functions Be Minimized via Graph Cuts?

Filip Malmberg$^{(\boxtimes)}$ and Robin Strand

Department of Information Technology, Uppsala University, Uppsala, Sweden
{filip.malmberg,robin.strand}@it.uu.se

Abstract. Techniques based on minimal graph cuts have become a standard tool for solving combinatorial optimization problems arising in image processing and computer vision applications. These techniques can be used to minimize objective functions written as the sum of a set of unary and pairwise terms, provided that the objective function is *submodular*. This can be interpreted as minimizing the l_1-norm of the vector containing all pairwise and unary terms. By raising each term to a power p, the same technique can also be used to minimize the l_p-norm of the vector. Unfortunately, the submodularity of an l_1-norm objective function does not guarantee the submodularity of the corresponding l_p-norm objective function. The contribution of this paper is to provide useful conditions under which an l_p-norm objective function is submodular for all $p \geq 1$, thereby identifying a large class of l_p-norm objective functions that can be minimized via minimal graph cuts.

Keywords: Minimal graph cuts · l_p norm · Submodularity

1 Introduction

Many fundamental problems in image processing and computer vision, such as image filtering, segmentation, registration, and stereo vision, can naturally be formulated as optimization problems [6]. Often, these optimization problems can be described as *labeling* problems, in which we wish to assign to each image element (pixel) an element from some finite set of labels. The interpretation of these labels depend on the optimization problem at hand. In image segmentation, the labels might indicate object categories. In registration and stereo disparity problems the labels represent correspondences between images, and in image reconstruction and filtering the labels represent intensities in the filtered image. We seek a label assignment configuration $\mathbf{x}$ that minimizes a given objective function E, which in the "canonical" case can be written as follows:

$$E(\mathbf{x}) = \sum_{i \in \mathcal{V}} \phi_i(x_i) + \sum_{i,j \in \mathcal{E}} \phi_{ij}(x_i, x_j). \tag{1}$$

In Eq. 1 above, $\mathcal{G} = (\mathcal{V}, \mathcal{E})$ is an undirected graph and x_i denotes the label of vertex $i \in \mathcal{V}$ which must belong to a finite set of integers $\{0, 1 \ldots, K - 1\}$.

© Springer Nature Switzerland AG 2018
R. P. Barneva et al. (Eds.): IWCIA 2018, LNCS 11255, pp. 112–117, 2018.
https://doi.org/10.1007/978-3-030-05288-1_9

We assume that both the *unary* terms $\phi_i(\cdot)$ and the *pairwise* terms $\phi_{ij}(\cdot, \cdot)$ are non-negative for all i, j. We seek a labeling $\mathbf{x} = (x_1, \ldots, x_{|\mathcal{V}|})$ for which $E(\mathbf{x})$ is minimal.

Finding a globally optimal solution to the labeling problem described above is NP-hard in the general case [6], but there are classes of objective functions for which efficient algorithms exist. Specifically, for the binary labeling problem, with $K = 2$, a globally optimal solution can be computed by solving a max-flow/min-cut problem on a suitably constructed graph, provided that all pairwise terms are *submodular* [3,6]. A pairwise term ϕ_{ij} is said to be submodular if

$$\phi_{ij}(0,0) + \phi_{ij}(1,1) \leq \phi_{ij}(0,1) + \phi_{ij}(1,0). \tag{2}$$

For $K > 2$, the optimization problem cannot in general be solved directly via graph cuts. The multi-label problem can, however, be reduced to a sequence of binary valued labeling problems using, e.g., the *expansion move* algorithm proposed by Boykov et al. [3]. The output of the expansion move algorithm is a labeling that is locally optimal in a strong sense, and that is guaranteed to lie within a multiplicative factor of the global minimum [3,6]. With this in mind, we here restrict our attention to the binary label case, i.e., $K = 2$.

Looking again at the labeling problem described above, we can view the objective function in Eq. 1 as consisting of two parts:

- A *local* error measure, in our case defined by the unary and pairwise terms.
- A *global* error measure, aggregating the local errors into a final score. In the case of Eq. 1, the global error measure is obtained by summing all the local error measures.

The choice of global error measure determines how local errors will be distributed in the optimal solution. Since we assume all terms to be non-negative, minimizing E can be seen as minimizing the l_1-norm of the vector containing all unary and pairwise terms. Here, we consider the generalization of this result to arbitrary l_p-norms, $p \geq 1$, and thus seek to minimize

$$\left(\sum_{i \in \mathcal{V}} \phi_i^p(x_i) + \sum_{i,j \in \mathcal{E}} \phi_{ij}^p(x_i, x_j) \right)^{1/p}, \tag{3}$$

where $\phi_i^p(\cdot) = (\phi_i(\cdot))^p$ and $\phi_{ij}^p(\cdot, \cdot) = (\phi_{ij}(\cdot, \cdot))^p$. The value p can be seen as a parameter controlling the balance between minimizing the overall cost versus minimizing the magnitude of the individual terms. For $p = 1$, the optimal labeling may contain arbitrarily large individual terms as long as the sum of the terms is small. As p increases, a larger penalty is assigned to solutions containing large individual terms. In the limit as p goes to infinity, the global error measure will approach the L_∞-norm, or max-norm, of the vector of local error measures. A labeling that minimizes Eq. 3 with p approaching infinity is a *strict minimizer* in the sense of Levi and Zorin [7].

It is easily seen that minimizing Eq. 3 is equivalent to minimizing

$$\sum_{i \in \mathcal{V}} \phi_i^p(x_i) + \sum_{i,j \in \mathcal{E}} \phi_{ij}^p(x_i, x_j), \tag{4}$$

i.e., minimizing the sum of all unary and pairwise terms raised to the power p. Again, this labeling problem can be solved using minimal graph cuts, provided that all pairwise terms ϕ_{ij}^p are submodular. Unfortunately, submodularity of ϕ_{ij} does not in general imply submodularity of ϕ_{ij}^p.[1]

The contribution of this paper is to provide useful conditions under which ϕ_{ij}^p is submodular. Specifically, we show that if ϕ_{ij} is submodular and

$$\max(\phi_{ij}(0,0), \phi_{ij}(1,1)) \leq \max(\phi_{ij}(1,0), \phi_{ij}(0,1)), \tag{5}$$

then ϕ_{ij}^p is submodular for all $p \geq 1$.

2   Related Work

Several authors have considered the use of graph cuts for solving l_p-norm optimization problems in image processing, mainly in the context of image segmentation. In this application, a cut is usually computed directly on a *pixel adjacency graph* – a graph whose vertex set is the image pixels and where adjacent pixels are connected by weighted edges – augmented with two vertices (s and t) representing object and background labels [2]. Compared to the objective function given in Eq. 1, this case only covers a simplified form of the pairwise terms: A fixed penalty is given when two adjacent pixels are assigned different labels, and zero penalty is assigned if the labels are the same. In this simplified case, the issue of submodularity is not important: To optimize the l_p norm of the cut, one may simply raise all *edge weights* to the power p and compute cut as usual. For more general optimization problems however, a pairwise term may assign different penalties to all possible label configurations (for K labels, there are K^2 possible label configurations for each pairwise term). This flexibility in assigning the penalties is important in many applications, e.g., stereo reconstruction and image registration.

Allène et al. [1] established links relating minimal graph cuts to optimal spanning forests, showing that when the power of the weights of the graph is above a certain number, the cut minimizing the graph cuts energy is a cut by maximum spanning forest. Similar results were independently derived by Miranda et al. [8]. Couprie et al. showed that both methods are instances of an even more general segmentation framework, which they refer to as *power watersheds* [4]. These interesting results all point to the choice of l_p-norm being a potentially important hyper-parameter to tune for optimization problems occurring in image analysis and computer vision. The results presented here facilitates the use of minimal graph cuts for solving more general l_p-norm problems, beyond the simplified case commonly considered in segmentation applications.

---

[1] As a counterexample, consider the two-label pairwise term ϕ given by $\phi(0,0) = 3$, $\phi(1,1) = 0$, and $\phi(0,1) = \phi(1,0) = 2$. It is easily verified that ϕ is submodular, while ϕ^2 is not.

3   Conditions for the Submodularity of ϕ^p

This section presents our main result; conditions for the submodularity of ϕ^p. We start by establishing a lemma that is central to the definition of this condition.

Lemma 1. *Let $a, b, c, d, p \in \mathbb{R}$, with $p > 1$ and $a, b, c, d \geq 0$. If $a + b \leq c + d$ and $\max(a, b) \leq \max(c, d)$ then $a^p + b^p \leq c^p + d^p$.*

Proof. Showing that $a^p + b^p \leq c^p + d^p$ is equivalent to showing that $a^p + b^p - c^p - d^p \leq 0$. We assume, without loss of generality, that $a \geq b$ and $c \geq d$ so that $\max(a, b) = a$ and $\max(c, d) = c$.

If $b < d$ then $b^p < d^p$ and, since also $a^p \leq c^p$, the lemma trivially holds. For the remainder of the proof, we will therefore assume that $b \geq d$. It then holds that $c \geq a \geq b \geq d$.

If $c = 0$, then also $a = b = c = 0$ and the lemma holds. For the remainder of the proof, we will therefore assume that $c > 0$.

If $a + b < c + d$, then $c + d - a - b > 0$ and so $a < a + (c + d - a - b) = c + d - b$. Let $A = c + d - b$. Since $d - b \leq 0$, it holds that $c \geq A$. Thus the numbers A, b, c, d satisfy the conditions given in the lemma: $A + b = c + d$ and $\max(A, b) \leq \max(c, d)$. Since $a^p + b^p \leq A^p + b^p$ it follows that if the lemma holds for A, b, c, d then it also holds for a, b, c, d. For the remainder of the proof, we will therefore assume that $a + b = c + d$. It follows that $b = c + d - a$ and so

$$a^p + b^p - c^p - d^p = a^p + (c + d - a)^p - c^p - d^p. \tag{6}$$

From the assumption $a \geq b$, it follows that $(c + d)/2 \leq a \leq c$. Let

$$f(x) = x^p + (c + d - x)^p \tag{7}$$

be a function defined on the domain $x \in [(c + d)/2, c]$. We have

$$f'(x) = px^{p-1} - p(c + d - x)^{p-1}. \tag{8}$$

and

$$f''(x) = (p - 1)px^{p-2} + (p - 1)p(c + d - x)^{p-2}. \tag{9}$$

Setting $f'(x) = 0$ yields

$$px^{p-1} - p(c + d - x)^{p-1} = 0 \tag{10}$$
$$\Leftrightarrow px^{p-1} = p(c + d - x)^{p-1} \tag{11}$$
$$\Leftrightarrow x = c + d - x \tag{12}$$
$$\Leftrightarrow x = (c + d)/2. \tag{13}$$

The function $f(x)$ thus has a single stationary point at $x = (c + d)/2$ which coincides with the lower bound of the function domain. Since

$$f''((c + d)/2) = 2(p - 1)p((c + d)/2)^{p-2} > 0 \tag{14}$$

this stationary point is a local minimum. Therefore, the maximum of $f(x)$ is attained at the upper bound of the domain $x = c$, and so $f(x) \leq f(c) = c^p + d^p$ on its domain.

Returning to Eq. 6, we now have

$$a^p + b^p - c^p - d^p = a^p + (c + d - a)^p - c^p - d^p \tag{15}$$
$$= f(a) - c^p - d^p \tag{16}$$
$$\leq c^p + d^p - c^p - d^p \tag{17}$$
$$= 0. \tag{18}$$

This concludes the proof.

Theorem 1. *Let ϕ be a submodular pairwise term. If $\max(\phi(0,0), \phi(1,1)) \leq \max(\phi(1,0), \phi(0,1))$, then ϕ^p is also submodular, for any real $p \geq 1$.*

Proof. Taking $a = \phi(0,0)$, $b = \phi(1,1)$, $c = \phi(1,0)$ and $d = \phi(0,1)$, the theorem follows directly from Lemma 1.

4   Conclusions

We have presented a condition under which a pairwise term ϕ^p is submodular for all $p \geq 1$, thereby identifying a large class of l_p-norm objective functions that can be minimized via minimal graph cuts. The conditions derived here are easy to verify for a given set of pairwise terms, and thus make it easier to apply minimal graph cuts for solving labeling problems with l_p-norm objective functions, without having to explicitly prove the submodularity of the pairwise terms for each specific p.

It should be noted that even when there are non-submodular pairwise terms, graph cut techniques may still be used to find approximate solutions [5]. Nevertheless, submodularity remains an important property for determining the feasibility of optimizing labeling problems via minimal graph cuts.

References

1. Allène, C., Audibert, J.Y., Couprie, M., Keriven, R.: Some links between extremum spanning forests, watersheds and min-cuts. Image Vis. Comput. **28**(10), 1460–1471 (2010)
2. Boykov, Y., Funka-Lea, G.: Graph cuts and efficient ND image segmentation. Int. J. Comput. Vis. **70**(2), 109–131 (2006)
3. Boykov, Y., Veksler, O., Zabih, R.: Fast approximate energy minimization via graph cuts. IEEE Trans. Pattern Anal. Mach. Intell. **23**(11), 1222–1239 (2001)
4. Couprie, C., Grady, L., Najman, L., Talbot, H.: Power watershed: a unifying graph-based optimization framework. IEEE Trans. Pattern Anal. Mach. Intell. **33**(7), 1384–1399 (2011)
5. Kolmogorov, V., Rother, C.: Minimizing nonsubmodular functions with graph cuts-a review. IEEE Trans. Pattern Anal. Mach. Intell. **29**(7), 1274–1279 (2007)

6. Kolmogorov, V., Zabin, R.: What energy functions can be minimized via graph cuts? IEEE Trans. Pattern Anal. Mach. Intell. **26**(2), 147–159 (2004)
7. Levi, Z., Zorin, D.: Strict minimizers for geometric optimization. ACM Trans. Graph. (TOG) **33**(6), 185 (2014)
8. Miranda, P.A., Falcão, A.X.: Links between image segmentation based on optimum-path forest and minimum cut in graph. J. Math. Imaging Vis. **35**(2), 128–142 (2009)

From Theory to Practice

Detection of Osteoarthritis by Gap and Shape Analysis of Knee-Bone X-ray

Sabyasachi Mukherjee[1], Oishila Bandyopadhyay[2]([✉]), Arindam Biswas[1], and Bhargab B. Bhattacharya[3]

[1] Indian Institute of Engineering Science and Technology, Shibpur, Howrah, India
[2] Indian Institute of Information Technology Kalyani, Kalyani, India
oishila@gmail.com
[3] Indian Statistical Institute, Kolkata, India

Abstract. Osteoarthritis in knee-joints of humans can be diagnosed by analyzing an X-ray image of the bone. The changes in the shape of the concerned bones (tibia and femur), and the variation in joint-gap, provide markers of such a bone disease. In this paper, digital-geometric techniques are deployed to analyze the X-ray image for identifying the change in shape and alignment of knee-bones, if any. The gap between the two sections of a knee-joint is checked for uniformity over the entire length. The shape of bone can also be correlated to the presence of osteophytes, if any. For automated diagnosis of osteoarthritis, the given X-ray image is analyzed to detect the presence of any abnormality in the bone-contour or gap. We use the concept of chain code and relaxed digital straight-line segments (RDSS) in our analysis.

Keywords: Bone X-ray image · Chain code · Osteoarthritis
Shape analysis

1 Introduction

Automated analysis of medical images for possible abnormality detection is one of the major components of a modern computer-aided diagnostic (CAD) system. Recent synergy between medical community and computer scientists has led to immense advances in this area. In particular, X-ray imaging provides a low-cost tool suitable for the diagnosis of fractures and other bone diseases. In this paper, we propose a CAD-tool for the detection of osteoarthritis in a patient based on the analysis of a few digital-geometric attributes present in the X-ray image of knee-bone.

In human anatomy, the cushion like structure between bone joints is called cartilage. When this cartilage wears away, the bones of the joint slide through each other with a reduced gap. As the main shock-absorbing layer of cartilage continues to diminish, rubbing of bones in joints results in pain, discomfort, swelling, stiffness, and in the worst case, jeopardizes the normal movement of the patient. This condition is called osteoarthritis (OA) [5]. It can happen in any

© Springer Nature Switzerland AG 2018
R. P. Barneva et al. (Eds.): IWCIA 2018, LNCS 11255, pp. 121–133, 2018.
https://doi.org/10.1007/978-3-030-05288-1_10

of the joints such as neck, fingers, lower back, hip, and knee. The area around a knee-joint is the most commonly found region affected by osteoarthritis. Since the impact of this disease is mostly seen in elderly people, accurate and timely detection is the key factor in controlling the disease. Doctors rely on X-ray or MR imaging of the affected part along with other physical examinations to diagnose osteoarthritis. During the past few years, several research groups have been active in developing automated diagnostic tools for OA in knee-joints. Ani-fahi et al. have proposed Gabor filter based morphological approach to identify the abnormality in gap between knee-bones [1]. Image features extracted from Wavelet, Fourier, and Chebyshev transformation have been utilized by Shamir et al. to diagnose the presence of OA in knee-joints [11]. They used Euclidean distance to measure the gap between two knee-bones. Variations in trabecular orientation in femur and tibia and its relationship with lower limb alignment are also investigated to detect the presence of osteoarthritis at knee-joints [10].

In this work, we analyze knee X-ray images for the diagnosis of osteoarthritis based on digital-geometric properties of bone-contours around a knee-joint. Two standard views of a knee X-ray image, namely antero-posterior (AP) and skyline or lateral, are used in our analysis. The AP-view is used for gap analysis, which in turn, identifies the narrowing of joint-space, if any; additionally, the lateral view is used for shape analysis that leads to the detection of osteophytes. Most of the approaches found in literature have considered the joint gap and knee atlas to detect the osteoarthritis affected knee-joint. As osteophytes appears at the initial stage of the disease before degeneration of knee-gap [5], the proposed approach has used osteophyte analysis along with knee-gap analysis for detecting osteoarthritis at the early stage.

2   Methodology

The proposed approach to osteoarthritis detection consists of various phases (shown in Fig. 1). The pre-processing stage includes contrast enhancement of edge pixels, identification of the region-of-interest (ROI) in the input image, and detection of the boundary of bone region. This stage is very important as the final outcome of the proposed diagnostic tool is heavily dependent on how effectively the input image has been processed.

Next, the analysis of bone-gap and contour-shape is performed concurrently. Gap analysis consists of ROI detection and checking for joint-space narrowing. Shape analysis is performed in order to find the presence of any growth on the bone (osteophyte) adjacent to the joint space. As an initial step, we perform contour tracing based on differential chain code, and further approximate it with a sequence of relaxed digital straight line segments (RDSS). Additionally, the internal angle between two consecutive RDSS along the contour is estimated. The analysis of chain code and angle-vector leads to the detection of any possible abnormality (bone-growth). We demonstrate that the proposed gap and shape analysis can be effectively used to detect the presence of osteoarthritis in tibia-femoral joint space.

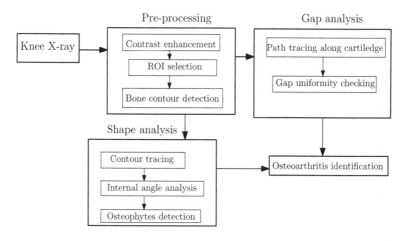

Fig. 1. Block diagram of the proposed method

2.1 Pre-processing

The given X-ray image is processed in this stage for better contrast enhancement. This stage is followed by contour detection to generate the bone boundary of the knee region.

Contrast Enhancement. Most of the knee X-ray images appear with overlapping bone and flesh region against the dark background. In this work, we have applied power law transformation to increase the contrast of the bone-flesh edge in the knee region (Fig. 3(b)). The intensity of high contrast output s is represented as a function of the intensity of the low contrast image [6] $s = C.r^\gamma$ where s is the output intensity level, r is the input intensity level, C is the +ve constant that is multiplied for further enhancement (value used is 1) and $\gamma > 1$ (value used is 3).

ROI Selection. The main objective of ROI selection is to identify the tibia-femoral joint space in a bone X-ray image. To detect the ROI, the center point and the axis of the bone X-ray image are computed (Fig. 2(a)). In knee-bone X-ray image (AP view), the knee-joint space between tibia and femur bone appears with relatively dark joint gap between two bright bone regions. The gray scale intensity along the bone-axis shows a sharp fall and rise at the knee-joint region. This low intensity region between two high intensity zones is considered as the ROI for further processing (Fig. 2(b)).

Bone Contour Detection. The last step of pre-processing stage deals with identifying the edge of the bone correctly. Edge detection using image gradient with Prewitt operator is used for this purpose. Both horizontal and vertical gradient values are computed and used to generate the new image with highlighted

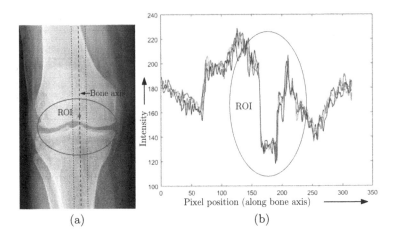

(a)   (b)

Fig. 2. (a) Bone axis, (b) Intensity variation along the bone axis

bone edges. Adaptive thresholding approach is applied on this newly generated image to detect the bone contour. In this approach, the threshold value for each pixel is computed from the median intensity value of the row to which the pixel belongs. In this way, the whole image is processed to generate the bone contour (Fig. 3(c)).

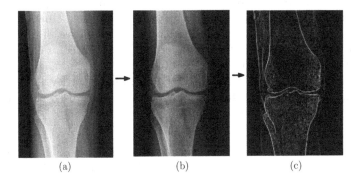

(a)   (b)   (c)

Fig. 3. (a) Input X-ray, (b) Power law transformation, (c) Bone-contour generation

2.2 Gap Analysis

In AP view of the knee X-ray image, the joint space between femur and tibia becomes visible. According to the medical literature [5], the joint space in a healthy person is symmetrical and uniformly maintained throughout the joint region. This indicates that the cartilage is protecting the bones from being rubbed with each other. The OA-affected bones usually have uneven joint space. If the severity of the disease is very high, the joint space between the bones is diminished, sometimes blocked, causing excessive pain. The Fig. 4 shows two AP-views, one for healthy and the other for a diseased knee X-ray image. In the image of a healthy person, the joint space is uniformly maintained while in the case of an OA-affected knee, the joint space on the left side has been reduced to an alarming level (marked on Fig. 4(b) by red circle).

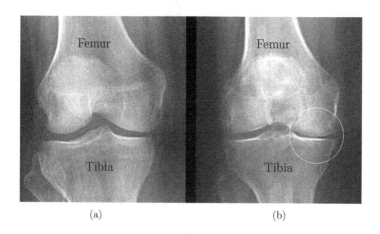

(a)   (b)

Fig. 4. (a) Healthy knee AP-view, (b) Diseased knee AP-view (Color figure online)

Trace Path Along the Joint Gap. In order to detect the gap in the tibia-femoral joint region, we have analyzed the connected components (CCA) and the joint space available for path tracing. In an image of a healthy knee-joint, two separate bone components are observed, whereas the image of an osteoarthritis-affected bone is likely appear as a single connected component (as one side of the joint space will have overlapping bones) (Fig. 4(b)). By performing connected component analysis on ROI of knee X-ray, the nature of the joint space (with uniform or nonuniform gap) can be ascertained. As per anatomical feature, the femur bone has two points that are closest to the tibia on both left and right side of the femur. The bottom-most points of femur on both left and right side are determined using standard image processing operations. Two perpendicular lines with respect to the horizontal direction are drawn from these points on tibia. The middle points of these line segments are calculated. Starting from the left middle point, a path is traversed along the right direction considering 8-connectivity. The traversal stops once the right-most point of tibia is crossed horizontally. The length of the path is denoted as L_right. Similar traversal is followed in the left direction (L_left). For healthy bones, the combined length of traversed paths must be greater than the maximum width of tibia (Fig. 5(a)). If the path exists, then it indicates that a gap exists throughout the joint region, otherwise it implies that the OA-stage is high enough to close the gap somewhere in the joint space (Fig. 5(b)).

$$max(tibia\_width) <= length(left\_path) + length(right\_path) \qquad (1)$$

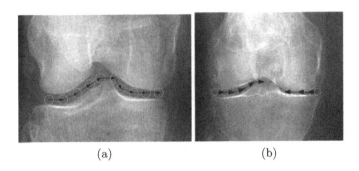

(a)   (b)

Fig. 5. (a) Path tracing through a healthy joint space, (b) path tracing through an OA-affected joint

Gap-Space Analysis. Once it is known that a gap exists throughout the entire length of the knee-joint, its uniformity along the joint is examined. This is necessary in order to check whether the gap has been narrowed somewhere in the joint ruling out the possibility of having osteoarthritis. In early stages of the disease, the gap may not be completely closed. In such cases, analyzing the variation of gap-width may provide conclusive evidence of the onset of OA.

For gap analysis, we simulate rolling of a disk-shaped object with a predefined radius through the joint space. The disk is moved through the joint gap of femur and tibia. The bounding circle of the disk is tangent to the topmost border tibia. If the gap is evenly distributed on both sides of knee-joint, the disk would slide with similar distance-attributes with respect to the femur bone. In the case of an image of a diseased person, the gap will be unevenly distributed on both sides of the joint, and hence, the overlap between the disk area and femur would vary greatly. This analysis is used to detect the presence of uneven joint space or its possible narrowing in an OA-affected bone image.

$$\Delta(overlap) = Area(femur) \cap Area(disk) \qquad (2)$$

2.3   Shape Analysis

Shape analysis is performed on the lateral view of a knee X-ray image. Osteophyte can be observed as small protrusions from the bones that grow within the joint-gap when the patient suffers from osteoarthritis. The protrusions become more prominent when the disease advances. In Fig. 6, the presence of osteophyte is marked with an arrow numbered 2 and the narrowing of joint-space is shown with an arrow labeled 1. The goal of shape analysis is to identify the location of protrusions caused by osteoarthritis.

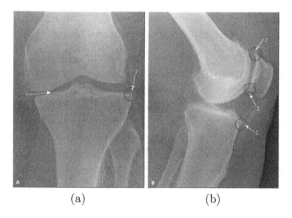

Fig. 6. (a) Presence of osteophyte as observed in an AP-view, (b) Presence of osteophyte as observed in a lateral-view

Contour Tracing Using Differential Chain Code. Chain codes [7] are used to represent a contour (or a boundary) as a connected sequence of pixels specifying the direction of traversal along its trajectory. The code varies depending on the nature of pixel connectivity (4- or 8-connected). Figure 7(a) shows chain code directions. The chain code of Fig. 7(b) is $0^5 1^5 7^4 6^4 4^1 2^3$. The first number indicates the element (directionality) of the chain code and its power indicates the number of consecutive pixels in that direction. In this work, the chain code representation with 8-connectivity is considered and the traversal of the contour is performed in counter-clockwise direction with top-left corner as the start point. The differential chain code represents the first difference of chain code. The difference is computed as the number of direction changes encountered while moving from one chain code to it's adjacent chain code. In this work, the con-

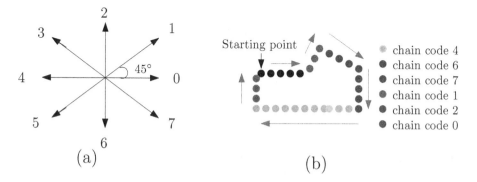

Fig. 7. (a) 8-connected chain code (45° direction change), (b) boundary representation with chain code, $0^5 1^5 7^4 6^4 4^1 2^3$

tours of femur, tibia, and patella are represented with differential chain codes for further analysis to detect the presence of osteophyte.

Tracking Angle Changes in Bone Contour. It is evident that the angles will also change with a change in chain code. The change in angle between two adjacent chain codes (like 0 and 1) is 45° (Fig. 7(b)). Along the boundary of an object, the change in angles can also be tracked looking at the change in chain code. However, the computation of angle and chain code for a contour-pixel may introduce some error as the contour itself is highly dependent on the accuracy of segmentation and the process of contour-generation. In order to mitigate such errors, we deploy the concept of *relaxed digital straight line segments* (RDSS) [2,3] while performing image analysis in our method for osteophytes detection.

Osteophytes Detection. The approximation of a curve-contour can be computed by applying the concept of digital straight line segment (DSS) [9], approximated digital straight line segment (ADSS) [4], and relaxed digital straight line segment (RDSS) [3]. RDSS defines digital straightness by relaxing certain requirements for being DSS or ADSS. In order to approximate the chain code representation of an object contour, RDSS considers the following rules:

(*Rule1*) The runs have at most two directions, differing by 45°;

(*Rule2*) Both directions can have at most three run lengths, which are consecutive integers.

Figure 8 shows examples of DSS, ADSS, and RDSS with chain-code directions '6' and '7'. Here $L1$ satisfies all properties of DSS, ADSS, and RDSS. In $L2$, both run lengths (4 and 5) have multiple occurrences. Thus, the property of single occurrence of one run length (3rd property of DSS [9]), is not satisfied. So $L2$ cannot be treated as a DSS; however, by definition, it will be recognized as an ADSS [4]). $L3$ has multiple occurrences of both directions. Therefore, it violates the basic property of both DSS and ADSS. Hence, $L3$ will neither be recognized as a DSS nor as an ADSS. Curve $L3$ has three run lengths for each of the two directions which are consecutive integers ('2', '3', '4' and '3', '4', '5' respectively). Hence, $L3$ satisfies both properties of RDSS. The definition of RDSS can be used to approximate a visibly straight-looking digital curve having a small curvature in a single straight line segment. In order to detect osteophytes, we represent the contour of the ROI of an input X-ray image (lateral view) using RDSS. The contour of the ROI is traversed in counter-clockwise direction to compute the differential chain code and RDSS (Fig. 9). Next, the angle between every two consecutive RDSS pairs representing the contour is computed. An acute angle between two consecutive RDSS pairs (marked in blue in Table 1) represents small curvature in the contour, whereas a right angle between two consecutive RDSS (R8, R9), and between (R19, R20) of Table 1 (marked in red) represents the presence of sharp growth (osteophytes) in the contour.

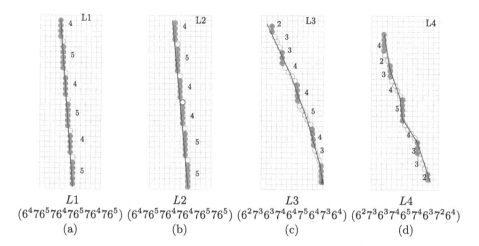

$$L1 \qquad L2 \qquad L3 \qquad L4$$
$(6^4 76^5 76^4 76^5 76^4 76^5) \quad (6^4 76^5 76^4 76^4 76^5 76^5) \quad (6^2 7^3 6^3 7^4 6^4 7^5 6^4 7^3 6^4) \quad (6^2 7^3 6^3 7^4 6^5 7^4 6^3 7^2 6^4)$
$\qquad$ (a) $\qquad\qquad$ (b) $\qquad\qquad\qquad$ (c) $\qquad\qquad\qquad$ (d)

Fig. 8. Illustration of DSS, ADSS, and RDSS: (a) $L1$ is a DSS, an ADSS, and a RDSS, (b) $L2$ is an ADSS but not a DSS, (c) $L3$ is a RDSS, but neither a DSS, nor an ADSS, (d) $L4$ does not belong to RDSS, or DSS, or ADSS

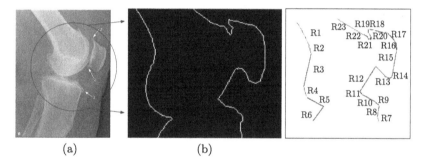

$\qquad$ (a) $\qquad\qquad\qquad\qquad$ (b)

Fig. 9. (a) Knee X-ray with osteophytes (marked as '2'), (b) Contour of ROI (marked as 'red' circle in (a)), (c) RDSS representation of (b) (Color figure online)

3 Experimental Results

The proposed approach is tested on an X-ray image dataset obtained from 30 osteoarthritis-affected patients and 20 healthy persons. The observations on joint space analysis with disk shape object are shown in Fig. 10. The values shown along the y-axis represent the diameter of the disk that is rolled through the joint gap. For an OA-affected image, as the disk moves towards the narrow joint space region, the diameter of the disk passing through the gap reduces. In a knee X-ray image with severe OA, the joint-space is narrowed to cause overlapping of femur and tibia bone. In such cases, the disk diameter covering the joint-space reduces to almost 0.

Table 1. RDSS analysis

RDSS (chain code)	Differential chain code	Angle between RDSS pair	Comments
R1 (6, 7), R2 (6)	7	315°	Reflex angle
R2 (6), R3 (5, 6)	7	315°	Reflex angle
R3 (5, 6), R4 (6, 7)	1	45°	Acute angle
R4 (6, 7), R5 (7)	1	45°	Acute angle
R5 (7), R6 (5)	6	270°	Reflex angle
R7 (2), R8 (1,2)	7	315°	Reflex angle
R8 (1, 2), R9 (3)	2	90°	Right angle
R9 (3), R10 (3, 4)	1	45°	Acute angle
R10 (3, 4), R11 (4)	1	45°	Acute angle
R11 (4), R12 (1)	5	225°	Reflex angle
R12 (1), R13 (7)	6	270°	Reflex angle
R13 (7), R14 (0)	1	45°	Acute angle
R14 (0), R15 (0, 1)	1	45°	Acute angle
R15 (0, 1), R16 (2)	1	45°	Acute angle
R16 (2), R17 (3)	1	45°	Acute angle
R17 (3), R18 (3, 4)	1	45°	Acute angle
R18 (3, 4), R19 (4, 5)	1	45°	Acute angle
R19 (4, 5), R20 (6, 7)	2	90°	Right angle
R20 (6, 7), R21 (5)	6	270°	Reflex angle
R21 (5), R22 (2)	5	225°	Reflex angle
R22 (2), R23 (3)	1	45°	Acute angle

It is observed that the analysis of OA-affected images yields different results with respect to gap-size and shape depending on the severity of the disease. Table 2 summarizes the observations.

Table 2. Shape and gap analysis

CCA in ROI	Gap path/femur contour	Overlapping area (pixel)	Right angle in contour	Comments
1	<1	✓	✓	OA with joint space partially closed (high severity)
>1	>1	✓	✓	OA with joint space not affected (low severity)
>1	>1	✗	✗	Healthy bone

Some of the X-ray images used to test the proposed approach are shown in Fig. 11. Table 3 shows the observations based on clinical findings and the proposed method. The results comply to the clinical inferences in most of the cases except for some X-rays (Fig. 11(g)), where due to improper illumination, either segmentation was not performed satisfactorily or disk-rolling failed to provide expected results (indicated in gray colour in Table 3). The ROC curve is generated using the experimental results with true positive, true negative, false positive, and false negative cases (Fig. 10(b)).

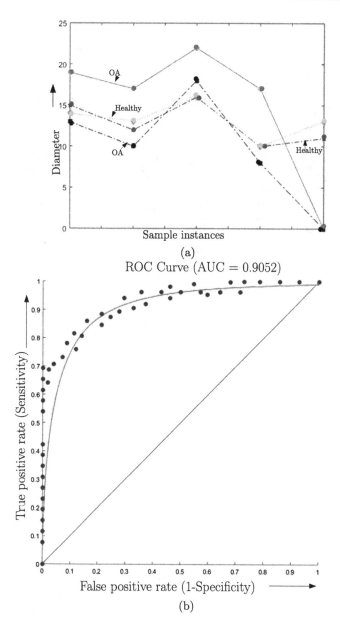

Fig. 10. (a) Joint space analysis for healthy and OA-affected knee X-ray images, (b) ROC curve based on experimental result with 50 X-ray images

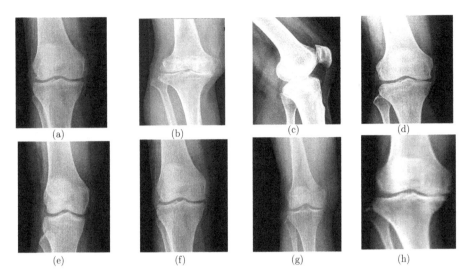

Fig. 11. Sample X-ray images of knee-bone taken from healthy and diseased persons

Table 3. Comparison of clinical decisions and the proposed method

Figure No.	Osteoarthritis Detection		Osteoarthritis Grade	
	Clinical	Proposed	Clinical	Proposed
A	Healthy	Healthy	No	No
B	Diseased	Diseased	High	High
C	Diseased	Diseased	High	High
D	Diseased	Diseased	High	High
E	Healthy	Healthy	No	No
F	Healthy	Healthy	No	No
G	Diseased	Healthy	Low	No
H	Diseased	Diseased	High	High

4   Conclusion

In this work, several digital-geometric concepts have been utilized to analyze the shape and gap of a knee-joint. The abnormality related to the narrowing of joint space in the tibia-femoral region is detected during gap analysis. During shape analysis, any abnormal sharpness or discontinuity in bone contour (osteophyte) is detected from the knee X-ray image. We use the concept of relaxed digital straight line to approximate the bone-contour in order to expedite the process. The study is performed on several X-ray images and the diagnostic outcome is cross-checked with the corresponding clinical findings. In most of the cases, automated diagnostics are found to be in good match with clinical inferences. The ROC curve shows the AUC value 0.9 (Fig. 10(b)). Since the method uses intensity based analysis, it works best with good quality images having better contrast between flesh and bone in the X-ray. A binary grading of osteoarthritis has been performed in this work based on simple X-ray image analysis, and diagnosis with more specificity spread over five classes as suggested by WHO [8] needs further study. Also, this work may be extended to investigate other features of osteoarthritis such as tracing the formation of subchondral sclerosis.

References

1. Anifah, L., Purnama, K.E., Hariadi, M., Purnomo, M.H.: Automatic segmentation of impaired joint space area for osteoarthritis knee on X-ray image using gabor filter based morphology process. J. Technol. Sci. **22**(3), 159–165 (2011)
2. Bandyopadhyay, O., Biswas, A., Bhattacharya, B.B.: Long-bone fracture detection in digital X-ray images based on concavity index. In: Barneva, R.P., Brimkov, V.E., Šlapal, J. (eds.) IWCIA 2014. LNCS, vol. 8466, pp. 212–223. Springer, Cham (2014). https://doi.org/10.1007/978-3-319-07148-0_19
3. Bandyopadhyay, O., Biswas, A., Bhattacharya, B.B.: Long-bone fracture detection in digital X-ray images based on digital-geometric techniques. Comput. Methods Programs Biomed. **123**, 2–14 (2016)
4. Bhowmick, P., Bhattacharya, B.B.: Fast polygonal approximation of digital curves using relaxed straightness properties. IEEE Trans. Pattern Anal. Mach. Intell. **29**(9), 1590–1602 (2007)
5. Buckland-Wright, C.: Subchondral bone changes in hand and knee osteoarthritis detected by radiography. Osteoarthr. Cartil. **12**, S10–S19 (2004)
6. Chanda, B., Majumdar, D.D.: Digital Image Processing and Analysis. Prentice Hall of India, New Delhi (2007)
7. Freeman, H.: On the encoding of arbitrary geometric configurations. IRE Trans. Electron. Comput. **10**, 260–268 (1961)
8. Kohn, M.D., Sassoon, A.A., Fernando, N.D.: Classifications in brief: Kellgren-Lawrence classification of osteoarthritis. Clin. Orthop. Relat. Res. **474**(8), 1886–93 (2016)
9. Rosenfeld, A.: Digital straight line segments. IEEE Trans. Comput. **23**, 1264–1269 (1974)
10. Sampath, S.A., Lewis, S., Fosco, M., Tigani, D.: Trabecular orientation in the human femur and tibia and the relationship with lower limb alignment for patients with osteoarthritis of the knee. J. Biomech. **48**, 1213–1218 (2015)
11. Shamir, L., et al.: Knee X-ray image analysis method for automated detection of osteoarthritis. IEEE Trans. Biomed. Eng. **56**(2), 407–415 (2009)

Registration of CT with PET: A Comparison of Intensity-Based Approaches

Gisèle Pereira[1], Inês Domingues[1,2], Pedro Martins[1], Pedro H. Abreu[1(✉)], Hugo Duarte[2], and João Santos[2]

[1] CISUC, Department of Informatics Engineering, University of Coimbra, Coimbra, Portugal
gispereira22@gmail.com, {icdomingues,pjmm,pha}@dei.uc.pt
[2] IPO-Porto Research Centre, Porto, Portugal
{hugo.duarte,joao.santos}@ipoporto.min-saude.pt

Abstract. The integration of functional imaging modality provided by Positron Emission Tomography (PET) and associated anatomical imaging modality provided by Computed Tomography (CT) has become an essential procedure both in the evaluation of different types of malignancy and in radiotherapy planning. The alignment of these two exams is thus of great importance. In this research work, three registration approaches (1) intensity-based registration, (2) rigid translation followed by intensity-based registration and (3) coarse registration followed by fine-tuning were evaluated and compared. To characterize the performance of these methods, 161 real volume scans from patients involved in Hodgkin Lymphoma staging were used: CT volumes used for radiotherapy planning were registered with PET volumes before any treatment. Registration results achieved 78%, 60%, and 91% of accuracy for methods (1), (2) and (3), respectively. Registration methods validation was extended to a corresponding landmarks points distance calculation. Methods (1), (2) and (3) achieved a median improvement registration rate of 66% mm, 51% mm and 70% mm, respectively. The accuracy of the proposed methods was further confirmed by extending our experiments to other multimodal datasets and in a monomodal dataset with different acquisition conditions.

Keywords: PET · CT · Registration · Cancer · Treatment planning

1 Introduction

Malignant lymphomas comprise a heterogeneous group of neoplasms which are divided into Hodgkin (HL) and non-Hodgkin lymphomas (NHL). Although HL is the most uncommon form of malignant lymphomas, 8260 people were diagnosed with the disease in 2017 and 1070 people were estimated to die in the United States only [22].

© Springer Nature Switzerland AG 2018
R. P. Barneva et al. (Eds.): IWCIA 2018, LNCS 11255, pp. 134–149, 2018.
https://doi.org/10.1007/978-3-030-05288-1_11

Computed tomography (CT) is normally used as the basis for radiotherapy. The reason is two-fold, (1) it contains density information that can be used to calculate treatment beam attenuation, and (2) it is reliable in representing shape and position. Positron-emission tomography (PET) is a nuclear imaging technique that enables the observation of metabolic processes using radiolabelled tracer molecules. With many applications in clinical practice, and in particular in oncology, it is currently used to diagnose, stage, and evaluate the effectiveness of the treatment [5,14]. In order to facilitate position estimation of regions with abnormal function, current procedures combine anatomical imaging modalities, such as CT with morphological information provided by PET. Medical imaging can benefit from computer-assisted tools [3].

The present line of work has as ultimate goal the automatic evaluation of the response to the treatment received, in order to assess the effectiveness of the cancer therapy and possibly change the course of action [17]. It is thus relevant to study the evolution of the areas that received treatment. While the planning of the treatment and the corresponding delimitation of the regions of interest are made using CT, the detection of abnormal activities at atypical sites is better performed in PET. The co-registration of these two types of information is, in this way, the main goal of the present work.

Three intensity-based approaches were tested. In the first, the CT is rescaled and then co-registration is attempted. In the second method, a fixed translation is done before performing co-registration. Finally, a novel adaptive technique is proposed to find an initial translation for each CT individually and provide a better initialization for registration. Results are presented in real volumes for 161 patients of Hodgkin lymphoma. The third method outperformed the other two, improving the accuracy in 31% when compared with the second method and in 13% when compared with the first.

The remainder of this paper is organized as follows. We start by overviewing relevant work in the field of medical image registration in Sect. 2. Then, the intensity-based proposed techniques are described in Sect. 3. The database details are given in Sect. 4 and results are shown in Sect. 5. Final conclusions and remarks are gathered in Sect. 6.

2   Related Work

Image registration has gained an important role in several medical specialties, such as neurosurgery and radiotherapy [27]. In particular, multimodal registration – registration of images from different modalities (e.g. PET/CT, PET/MRI, CT/MRI) – has been a very active research topic, which is corroborated by the number and diversity of solutions proposed in the literature [15,27]. For an exhaustive review of medical image registration methods, we refer to the survey in [15].

In the context of radiotherapy planning, the integration of PET and CT information has become an essential procedure to evaluate different types of malignancies [7]. Mutual information and normalized mutual information are common measures for performing PET/CT registration, as they have the advantage of providing more accurate, robust, and reliable results [6]. A number of intensity-based PET/CT registration methods is built on the aforementioned metrics, with the main difference among them being the optimization algorithm. Additionally, most methods propose a deformable registration (e.g., [12,21]) rather than a rigid one, as it can model anatomic changes resulting from tumor shrinkage, weight loss or organ deformation [18].

Examples of PET/CT registration methods based on mutual information include the work of Marinelli et al. [11], which is a two-step method for aligning PET and CT cardiac images based on mutual information and a genetic algorithm. The first step consists in identifying a global maximum for the mutual information by using a genetic algorithm on downsampled data. The final step concludes the registration process by performing a high resolution local optimization based on the downhill simplex algorithm. Another example is the work of Jin et al. [8], which uses mutual information and the demon algorithm to register PET and CT scans of esophageal cancer patients. Suh et al. [23] propose a deformable registration based on a weighted demon algorithm to align whole-body rat CT and PET images, using the maximum likelihood Hausdorff distance as similarity measure. The experimental results showed a better performance as compared to a symmetric demon algorithm [24] and a normalized mutual information-based method [19].

Overall, one can say that current deformable intensity-based registration techniques are the most suitable for radiotherapy planning. While they tend to be computationally expensive, these techniques can model severe anatomic changes and, consequently, achieve high-accuracy registration.

3   Intensity-Based Registration

Three different registration methods were applied, (1) intensity-based registration, (2) rigid translation followed by intensity-based registration and (3) coarse registration followed by fine-tuning. All the methods are preceded by pixel size homogenization (re-slicing). The block diagrams for each method are given in Fig. 1.

Pixel size homogenization (re-slicing) is performed using the pixel spacing and patient image position information on the DICOM headers, as illustrated in Fig. 2.

In the intensity-based image registration, Mattes mutual information is optimized with one-plus-one evolutionary optimization with 100 maximum iterations, an initial size of search radius of 6.25^{-3}, growth factor of the search radius of 1.05, and minimum size of the search radius of 1.5^{-6}. The number of spatial samples used to compute the mutual information metric is 500, and histograms of 50 bins are used. All pixels in the overlap region of the images are used when computing the mutual information metric. This is illustrated in Fig. 3.

When further analyzing the volumes, it was observed that most of the CT images correspond to a subset of the body region represented in the PET. Supplementary analysis lead to the conclusion that translations of 17, 8 and 18 on

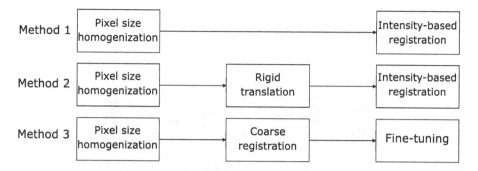

Method 1 | Pixel size homogenization | → | Intensity-based registration

Method 2 | Pixel size homogenization | → | Rigid translation | → | Intensity-based registration

Method 3 | Pixel size homogenization | → | Coarse registration | → | Fine-tuning

Fig. 1. Block diagrams of the three intensity-based registration methods.

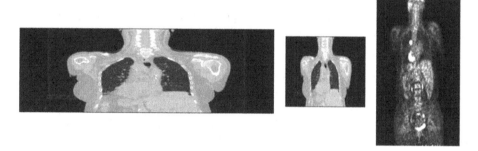

Fig. 2. Exemplification of the resize of a CT to match the PET (coronal slices). Left figure represents the original CT, middle the resized CT, and right the original PET.

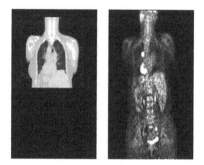

Fig. 3. Illustration of method 1 on the example given in Fig. 2. Registered CT on the left, PET on the right.

x, y and z-axis respectively were a good initialization for the registration. In this way, in method 2, CT is first translated and then intensity registration is performed as described above. Figure 4 illustrates this method. Note that the slice shown is the center one and thus the differences, not only in the x and y axis positioning, but also in the z-axis.

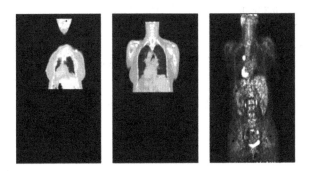

Fig. 4. Illustration of method 2 on the example given in Fig. 2. CT after rigid translation on the left, final registered CT on the middle, PET on the right.

The second method allowed the intensity based registration to converge in cases where it diverged when attempting at the registration without the translation. However, the fixed translation does not have the most appropriate parameters for every case. An adaptive technique was thus developed, and its flow is shown in Fig. 5.

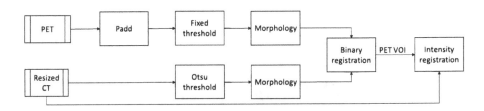

Fig. 5. Fluxogram of the registration method 3.

In short, method 3 starts by padding the PET volume with 50 black pixels in every dimension (25 on each side). Next, an empirically selected fixed threshold of 0.004 (intensities are previously normalized to $[0, 1]$) is applied. The morphological operations consist in retrieving the biggest connected component (considering a 6-connected neighborhood) and filling holes (where a hole is defined as an area of black pixels surrounded by white pixels considering a 6-connected neighborhood). For CT, the volume is binarized with the Otsu [16] threshold and the biggest connected component is also selected. Binary PET and CT volumes are then registered through a volumetric sliding window scheme, by minimizing the average number of pixels with the same value (a step of 10 was chosen to improve computational efficiency). The volumetric sliding window algorithm returns a translation that is used to extract a volume of interest (VOI) of the PET. This VOI is intensity registered with the CT. This procedure is illustrated in Fig. 6.

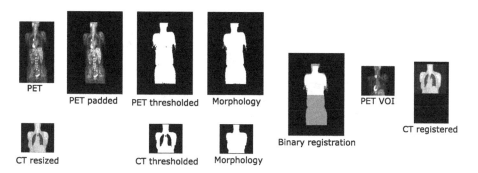

Fig. 6. Illustration of method 3. In the binary registration figure, a composite image is given where white regions represent regions where both masks are 1, green where PET is 1 and CT is 0, and magenta where CT is 1 and PET 0. (Color figure online)

4   Database

The dataset used in this work includes pre-treatment PET volumes, CT volumes used for treatment planning, and post-treatment PET volumes from 161 patients (see Fig. 7), provided by Institute of Oncology of Porto (IPO).

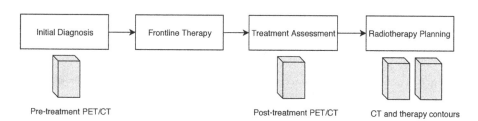

Fig. 7. Temporal diagram of data acquisition of the dataset used in this work. At the initial diagnosis, before any treatment for the Hodgkin Lymphoma, a PET/CT scan was acquired. The frontline therapy was usually composed of 2 cycles of chemotherapy and after, a PET/CT scan was acquired to assess the effectiveness of the treatment. Lastly, CT scans were acquired for radiotherapy planning and the regions for dose distribution were delineated by experts.

Our dataset is classified into the Five-point Deauville scale [20] by an expert thought the comparison of pre and post treatment PET volumes and its distribution is represented in Fig. 8. This is important to study the robustness of the algorithms on images with different characteristics. PET volumes were acquired with a pixel spacing of 4.1 mm and a difference of patient position between adjacent slices of 2.0 or 3.0 mm. CT volumes were acquired with a pixel spacing of 1.0, 1.1, 1.2 or 1.3 mm and a difference of patient position between adjacent slices of 2.0, 2.5 or 5.0 mm.

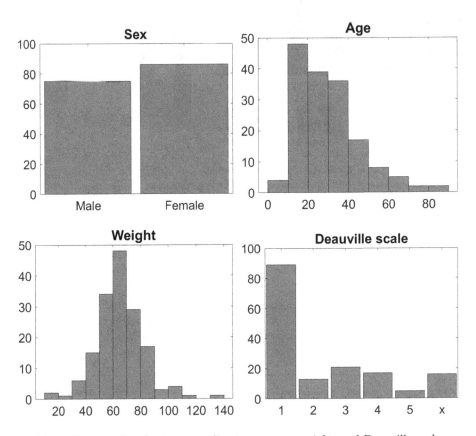

Fig. 8. Dataset distribution according to sex, age, weight, and Deauville scale.

5   Results

The results were first visually inspected in order to access the number of successful registrations versus unsuccessful ones (Sect. 5.1). Next, distances were studied through the placement of landmarks in the volumes (Sect. 5.2). Further quantification of the results is presented in Sect. 5.3 by using (dis)similarity parameters.

Finally, the generalization behavior of the algorithms is studied in Sect. 5.4 by testing on different datasets.

5.1 Manual Inspection

Registration results were visually inspected, achieving 78%, 60%, and 91% of accuracy for method 1, 2 and 3, respectively. There are 5 cases for which all the methods fail and 81 where all the methods succeed. Since shoulders are an important anatomic landmark, a preponderance was found for the methods to fail when these are not present in the CT scan, or when the patient had the arm up in one of the acquisitions and down in the other.

When looking at the distribution of the success/failure cases, several interesting observations can be made. The patient sex does not seem to have influence on the success rate of the methods. For Method 2, the rate of unsuccessful cases increases with the patient age. Method 1 does not fail for any patient older than 56 and Method 3 does not fail for any patient aged between 53 and 82 years. Method 1 and 2 fail for all patients heavier than 100 kg. Method 3 fails for patients weighting between 105 and 125 kg. Method 1 was successful in all Deauvile 5 cases, while Method 2 was successful in all Deauvile 4 and 5 cases.

5.2 Semi-automatic Inspection

Validation of registration methods and results is currently considered to be a non-trivial task [27]. Despite image registration being formulated as an optimization exercise (i.e. minimizes or maximizes a similarity measure), most similarity measures have not a direct physical interpretation and do not ensure the biological trustworthiness of the mapping [15].

A reliable solution to access co-registration results is through the use of landmarks. As stated in [13], corresponding landmarks points provide useful information to evaluate results between registration algorithms. In our work, we appointed the easily defined lungs through visual assessment as our reference organ.

First the coronal and transversal slices where the lungs are bigger were identified. Next, four landmarks are placed in each lung corresponding to the maximum and minimum, vertical and horizontal, lung limits, as shown in Fig. 9. Based on landmarks correspondence, the registration accuracy is evaluated in terms of Euclidean distance, which has a physical meaning. The mean distance of each of the 16 correspondent landmarks distances was obtained within each data sample.

From the 161 patients on the dataset, the CT of 14 patients did not include the totality of the lungs and were thus excluded from this part of the evaluation. It should be noted that the cases for which the registration diverged were not included in this statistics (8 cases for method 1, 9 cases for method 2 and 10 cases for method 3).

In Fig. 10a, the distribution of the original distances of the landmarks (i.e. without any registration transformation), after the application of method 1,

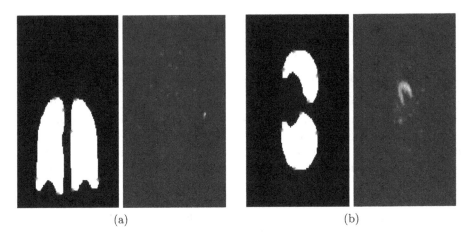

(a)   (b)

Fig. 9. Exemplification of landmarks positions represented by red asterisks: (a) coronal slice of the CT mask (left) and PET (right); (b) transversal slice of the CT mask (left) and PET (right). (Color figure online)

2 and 3 is presented. The minimum original distance is about 39.77 mm, the maximum is 224.68 mm and the median is 140.74 mm. It is visible that the initial dataset was heterogeneous in terms of original landmarks distances and most of the points in the data samples were considerably deviated, which means that they were not initially registered and therefore there was a need to register them. The minimum distance of method 1 was 12.77 mm, the maximum was 459.39 mm and the median 39.03 mm. The minimum distance of method 2 was 16.54 mm, the maximum was 522.03 mm and the median 47.99 mm. The minimum distance of method 3 was 18.22 mm, the maximum was 403.41 mm and the median 37.54 mm. As expected, the registration process made a decreased shift in the distances of the landmarks and as verified in our initial evaluation, the method 2 provides the biggest range of distances and method 3 provides the best results.

To obtain a better notion of the improvement provided by the registration methods, an improvement rate was calculated. For each instance, the baseline distance considered was the original distance. The improvement rate was calculated dividing the difference between the baseline distance and the final distance after registration by the baseline distance. The median improvement rate was 66.01% mm, 51.25% mm and 69.83% mm for method 1, 2 and 3 respectively. Method 1 and 2 are significantly different as well as method 2 and 3 (p values of .003 and <.001 respectively).

On the whole, method 1 achieved better performance results for 45 cases, method 2 was the best for other 45 cases and method 3 for 57 cases. Figure 10b enables to distinguish the range of distances for which each method is better. We can conclude that method 3 is better for initially higher spaced landmarks.

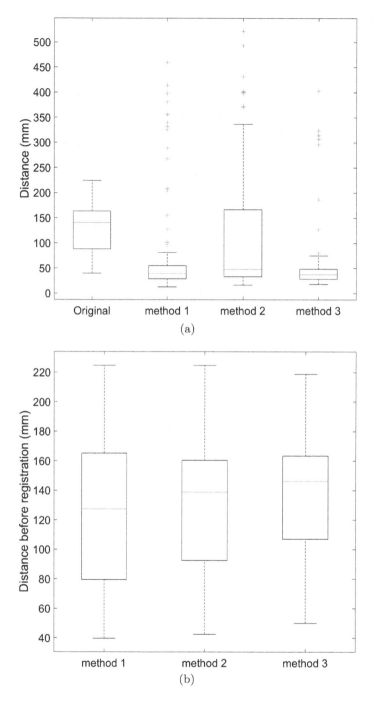

Fig. 10. Evaluation per landmarks results: (a) distribution of the mean distances of corresponding landmarks in millimeters of all the data samples: in the original dataset, after method 1, 2 and 3; (b) ranges of original distances in millimeters in which method 1, 2 and 3 performed better.

5.3   Automatic Evaluation

Even with the drawbacks of the (dis)similarity measures pointed out in Sect. 5.2, four parameters were calculated in an attempt to further compare and quantify the attained results. These are: Mean-squared error (MSE), Mutual Information (MI), Structural Similarity Index (SSIM), and Peak Signal-to-Noise Ratio (PSNR). Overall results are given in Fig. 11. All the methods confirm that method 2 behaves worse than method 1 and method 3 behaves better than method 2. According to a two-sample t-test, results are significantly different, when considering MI and SSIM, for Method 3 when compared both with Method 1 and Method 2 (p values of .044, <.001, .009, and <.001 respectively).

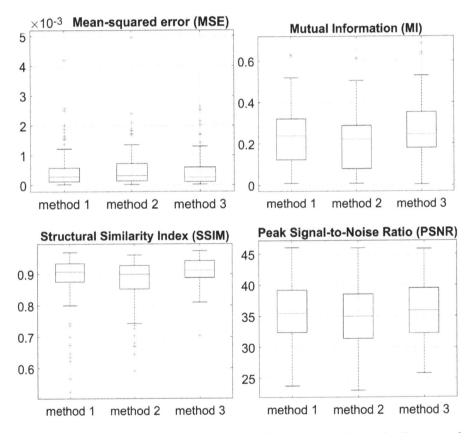

Fig. 11. Results quantification with MSE, MI, SSIM and PSNR for the three tested techniques.

Figure 12 quantifies results splitting by success *versus* unsuccessful cases. Only MI and SSIM are shown for brevity. As expected, results for unsuccessful are always worse than successful ones, these differences are statistically significant when considering MI for the first and second methods (p values <.001), or when using SSIM for all methods (p values of $<.001$ for method 1 and 2 and .006 for method 3).

Looking at the differences between unsuccessful cases, MI determines that Method 3 performs different than Methods 1 and 2; while SSIM, highlights differences between Method 2 and 3.

Results were also studied when grouped by sex, age, weight and Deauville scale. Both MI and SSIM were observed to be higher for female patients when compared with male ones. Age was positively correlated with MI and weight

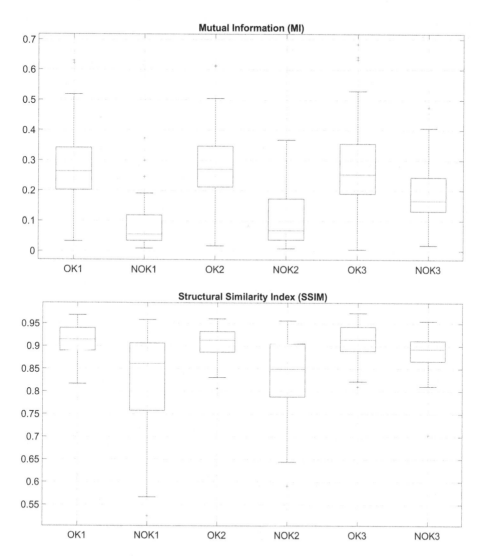

Fig. 12. Results quantification with MI and SSIM for the three tested techniques, divided by success (OK) and unsuccessful (NOK) results.

negatively correlated with SSIM. Deauville scale did not seem to have any impact in the registration results.

5.4   Results on Other Datasets

To access the generalization ability of the methods, we validated the registration methods on publicly available datasets from The Cancer Imaging Archive [4]. We narrowed down our selection to Collections that contained PET and CT data: APOLLO, NaF Prostate, Soft-tissue Sarcoma and a large number of Collections from the Cancer Genome Atlas: TCGA-LUSC, TCGA-PRAD, TCGA-THCA, TCGA-LUAD, TCGA-KRIP, TCGA-LIHC. In total, 120 patients were extracted. Registration results were 95%, 80.83%, and 94.17% of accuracy for method 1, 2 and 3, respectively. There was no case where at least one of the methods did not register successfully and 90 cases where all the methods succeed. Additionally, there were two cases where only method 1 succeeded, two cases where only method 3 succeeded and one case where only method 2 succeeded.

Moreover, the three registration methods were tested on pre and post treatment PET/CT volumes. Although they are of the same modality, the purpose is to validate its robustness in different acquisition conditions. Pre and post volumes have an average acquisition spacing of 120.39 days, approximately 4 months. Registration results were inspected on the 163 patients also provided by IPO-Porto, achieving 92.63%, 81.59%, and 96.93% of accuracy for method 1, 2 and 3, respectively. There was no case where at least one of the methods did not register successfully and 123 cases where all the methods succeed. Additionally, there were seven cases where only method 3 succeeded.

6   Conclusion

PET can detect sites of disease in structures that do not appear abnormal on CT. Ideally for PET-CT visualization, a region of interest on PET, such as a tumor, is shown while the underlying anatomy from CT is preserved, without compromising the focus of interest, to provide precise localization of the tumor [9]. It is thus of great importance that these two exams are aligned.

Fusion is, however, difficult and often unsuccessful because of the many degrees of freedom accessible to the human body when imaged by two different modalities on two different occasions, as noted in [25]. In the present work, three intensity-level techniques are tested. The first starts by resizing the volumes so that exams from a given patient have the same pixel size, this is followed by intensity-based registration. When analyzing some results with the previous method, it was observed that, for some cases, the optimization failed. The second technique tries to give a better initialization by performing a fixed translation. The fixed translation has shown not to be generalizable, and thus, in the last method, an adaptive translation method is proposed.

In the present work, CT volumes used for radiotherapy planning are co-registered with PET volumes at baseline (before any treatment) for 161 patients with Hodgkin lymphoma. Chemotherapy has been performed between the two exams and thus tumors may have increased size if they did not respond to the chemotherapy or decreased in case they respond positively to the chemotherapy, making the problem even more changeling. The third method here proposed has shown to be significantly better than the other two tested techniques when considering Mutual Information (MT) and Structural Similarity Index (SSI). Registration was additionally evaluated based on landmarks correspondence metrics. That way, we confirmed that the novel adaptive method 3 is the more suitable method for data with initially higher spaced correspondent landmarks.

Co-registration parameters will be used in the future to transform volumes defined by the specialists on the CT during radiotherapy treatment planning (such as the gross tumor volume (GTV), clinical target volume (CTV), and planning target volume (PTV) [2]) into the pre and post treatment PET, in order to automatically evaluate the response to treatment.

In this research work, it was observed that the shoulders are an important anatomic feature used by the studied intensity-based methods. When these are not present in one of the modalities, or the patient has the arms up in one volume and down in the other, all of the methods behave poorly. Future work will focus on the development of different techniques for these cases. The user can be prompted to answer if shoulders are present and if the patient has arms down in both exams. Being truth, the methods given here are tested. Otherwise, other, more complex and computationally demanding methods can be applied such as the ones based on points of interest (e.g. SIFT [10], SURF [1], FAST [26], etc.) or others as the ones referred to in the state of the art section (Sect. 2).

While the focus of this research work has been on the registration of PET and CT volumes, we believe that the same proposed methods can be used in the alignment of different modalities. To assess this hypothesizes will be a focus of future work.

Acknowledgment. This article is a result of the project NORTE-01-0145-FEDER-000027, supported by Norte Portugal Regional Operational Programme (NORTE 2020), under the PORTUGAL 2020 Partnership Agreement, through the European Regional Development Fund (ERDF).

References

1. Bay, H., Ess, A., Tuytelaars, T., Van Gool, L.: Speeded-up robust features (SURF). Comput. Vis. Image Underst. **110**(3), 346–359 (2008)
2. Burnet, N., Thomas, S., Burton, K., Jefferies, S.: Defining the tumour and target volumes for radiotherapy. Cancer Imaging **4**(2), 153–161 (2004)
3. Chen, C., Chou, Y., Tagawa, N., Do, Y.: Computer-aided detection and diagnosis in medical imaging. Comput. Math. Methods Med. **2013**, 2 p. (2013)
4. Clark, K., et al.: The cancer imaging archive (TCIA): maintaining and operating a public information repository. J. Digit. Imaging **26**(6), 1045–1057 (2013)

5. Domingues, I., Amorim, J., Abreu, P., Duarte, H., Santos, J.: Evaluation of over-sampling data balancing techniques in the context of ordinal classification. In: International Joint Conference on Neural Networks (IJCNN) (2018)
6. El-Gamal, F., Elmogy, M., Atwan, A.: Current trends in medical image registration and fusion. Egypt. Inform. J. **17**(1), 99–124 (2016)
7. Jelercic, S., Rajer, M.: The role of PET-CT in radiotherapy planning of solid tumours. Radiol. Oncol. **49**(1), 1–9 (2015)
8. Jin, S., Li, D., Wang, H., Yin, Y.: Registration of PET and CT images based on multiresolution gradient of mutual information demons algorithm for positioning esophageal cancer patients. J. Appl. Clin. Med. Phys. **14**(1), 50–61 (2013)
9. Jung, Y.: Feature driven volume visualization of medical imaging data. Doctor of philosophy, University of Sydney (2015)
10. Lowe, D.: Distinctive image features from scale-invariant keypoints. Int. J. Comput. Vis. **60**(2), 91–110 (2004)
11. Marinelli, M., Positano, V., Tucci, F., Neglia, D., Landini, L.: Automatic PET-CT image registration method based on mutual information and genetic algorithms. Sci. World J. **2012**, 12 p. (2012)
12. Mattes, D., Haynor, D., Vesselle, H., Lewellen, T., Eubank, W.: PET-CT image registration in the chest using free-form deformations. IEEE Trans. Med. Imaging **22**(1), 120–128 (2003)
13. Murphy, K., et al.: Evaluation of registration methods on thoracic CT: the EMPIRE10 challenge. IEEE Trans. Med. Imaging **30**(11), 1901–1920 (2011)
14. Nogueira, M., Abreu, P., Martins, P., Machado, P., Duarte, H., Santos, J.: An artificial neural networks approach for assessment treatment response in oncological patients using PET/CT images. BMC Med. Imaging **17**(1), 13 (2017)
15. Oliveira, F., Tavares, J.: Medical image registration: a review. Comput. Methods Biomech. Biomed. Eng. **17**(2), 73–93 (2014)
16. Otsu, N.: A threshold selection method from gray-level histograms. IEEE Trans. Syst. Man Cybern. **9**(1), 62–66 (1979)
17. Pereira, G.: Deep Learning techniques for the evaluation of response to treatment in Hodgkin Lymphoma. M.Sc. in biomedical engineering, University of Coimbra (2018)
18. Qi, X.S.: Image-guided radiation therapy. In: Maqbool, M. (ed.) An Introduction to Medical Physics. BMPBE, pp. 131–173. Springer, Cham (2017). https://doi.org/10.1007/978-3-319-61540-0_5
19. Rueckert, D., Sonoda, L., Hayes, C., Hill, D., Leach, M., Hawkes, D.: Nonrigid registration using free-form deformations: application to breast MR images. IEEE Trans. Med. Imaging **18**(8), 712–721 (1999)
20. Sheikhbahaei, S., Mena, E., Pattanayak, P., Taghipour, M., Solnes, L., Subramaniam, R.: Molecular imaging and precision medicine: PET/CT and therapy response assessment in oncology. PET Clin. **12**(1), 105–118 (2017)
21. Shekhar, R., et al.: Automated 3-dimensional elastic registration of whole-body PET and CT from separate or combined scanners. J. Nucl. Med. **46**(9), 1488–1496 (2005)
22. Siegel, R., Miller, K., Jemal, A.: Cancer statistics, 2017. CA: Cancer J. Clin. **67**(1), 7–30 (2017)
23. Suh, J., Kwon, O., Scheinost, D., Sinusas, A., Cline, G., Papademetris, X.: CT-PET weighted image fusion for separately scanned whole body rat. Med. Phys. **39**(1), 533–542 (2012)
24. Thirion, J.: Image matching as a diffusion process: an analogy with Maxwell's demons. Med. Image Anal. **2**(3), 243–260 (1998)

25. Townsend, D., Carney, J., Yap, J., Hall, N.: PET/CT today and tomorrow. J. Nucl. Med. **45**(1), 4–14 (2004)
26. Trajkovii, M., Hedley, M., Trajkovic, M., Hedley, M.: FAST corner detection. Image Vis. Comput. **16**(2), 75–87 (1998)
27. Viergever, M., Maintz, J., Klein, S., Murphy, K., Staring, M., Pluim, J.: A survey of medical image registration-under review. Med. Image Anal. **33**, 140–144 (2016)

Iterative High Resolution Tomography from Combined High-Low Resolution Sinogram Pairs

László Varga[1(✉)] and Rajmund Mokso[2]

[1] Department of Image Processing and Computer Graphics, University of Szeged, Szeged, Hungary
vargalg@inf.u-szeged.hu
[2] Max IV Laboraroty, Lund University, Lund, Sweden
rajmund.mokso@maxiv.lu.se

Abstract. In some cases of tomography we can only gain high resolution projections of the object with only partial coverage, whereas only a small part of the object – a given Region of Interest (ROI) – is fully covered by high resolution projections. In such cases the structures outside the region of interest cause artefacts to appear in the reconstructed image and degrade the image quality of the tomogram. We proposed three new iterative approaches for the accurate reconstruction of the ROI by combining a high resolution set of projections, with low resolution full field of view projections and prior information. We also evaluate our methods reconstructing software phantoms, and compare their performance to other methods in the literature.

Keywords: Tomography · Reconstruction · Region of interest
ROI · Sinogram combination · GPGPU

1 Introduction

Roughly speaking, transmission tomography is the 2D imaging of cross sections of an object of interest from its 1D projections.

One serious limitation in transmission tomography is for the high resolution imaging of large objects. Whereas it is possible to get images on μm spacial resolution and we can also image objects with a diameter of 1 m (or larger), the combination of the two tasks raise new problems. This is because imaging techniques and computation image processing tools can only handle image sizes of a few thousand (say, up to 4096 by 4096) pixels in width and depth which can either be a high resolution image of a small volume or the low resolution image of a large part of space. Combining the two is, however, challenging beyond current means as imaging a 1 μm resolution slice of an object of 10 cm would require 100000 by 100000 pixels.

Still high resolution imaging of large objects is necessary in many fields like (among others) industry and material science [7,18], biology [5] or medicine

© Springer Nature Switzerland AG 2018
R. P. Barneva et al. (Eds.): IWCIA 2018, LNCS 11255, pp. 150–163, 2018.
https://doi.org/10.1007/978-3-030-05288-1_12

[2,3,17]. Fortunately, these application usually only need the high resolution image of a small part of the larger object.

Region of Interest (ROI) tomography is a set of tools for imaging only a part of the object of study. In such measurements only the ROI is fully covered by high resolution projections while a large portion of the object is outside the field of view. The goal here is to get a highly accurate image of the region of interest, that can be deep inside a large er object.

Such methods have various possible applications. For example in industrial studies one can analyse the structure of mechanical parts looking for small degradation in the material (i.e. fractures). In biology researchers can use ROI tomography for examining the fine tissue structures in live animals. In medicine one can look for small malformations, i.e. see small remainders of tumours after operation.

The above task was already addressed in the literature. Some methods perform reconstruction from one single set of projections [4,6,9,13,14,19]. Another set of results are gathered around taking two sets of projections – a high resolution limited view one, and a low resolution set of projections of the full object – and combining the two sets before or during filtered backprojection [10,16]. Some other techniques apply compressed sensing tools for iterative reconstruction [22,23].

In this paper, we present three reconstruction methods for ROI tomography which are based on the algebraic formulation of the reconstruction problem. The new approaches contain different types of (non-negativity, discreteness, smoothness) prior information some of which are beneficial for the accuracy of the results. With these proir information we could reach a significant improvement of image quality compared to a state of the art technique in the literature.

The paper is structured as follows. In Sect. 2 we are presenting the mathematical background of the problem and our approach. Then, in Sect. 3 we give three reconstruction methods for performing ROI tomography. In Sect. 4 we outline a test environment we used for evaluating out algorithms and comparing them to a state of the art method from the literature, and finally in Sect. 5 we conclude our findings.

2 Preliminaries

Our presented methods assume, that we want to reconstruct the 2 dimensional cross-sections of an object of study. Although, we will give the methods for 2-dimensional parallel-beam reconstruction, we must note, that the findings can be extended to any (including fan-beam and cone-beam) reconstruction geometry, that can be formulated by a linear system of equations.

We represent the cross-section of the image by an $f(u, v) : \mathbb{R}^2 \mapsto \mathbb{R}$ function. The function f itself is considered to be unknown, but we can produce its projections given by a set of its line integrals determined by the Radon-transform [8,11] as

$$[\mathcal{R}f](\alpha, t) = \int_{-\infty}^{\infty} f(t\cos(\alpha) - q\sin(\alpha), t\sin(\alpha) + q\cos(\alpha)) \, dq \ . \tag{1}$$

In the above formulation the α and t values, respectively, describe the direction and the position of a line with its points parametrized by q. The task of tomographic reconstruction is to find an $f' : \mathbb{R}^2 \to \mathbb{R}$ function that satisfies $[\mathcal{R}f](\alpha, t) = [\mathcal{R}f'](\alpha, t)$ for a set of predetermined (α, t) pairs, i.e., which has the same projections as the unknown f function in a specific set of directions.

We also define a centred version of the radon transform

$$[\mathcal{R}_\sigma f](\alpha, t) = \int_{-\infty}^{\infty} f(\sigma_u + t\cos(\alpha) - q\sin(\alpha), \sigma_v + t\sin(\alpha) + q\cos(\alpha)) \, dq \ , \tag{2}$$

that has a rotation centre in a predetermined $\sigma = (\sigma_u, \sigma_v)$ point.

Of course, in a practical computer implementation we have to perform reconstruction on a discrete domain, therefore, we define pixels on finite grids as a set of indices

$$\Phi_{\theta,\omega,\sigma}(i, j) = \begin{cases} \phi_{\theta,\omega,\sigma}(i, j) & , \text{if } i, j \in \mathbb{Z} \cap [1, \omega] \\ \emptyset & , \text{otherwise}, \end{cases} \tag{3}$$

where

$$\phi_{\theta,\omega,\sigma}(i, j) = \left\{ \theta \cdot \left((i-1, j-1) - \frac{\omega}{2} + (u, v) \right) + \sigma \mid (u, v) \in [0, 1)^2 \right\} \ . \tag{4}$$

Here i and j are pixel coordinates, $\sigma = (\sigma_u, \sigma_v)$ is the centre of the grid, θ is the size of the pixels, and ω is the maximal number of grid elements in the horizontal and vertical direction.

Although, the real object might not satisfy this criteria, but in the reconstruction we assume, that each pixel of the reconstructed $f(u, v)$ function is homogeneous, i.e.,

$$f(u, v) = f(x, y) \ , \quad \forall (u, v), (x, y) \in \Phi_{\theta,\omega,\sigma}(i, j) \ , \quad \forall i, j \in \mathbb{Z} \ . \tag{5}$$

In some cases, we will further assume, that the reconstruction has a bounded support, therefore,

$$f(u, v) = 0 \ , \quad \text{if } \nexists (i, j) : \ (u, v) \in \Phi_{\theta,\omega,\sigma}(i, j) \ . \tag{6}$$

Using (3), (5) and (6) we can substitute the function to be reconstructed by an

$$I_{\theta,\omega}(u, v) \in \mathbb{R}^{\omega \times \omega} \ , \tag{7}$$

digital image of size ω and pixel size θ.

As for formalizing the projections we define the set of projection lines as a set of α, t pairs

$$\Lambda_{\xi,\tau,\omega\theta} = \left\{ (\alpha, t) \ : \ \alpha \in \left\{ \frac{i\pi}{\xi} \ : \ i \in \mathbb{Z} \cap [0, \xi) \right\} \ , \right.$$

$$\left. t \in \left\{ (k + 1/2)\tau \ : \ k \in \mathbb{Z}, (k + 1/2)\tau \in \left[-\frac{\omega\theta}{\sqrt{2}}, \frac{\omega\theta}{\sqrt{2}} \right] \right\} \right\} \ . \tag{8}$$

In practice, this is a ξ number of projections equally distributed in the $[0, \pi)$ angle range, each projection having equally spaced parallel projection lines, which can fully cover an image of size $\omega\theta$.

Finally, we define a $\mathcal{P}_{\Lambda,f,\sigma} : \{k \in \mathbb{N}^+ : k \leq |\Lambda|\} \mapsto \{[\mathcal{R}_\sigma f](\alpha, t) : (\alpha, t) \in \Lambda\}$ as a bijective function mapping indices to the projection values defined in a $\Lambda_{\xi,\tau,\omega\theta}$ set of projection lines.

Furthermore, we can now transform our model to be represented by a system of equations. Let $\mathbf{p}$ be a vector of $\mathcal{P}_{\Lambda,f,\sigma}(i)$ values. For an easier notation, we will denote the elements of $\mathbf{p}$ as $p_i = \mathcal{P}_{\Lambda,f,\sigma}(i)$. Also, let $\mathbf{x}$ be a vector gained as a sequence of the pixels of an (7) image (as illustrated in Fig. 1). To make this more exact, let

$$\varphi_\omega : \mathbb{N} \cap [1, \omega^2] \mapsto (\mathbb{N} \cap [1, \omega])^2 , \tag{9}$$

be a bijective mapping that assigns a pixel coordinate to the integers between 1 and ω^2. Therefore, for each ω sized grid we can directly connect the x_i values to the I image as $x_i = I(\varphi(i))$.

With $\mathbf{x}$ and $\mathbf{p}$, let $\mathbf{R}$ be a matrix, such that

$$\mathbf{Rx} = \mathbf{p} , \tag{10}$$

is equivalent with $\mathcal{P}_{\Lambda,f,\sigma}(i)$ of f. Later in the paper, we will clarify the parameters of the Φ grid, the Λ set of projections and the σ centre of rotation in the context.

Given a set of $\mathbf{p}$ projection values, and an $\mathbf{R}$ projection matrix, we can perform the reconstruction by solving (10) (for some approaches see, e.g., [8,11, 20]).

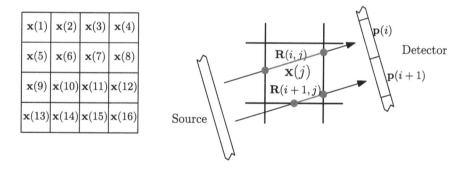

Fig. 1. Illustration of the equation system-based representation of the reconstruction problem.

Now we can get to the multi-resolution extension of the reconstruction task. Assume, that we have two sets of projections of the same object (i.e., the same f function), with different geometries $\Lambda_{\xi_l,\tau_l,\omega_l\theta_l,\sigma_l}$ (we denote this Λ_l) and $\Lambda_{\xi_r,\tau_r,\omega_r\theta_r,\sigma_r}$ (which we denote Λ_r). Λ_l is a low resolution projection set covering the full object, while Λ_r is a high resolution set of projections with limited field of view. In the above formulation this means, that $\tau_l > \tau_r$ and $\omega_l\theta_l > \omega_r\theta_r$.

We can also define two grids $\Phi_{\theta_l,\omega_l,\sigma_l}$ which is a set of larger pixels covering the full object and a $\Phi_{\theta_r,\omega_r,\sigma_r}$ region of interest that is a fine resolution grid covering a smaller ROI (in short Φ_l and Φ_r). We make a restriction, that the pixels of Φ_l cannot be partially covered by Φ_r, i.e., $\Phi_l(i,j) \subseteq \bigcup_{(k,l)\in\mathbb{Z}^2} \Phi_r(k,l)$, or $\Phi_l(i,j) \cap (\bigcup_{(k,l)\in\mathbb{Z}^2} \Phi_r(k,l)) = \emptyset$.

The image of the region of interest will be denoted by a new function

$$f_r(u,v) = \begin{cases} f(u,v) & , \text{if } \exists (i,j) \in \Phi_r \text{ such that } (u,v) \in (i,j) , \\ 0 & , \text{otherwise} . \end{cases} \quad (11)$$

In a discrete context, $\mathbf{x}_l$ and $\mathbf{x}_r$ will represent, respectively, f on the Φ_l gird and f_r on the Φ_r grid.

Furthermore, we define four types of projections, with four equation systems:

- Let $\mathbf{p}_{ll}$ be a sequence of $\mathcal{P}_{\Lambda_l,f,\sigma_l}$ values, and $\mathbf{R}_{ll}$ be a matrix, such that $\mathbf{R}_{ll}\mathbf{x}_l = \mathbf{p}_{ll}$ is equivalent with $\mathcal{P}_{\Lambda_l,f,\sigma_l}$ on the Φ_l grid;
- Let $\mathbf{p}_{lr}$ be a sequence of $\mathcal{P}_{\Lambda_r,f,\sigma_l}$ values, and $\mathbf{R}_{lr}$ be a matrix, such that $\mathbf{R}_{lr}\mathbf{x}_l = \mathbf{p}_{lr}$ is equivalent with $\mathcal{P}_{\Lambda_r,f,\sigma_l}$ on the Φ_l grid;
- Let $\mathbf{p}_{rr}$ be a sequence of $\mathcal{P}_{\Lambda_r,f_r,\sigma_r}$ values, and $\mathbf{R}_{rr}$ be a matrix, such that $\mathbf{R}_{rr}\mathbf{x}_r = \mathbf{p}_{rr}$ is equivalent with $\mathcal{P}_{\Lambda_r,f_r,\sigma_r}$ on the Φ_r grid;
- And let $\mathbf{p}_{rl}$ be a sequence of $\mathcal{P}_{\Lambda_l,f_r,\sigma_r}$ values, and $\mathbf{R}_{rl}$ be a matrix, such that $\mathbf{R}_{rl}\mathbf{x}_r = \mathbf{p}_{rl}$ is equivalent with $\mathcal{P}_{\Lambda_l,f_r,\sigma_r}$ on the Φ_r grid.

This is represented in Fig. 2.

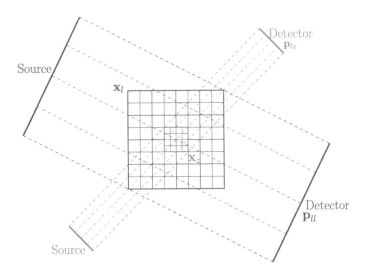

Fig. 2. Illustration of using multiple projection geometries.

Note, that in practical projection acquisition we can only measure the $\mathbf{p}_{ll}$ and $\mathbf{p}_{lz}$ vectors.

We can also define an intersection matrix determining the connection between $\mathbf{x}_z$ and $\mathbf{x}_l$. Let $\mathbf{A} \in \mathbb{R}^{\omega_l \times \omega_r}$ be a matrix such that

$$\mathbf{A}(i,j) = Area\left(\Phi_l(\varphi_{\omega_l}(i)) \cap \Phi_r(\varphi_{\omega_r}(j))\right) \ . \tag{12}$$

Here, $Area(.)$ denotes the area of the intersection of two pixels.

3 Reconstruction from Hybrid Geometries

Given the formulation of Sect. 2 we define different reconstruction methods for the high resolution reconstruction of the ROI.

3.1 Two-Round Iterative Reconstruction

The first method performs the reconstruction by first reconstructing a low resolution full image, then using this first reconstruction approximate the $\mathbf{p}_{rr}$ projections of only the ROI. Then, from $\mathbf{p}_{rr}$, we can calculate $\mathbf{x}_r$ by solving $\mathbf{R}_{rr}\mathbf{x}_r = \mathbf{p}_{rr}$.

The difficulty behind this idea, is that we do not have $\mathbf{p}_{rr}$. On the other hand, in the formulation of Sect. 2, $\mathbf{p}_{rr}$ is the equivalent of $\mathcal{P}_{\Lambda_r, f_r}$, and we know that

$$\mathcal{P}_{\Lambda_r, f} = \mathcal{P}_{\Lambda_r, f_r} + \mathcal{P}_{\Lambda_r, f-f_r} \ , \tag{13}$$

e.i., because the projection of the full object is the projection of the ROI, plus the projection of the material outside the ROI. From this

$$\mathcal{P}_{\Lambda_r, f_r} = \mathcal{P}_{\Lambda_r, f} - \mathcal{P}_{\Lambda_r, f-f_r} \ . \tag{14}$$

From the (11) definition of f_r we also know that

$$(f - f_r)(u,v) = \begin{cases} 0 & \text{, if } \exists (i,j) \in \Phi_r \text{ such that } (u,v) \in (i,j) \\ f(u,v) & \text{, otherwise } . \end{cases} \tag{15}$$

Therefore, if we had an $\hat{f}$ approximation of f, we can get an approximation of $f - f_r$ by setting the regions of $\hat{f}$ covered by the ROI to 0.

For this we calculate an $\mathbf{z}_l$ reconstructions with a reconstruction algorithm, set $\mathbf{z}_l(i)$ values corresponding to the ROI to zero and simulate $\mathcal{P}_{\Lambda_r, f-f_r, \sigma_r}$ as $\mathbf{c} = \mathbf{R}_{lz}\mathbf{z}_l$. Afterwards, we can approximate $\mathbf{p}_{rr}$ as $\mathbf{p}_{rr} \approx \mathbf{p}_{lr} - \mathbf{c}$, and perform the reconstruction from the resulting projection value.

For calculating $\mathbf{z}_l$ and performing the final reconstructions we used two different reconstruction techniques. The pseudo-code of this two-rounded reconstruction method can be found in Algorithm 1. We denote $Recon(\mathbf{R}, \mathbf{p})$ the result of a reconstruction performed by a given "$Recon$" algorithm. In our case, we tried two reconstruction methods. One was the SIRT [20], and the other one was the DART [1] algorithm.

Algorithm 1. Two-round reconstruction by

Input: $\mathbf{R}_{ll}$, $\mathbf{R}_{zz}$, $\mathbf{R}_{lz}$ projection coefficient matrices; $\mathbf{A}$ resolution connection matrix; $\mathbf{p}_{ll}$, $\mathbf{p}_{lz}$ projection values.
Output: $\mathbf{x}_l$ low resolution full reconstruction, and $\mathbf{x}_r$ high resolution reconstructed ROI.

1: $\mathbf{x}_l \leftarrow Recon(\mathbf{R}_{ll}, \mathbf{p}_{ll})$
2: $\mathbf{z}_l \leftarrow \mathbf{x}_l$
3: **for each** $\{i \in \{1, \ldots, \omega_l^2\} \ : \ \sum_{j=1}^{\omega_r^2} \mathbf{A}(i,j) = 0\}$ **do**
4:     $\mathbf{z}_l(i) \leftarrow 0$
5: **end for**
6: $\mathbf{c} \leftarrow \mathbf{R}_{lr} \mathbf{z}_l$
7: $\mathbf{x}_r \leftarrow Recon(\mathbf{R}_{rr}, \mathbf{p}_{lr} - \mathbf{c})$
8: **return** $(\mathbf{x}_l, \mathbf{x}_r)$

3.2 Multi-resolution Tomography by Energy Minimization

Our second proposed method performs the reconstruction by minimizing a suitable energy function. The energy function has the form

$$\mathcal{E}(\mathbf{x}_l, \mathbf{y}_r) = \|\mathbf{R}_{ll}\mathbf{x}_l + \mathbf{R}_{rl}\mathbf{y}_r - \mathbf{p}_{ll}\|_2^2 + \|\mathbf{R}_{lr}\mathbf{x}_l + \mathbf{R}_{rr}\mathbf{y}_r - \mathbf{p}_{lr}\|_2^2 +$$

$$\gamma\|g(\mathbf{x}_l)\|_1 + \delta\|g(\mathbf{x}_r)\|_1 + \mu\|\mathbf{y}_r\|_1 + \nu \sum_{i=1}^{\omega_r^2} \sum_{j \in N_4(i)} |\mathbf{x}_r(i) - \mathbf{x}_r(j)| \ , \tag{16}$$

where $\mathbf{y}_r$ is not the reconstruction of the high resolution ROI by itself, but a difference image refining the low resolution reconstruction, i.e.,

$$\mathbf{x}_r = \mathbf{y}_r + \mathbf{A}^T \mathbf{x}_l \ , \tag{17}$$

$g(\mathbf{x})$ is a non-negativity function

$$g(\mathbf{x}) = min(-\mathbf{x}, 0) \ , \tag{18}$$

$N_4(i)$ is the set of indices of the pixels 4-adjacent to the i-th pixel in $\mathbf{x}_r$, and γ, δ, μ, ν are constants setting the importance of the parts of (16).

In a more intuitive description, the first $\|\mathbf{R}_{ll}\mathbf{x}_l + \mathbf{R}_{rl}\mathbf{y}_r - \mathbf{p}_{ll}\|_2^2$ term is only a data fidelity term of the low resolution sinogram while the second $\|\mathbf{R}_{lr}\mathbf{x}_l + \mathbf{R}_{rr}\mathbf{y}_r - \mathbf{p}_{lr}\|_2^2$ term stands for the data fidelity of the high resolution projections. As the high resolution reconstruction is performed by the refinement of the low-resolution reconstruction we need to simulate the LR and HR projections of both $\mathbf{x}_l$ and $\mathbf{y}_r$. The sum of the two gives the projections of the actual reconstructions that should be the same as the $\mathbf{p}_{ll}$ and $\mathbf{p}_{lr}$ projections.

The next two terms stand for the positivity of the data. We should note, that both the hight resolution and low resolution reconstructions should contain positive values (since, in transmission tomography we do not have negative absorption coefficients). For the low resolution term this is simply done by adding

$\|g(\mathbf{x}_l)\|_1$, where $g(\mathbf{x})$ is a function taking positive values if $\mathbf{x}_l(i)$ is negative, and 0 values otherwise. Taking the L_1 norm of this punishes negative values in the results. As for the high resolution reconstruction, we have to apply the non-negativity term to the final high resolution image, that is given by combining the low-resolution image and the high resolution refinement

$$\|g(\mathbf{x}_r)\|_1 = \|g(\mathbf{y}_r + \mathbf{A}^T\mathbf{x}_l)\|_1 \ . \tag{19}$$

The next $\|\mathbf{y}_r\|_1$ term is a simple regularization of the refinement image, suppressing noise. This term punishes high variance of the refinement, therefore propagates smooth areas. It also makes sure to have a good low resolution reconstruction. Without this term, the $\mathbf{x}_l$ reconstruction tends to be homogeneous on the region of interest while all the details are stored in $\mathbf{y}_r$.

Finally, the last $\sum_{i=1}^{\omega_r^2}\sum_{j\in N_4(i)}|\mathbf{x}_r(i) - \mathbf{x}_r(j)|$ term is an L_1 smoothness regularization between the 4-adjacent pixels of $\mathbf{x}_r$.

Given the energy function, the reconstruction can be performed by many different approaches. One should note that the energy function is convex and can be optimized by advanced gradient descent methods. Here, we decided to used the Adam [12] optimizer, that is best known in artificial deep learning but also works perfect for minimizing (16).

4   Validation and Results

For the validation of the results we performed simulated reconstructions of software phantoms. These phantoms can be seen in Fig. 3.

Our first phantom was a 2048 by 2048 pixel sized slice of the Forbild Head phantom [15], which is a simulated head object, containing various structures resembling structures in the human skull. In case of this phantom we performed reconstructions with two defined regions of interests, which are highlighted in Fig. 3.

We also wanted to test the compared methods on more complex images. As complex structures outside the region of interest can appear as noise in the ROI, we wanted to have test images having highly modular structures in the outside regions. This lead to the construction of two new phantoms. Phantom 2 is a simple structure in a size of 1024 by 1024 pixels. This image contained three intensities, granular structures and cavities. Phantom 3, on the other hand, is a highly modular image in a size of 2048 by 2048 pixels having only refined granular structures.

4.1   Geometric Parameters of the Experiments

We performed the evaluations by simulating the low resolution full coverage, and high resolution partial coverage sinograms of the phantoms. Both the high- and low resolution sinograms contained 180 projections with parallel line beam geometry. The low-resolution projections were gained by decreasing the resolution of the full sinogram by two downscaling factors (4 and 8).

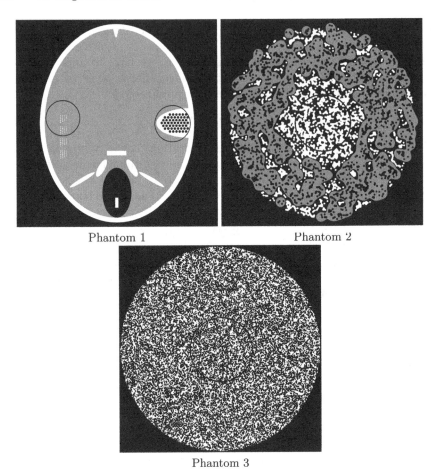

Phantom 1   Phantom 2

Phantom 3

Fig. 3. Phantoms used in the testing. The regions of interest are indicated by red circles. (Color figure online)

In case of 4-times downscaling – using the notation of Sect. 2 – we set the parameters of the Φ_l, Φ_r grids and Λ_l, Λ_r projection geometries to be $\theta_l = 4$, $\xi_l = 180$, $\tau_l = 4$ and $\theta_r = 1$, $\xi_r = 180$, $\tau_r = 1$. The σ_l centre of image and rotation was placed into the centre of the image and σ_r into the centre of the ROI. With phantoms Phantom 1 and 3 we set $\omega_l = \omega_r = 512$ and for Phantom 2 we used $\omega_l = \omega_r = 256$.

In the second set of tests with 8-times downscaling we used the parameters $\theta_l = 8$, $\xi_l = 180$ $\tau_l = 8$ and $\theta_r = 1$, $\xi_r = 180$ $\tau_r = 1$. The σ_l centre of image and rotation was again placed into the centre of the image and σ_r into the centre of the ROI. With Phantom 1 and 3 we set $\omega_l = \omega_r = 256$ and for Phantom 2 we used $\omega_l = \omega_r = 128$.

Table 1. Reconstruction Errors (mean absolute error in percent) in the region if interests performed on the 4 algorithms with two downscaling factors. (smaller is better)

	Phan. 1a	Phan. 1b	Phan. 2	Phan. 3
Downscale factor: 4				
Alg. from [16]	3.89	3.25	11.21	18.68
2-round SIRT	3.40	5.45	10.86	20.50
2-round DART	0.74	2.90	9.00	8.98
Energy min	1.36	3.39	8.39	18.82
Downscale factor: 8				
Alg. from [16]	4.60	6.32	12.08	20.47
2-round SIRT	8.28	8.92	17.07	29.72
2-round DART	0.63	6.72	7.41	14.38
Energy min	5.62	8.88	8.06	18.61

In all cases we simulated the $\mathbf{p}_{ll}$ and $\mathbf{p}_{lr}$ projections using the original phantoms.

4.2 Parameters of the Reconstruction Algorithms

In the validation we set the parameters of the reconstruction methods empirically. In case of the algorithms of Sect. 3.1 the SIRT method was stopped if the L_2 change between consecutive steps was smaller then 0.01 or the algorithm reached 1000 iterations. We used a projected variant of the SIRT method which does not allow negative values in the result. In case of the DART method we ran 500 DART iterations each containing 10 SIRT iterations. As for the algorithm of Sect. 3.2 the parameters of the energy function were chosen to be $\gamma = \delta = 1000$, $\mu = 100$ and $\nu = 10$. The parameters of the Adam optimizer were $\alpha = 0.01$, $\beta_1 = 0.99$, $\beta_2 = 0.9999$ and $\epsilon = 10^{-8}$.

4.3 Results

For a ground-truth comparison, we compared our methods to another algorithm from the literature, that was the data weighting method of [16].

Some of the regions of interest of the reconstructions can be seen in Figs. 4 and 5. We also performed a numerical evaluation of the images by calculating the Mean Absolute Errors of the reconstructions in the ROI. The accuracy statistics can be found in Table 1.

Regarding the results we can see that apart from one occasion the two-round DART method gave the best results. This is likely due to its advanced discreteness prior that already showed to bring significant improvement to the reconstruction accuracy [1,21]. Regarding the other algorithms the energy minimization-based method usually gave better results then the other two, followed

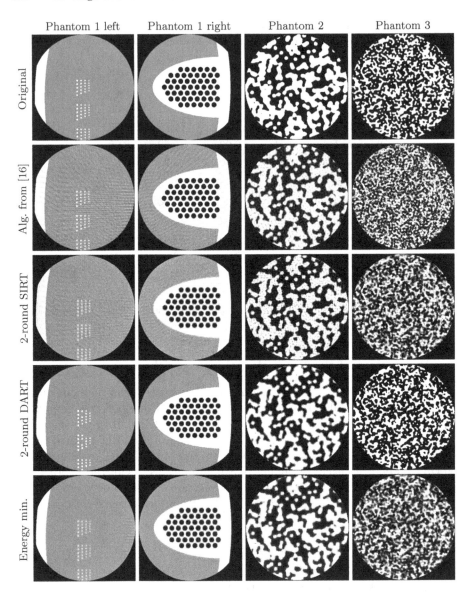

Fig. 4. High-resolution reconstructions, with 4 times downscaling factor.

by the algorithm of [16] and the two round SIRT. This might be because the energy function also uses various prior information for the reconstruction leading to better results. As for the SIRT and the reference algorithm they do not use any prior knowledge but the filtered back projection method giving the foundation of the reference is proved to be robust in ROI tomography.

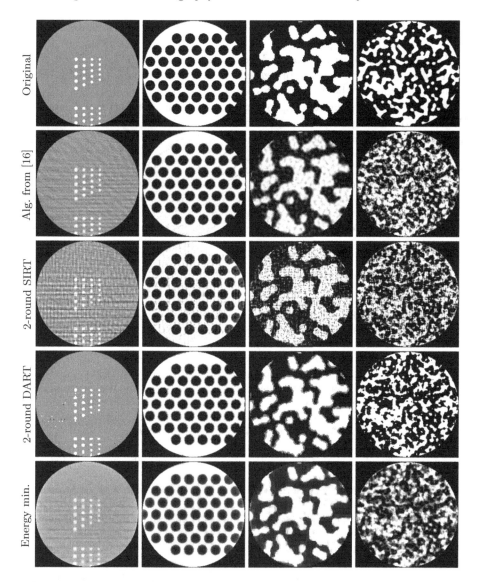

Fig. 5. High-resolution reconstructions, with 8 times downscaling factor.

5   Conclusion and Future Plans

The paper represented new methods for Region of Interest tomography from two projection sets. One projection set contains high resolution projection with limited field of view only covering the ROI, while the other set is a low resolution projection set covering the whole image. Our given algorithms are various techniques based on the algebraic formulation of the reconstruction problem. They also hold various types of prior informations like smoothness priors, discretenes, smoothness and non-negativity.

We also evaluated our proposed methods in simulation data. Using these piror information, some of the presented methods were capable of giving better results than state of the art algorithms in the literature.

In the future, we plan on improving the algorithms for better performance. We are also working on placing the methods into practical use by imaging the lung tissue of small animals.

Acknowledgement. This research was supported by the project "Integrated program for training new generation of scientists in the fields of computer science", no EFOP-3.6.3-VEKOP-16-2017-0002. The project has been supported by the European Union and co-funded by the European Social Fund. We gratefully acknowledge the support of NVIDIA Corporation with the donation of a Tesla K40 GPU used for this research.

References

1. Batenburg, K.J., Sijbers, J.: Dart: a practical reconstruction algorithm for discrete tomography. IEEE Trans. Image Process. **20**(9), 2542–2553 (2011)
2. Chen, L., et al.: Dual resolution cone beam breast CT: a feasibility study. Med. Phys. **36**(9Part1), 4007–4014 (2009)
3. Chityala, R., Hoffmann, K.R., Rudin, S., Bednarek, D.R.: Region of interest (ROI) computed tomography (CT): comparison with full field of view (FFOV) and truncated CT for a human head phantom. In: Flynn, M.J. (ed.) Medical Imaging 2005: Physics of Medical Imaging. SPIE, April 2005
4. Cho, P.S., Rudd, A.D., Johnson, R.H.: Cone-beam CT from width-truncated projections. Comput. Med. Imaging Graph. **20**(1), 49–57 (1996)
5. Chun, I.K., Cho, M.H., Lee, S.C., Cho, M.H., Lee, S.Y.: X-ray micro-tomography system for small-animal imaging with zoom-in imaging capability. Phys. Med. Biol. **49**(17), 3889–3902 (2004)
6. Courdurier, M., Noo, F., Defrise, M., Kudo, H.: Solving the interior problem of computed tomography using a priori knowledge. Inverse Prob. **24**(6), 065001 (2008)
7. Gentle, D.J., Spyrou, N.M.: Region of interest tomography in industrial applications. Nucl. Instrum. Methods Phys. Res. Sect. A Accel. Spectrometers Detect. Assoc. Equip. **299**(1), 534–537 (1990)
8. Herman, G.T.: Fundamentals of Computerized Tomography: Image Reconstruction from Projections. Springer, Heidelberg (2009). https://doi.org/10.1007/978-1-84628-723-7
9. Huesman, R.H.: A new fast algorithm for the evaluation of regions of interest and statistical uncertainty in computed tomography. Phys. Med. Biol. **29**(5), 543–552 (1984)
10. Kadrmas, D.J., Jaszczak, R.J., McCormick, J.W., Coleman, R.E.: Truncation artifact reduction in transmission CT for improved SPECT attenuation compensation. Phys. Med. Biol. **40**(6), 1085–1104 (1995)
11. Kak, A.C., Slaney, M.: Principles of Computerized Tomographic Imaging. IEEE Press, New York (1999)
12. Kingma, D.P., Ba, J.: Adam: a method for stochastic optimization. arXiv:1412.6980 (2014)

13. Kudo, H., Courdurier, M., Noo, F., Defrise, M.: Tiny a prioriknowledge solves the interior problem in computed tomography. Phys. Med. Biol. **53**(9), 2207–2231 (2008)
14. Kyrieleis, A., Titarenko, V., Ibison, M., Connolley, T., Withers, P.J.: Region-of-interest tomography using filtered backprojection: assessing the practical limits. J. Microsc. **241**(1), 69–82 (2010)
15. Lauritsch, G., Bruder, H.: Technical report: head phantom. Technical report, Institute of Medical Physics, Friedrich-Alexander-University Erlangen-Nrnberg (2009)
16. Maaß, C., Knaup, M., Kachelrieß, M.: New approaches to region of interest computed tomography. Med. Phys. **38**(6Part1), 2868–2878 (2011)
17. Patel, V., Hoffmann, K.R., Ionita, C.N., Keleshis, C., Bednarek, D.R., Rudin, S.: Rotational micro-CT using a clinical C-arm angiography gantry. Med. Phys. **35**(10), 4757–4764 (2008)
18. Reimers, P., Kettschau, A., Goebbels, J.: Region-of-interest (ROI) mode in industrial X-ray computed tomography. NDT Int. **23**(5), 255–261 (1990)
19. Sourbelle, K., Kachelriess, M., Kalender, W.A.: Reconstruction from truncated projections in CT using adaptive detruncation. Eur. Radiol. **15**(5), 1008–1014 (2005)
20. van der Sluis, A., van der Vorst, H.A.: SIRT- and CG-type methods for the iterative solution of sparse linear least-squares problems. Linear Algebra Appl. **130**, 257–303 (1990)
21. Weber, S., Nagy, A., Schüle, T., Schnörr, C., Kuba, A.: A benchmark evaluation of large-scale optimization approaches to binary tomography. In: Kuba, A., Nyúl, L.G., Palágyi, K. (eds.) DGCI 2006. LNCS, vol. 4245, pp. 146–156. Springer, Heidelberg (2006). https://doi.org/10.1007/11907350_13
22. Yu, H., Wang, G.: Compressed sensing based interior tomography. Phys. Med. Biol. **54**(9), 2791–2805 (2009)
23. Yu, H., Yang, J., Jiang, M., Wang, G.: Supplemental analysis on compressed sensing based interior tomography. Phys. Med. Biol. **54**(18), N425–N432 (2009)

A Multi-channel DART Algorithm

Mathé Zeegers[1]([✉]), Felix Lucka[1,2], and Kees Joost Batenburg[1]

[1] Computational Imaging, Centrum Wiskunde & Informatica (CWI), Amsterdam,
The Netherlands
`m.t.zeegers@cwi.nl`
[2] Department of Computer Science, University College London, London, UK

Abstract. Tomography deals with the reconstruction of objects from
their projections, acquired along a range of angles. Discrete tomography
is concerned with objects that consist of a small number of materials,
which makes it possible to compute accurate reconstructions from highly
limited projection data. For cases where the allowed intensity values
in the reconstruction are known a priori, the discrete algebraic reconstruction technique (DART) has shown to yield accurate reconstructions
from few projections. However, a key limitation is that the benefit of
DART diminishes as the number of different materials increases. Many
tomographic imaging techniques can simultaneously record tomographic
data at multiple *channels*, each corresponding to a different weighting
of the materials in the object. Whenever projection data from more
than one channel is available, this additional information can potentially be exploited by the reconstruction algorithm. In this paper we
present Multi-Channel DART (MC-DART), which deals effectively with
multi-channel data. This class of algorithms is a generalization of DART
to multiple channels and combines the information for each separate
channel-reconstruction in a multi-channel segmentation step. We demonstrate that in a range of simulation experiments, MC-DART is capable
of producing more accurate reconstructions compared to single-channel
DART.

Keywords: Computed tomography · Discrete tomography
Discrete algebraic reconstruction technique (DART)
Multi-channel segmentation

1 Introduction

Tomography is a non-invasive technique for creating 2D or 3D images of the
inner structure of an object. Projections of the object are acquired by sending
photonic or particle beams (e.g. X-rays, electrons, neutrons) through the object
in a particular direction and measuring the signal resulting from interaction of
the beam and the object at a detector. By acquiring this data from multiple
positions and under various angles, a collection of projections is obtained. An
image of the interior of the object is then reconstructed by applying a reconstruction algorithm to this projection data. Tomography is successfully used in

ⓒ Springer Nature Switzerland AG 2018
R. P. Barneva et al. (Eds.): IWCIA 2018, LNCS 11255, pp. 164–178, 2018.
https://doi.org/10.1007/978-3-030-05288-1_13

many fields, including medical imaging [10] and electron tomography in materials science [9,14]. If a large number of accurate projection images are available, solving the reconstruction problem is straightforward by a closed-form inversion formula [7]. Practical constraints on the dose, acquisition time or available space can impose limitations on the number of projections that can be taken, the angular range, or the noise level of the data, resulting in artefacts in the reconstructed images if standard reconstruction methods are used [10].

Discrete tomography is a powerful technique for dealing with such limited tomographic data. It can be applied if the object consists of only a limited number of materials with homogeneous densities. The Discrete Algebraic Reconstruction Technique (DART) [4,5] is an algebraic reconstruction method for discrete tomography that alternates between continuous reconstruction steps and discretization of the image intensities by segmentation. The DART algorithm has demonstrated to obtain higher image quality reconstructions with limited projections and angles compared to standard reconstruction methods. Numerous successive studies have improved the DART algorithm, which include automatic parameter estimation (PDM-DART [1] and TVR-DART [18]), multi-resolution reconstruction (MDART [8]), relaxing voxel constraints (SDART [6]) and adaptive boundary reconstructions (ADART [13]). Nevertheless, a key limitation of DART is that it can only improve reconstruction quality if the number of different materials in the object is relatively small. The main reason is that for a larger number of materials, the segmentation step is no longer effective [4,5].

In some cases it is possible to obtain tomographic information in multiple measurements channels. For instance, in X-ray imaging the beams are typically polychromatic, i.e. X-ray photon energies are distributed over a spectrum. Each material in the object has different attenuation properties for different X-ray energy levels. Whenever a single X-ray energy value is desired the range of energies within the beam can be narrowed by applying filters at the X-ray source [7]. Some detectors are capable of separating the incoming photons into energy bins while counting (e.g. HEXITEC [17]). In these cases spectral or multi-channel projection data is acquired, providing additional information about the object at different energies. Compared to the single-channel setting, where each material has a single attenuation value in the reconstructed image, in the multi-channel setting the attenuation value for each material varies along the channels. In this way, a tomographic dataset of the object is acquired for each channel, where the attenuation value of the materials changes throughout these datasets. This multi-channel imaging can potentially yield extra information about the materials. With more materials in the object, especially with similar attenuation features at a fixed energy, having data from multiple channels enables a better separation during segmentation. A conceptual example of this is shown in Fig. 1. It is hard to separate points based on their attenuation values in a one-dimensional energy space. For instance, the right side of the blue area might as well be assigned to the green or yellow material during segmentation. With two energy dimensions the points are easily separable, since each voxel value lies close to its attenuation cloud center. Note that these spectra are artificial and not likely to occur in real-world examples.

In this paper we present a new class of algorithms that combines DART with multi-channel imaging for solving discrete multi-channel reconstruction problems. Our algorithm can combine the information from multiple channels to produce a final segmentation that is superior to that of the (single-channel) DART algorithm. Note that since this new method is designed by means of modules or subroutines that are interchangeable (as with DART), the method is essentially a class of algorithms providing a framework for dealing with multichannel data. For simplicity, however, we will frequently call this framework an algorithm.

This paper is structured as follows. Section 2 introduces the multi-channel discrete tomography problem. In Sect. 3 the DART algorithm is restated and the Multi-Channel DART (MC-DART) algorithm is introduced. Results of experiments with this algorithm are reported in Sect. 4. Finally, Sect. 5 presents the conclusions of this study.

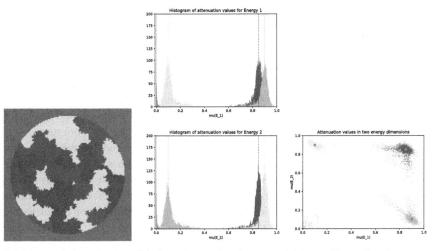

(a) Material distribution (b) One-dimensional atten- (c) Two-dimensional attenua-
                              uations   tions

Fig. 1. Elementary example of separation difficulties during segmentation. (a) Distribution of the three materials (blue, yellow, green) in the object. The background is indicated in red. (b) Histogram of attenuation values of pixels at energy E_1 (above) and E_2 (below). Vertical lines show true material attenuations. (c) Attenuations of the materials (red dots) and computed attenuations by a reconstruction algorithm for each voxel (colors indicate the material they belong to). (Color figure online)

2   Problem Formulation

The standard (single-channel) tomography problem can be modeled as a system of linear equations. The image is characterized by a vector of voxel attenuation values $\boldsymbol{x} \in \mathbb{R}^n$, where n is the number of voxels. We will work with 2D images, but the problem formulation and methods in this paper can easily be extended to the 3D setting. We will refer to the image pixels as *voxels* to distinguish these from detector pixels. We will often interchangeably speak of voxels and their corresponding indices. The projection values (also called data) are given as the vector $\boldsymbol{p} \in \mathbb{R}^l$, where l is the number of projection angles times the number of detector pixels. The reconstruction problem can then be described by solving the following set of linear equations for $\boldsymbol{x}$:

$$\boldsymbol{W}\boldsymbol{x} = \boldsymbol{p}. \tag{1}$$

Here $\boldsymbol{W}$ is the projection matrix, also called the forward operator [11]. This matrix incorporates the contribution of each voxel to each projection, where element w_{ij} indicates the contribution of voxel j to projection i. Applying the operator $\boldsymbol{W}$ on a vector $\boldsymbol{x}$ results in the forward projection (also called sinogram). Since inverting the matrix $\boldsymbol{W}$ is computationally too expensive (or not even possible, for example when the problem is ill-posed) the reconstruction problem is to find a solution $\boldsymbol{x}^*$ whose forward projection $\boldsymbol{W}\boldsymbol{x}^*$ matches the projection data best with respect to some norm $|| \cdot ||$.

$$\boldsymbol{x}^* = \operatorname*{arg\,min}_{\boldsymbol{x} \in \mathbb{R}^n} ||\boldsymbol{W}\boldsymbol{x} - \boldsymbol{p}|| \tag{2}$$

Since this is a least squares problem over $\mathbb{R}^n$, a solution always exists. For simplicity of notation we also assume that it is unique. A vector that encapsulates noise from real-world examples can also be modeled with (2). In our experiments with phantom examples in Sect. 4 there is no noise.

In the *discrete tomography problem*, the image to be reconstructed consists of a limited number of materials with homogeneous densities, each having an attenuation which is known beforehand by means of the set $\mathcal{R} = \{\rho_1, \ldots, \rho_m\}$, where m is the number of different materials in the object. Therefore the problem to be solved becomes finding a vector $\boldsymbol{x} \in \mathcal{R}^n$ that matches the data best:

$$\boldsymbol{x}^* = \operatorname*{arg\,min}_{\boldsymbol{x} \in \mathcal{R}^n} ||\boldsymbol{W}\boldsymbol{x} - \boldsymbol{p}||. \tag{3}$$

Note that this is a minimization problem over a non-empty finite set. Hence, a minimum always exists. Again, it does not need to be unique but we use this notation throughout the paper for simplicity.

In the *multi-channel* setting different properties of the target can be individually interrogated and measured. The information of each property is obtained through a separate channel. An example of channel is an energy level, as in the example in Sect. 1. In Fig. 1b, the channels are the two energy levels revealing attenuations of the object at different energies. In a more abstract way the object is described as set a of voxels with labels instead of attenuation values, since each material has different attenuation values in different channels. The material labels are values in the set $\mathcal{M} = \{1, 2, \ldots, m\}$. The channel indices are given by $\mathcal{E} = \{E_1, E_2, \ldots, E_C\}$ where the number of channels is given by C. Again, the attenuations are known beforehand in the sets $\mathcal{R}_{E_1} = \{\rho_{1,1}, \ldots, \rho_{1,m}\}, \mathcal{R}_{E_2} = \{\rho_{2,1}, \ldots, \rho_{2,m}\}, \ldots, \mathcal{R}_{E_C} = \{\rho_{C,1} \ldots, \rho_{C,m}\}$. In this setting, let $\mathcal{R} = \cup \mathcal{R}_{E_c}$. The function $\mu : \mathcal{M} \times \mathcal{E} \mapsto \mathcal{R}$ maps the label-channel combinations to their attenuation value, so the attenuation of a material with label s at channel E_c is given by $\mu(s, E_c)$. Note that there is not necessarily a one-to-one correspondence between the attenuation values and the material-channel combinations, because some combinations can have the same attenuation value. In this multi-channel case the projection data is given by a vector of projection data vectors at various channels:

$$P = (p_{E_1}, \ldots, p_{E_C}) \in \mathbb{R}^{n \times C}. \tag{4}$$

For each channel E_c the reconstruction problem for x_{E_c} is given by the following set of linear equations:

$$W x_{E_c} = p_{E_c}, \qquad E_c \in \{E_1, \ldots E_C\}. \tag{5}$$

For $y \in \mathcal{M}^n$, define $\mu(y, E_h) = (\mu(y_1, E_h), \ldots, \mu(y_n, E_h))^\top$ as the vector of voxel attenuation values at channel E_h. The multi-channel problem is now defined as follows. Given data vector P and projection matrix W, find a labeling vector $y^* \in \mathcal{M}^n$ such that for each channel E_c the difference between forward projection $W\mu(y^*, E_h)$ and data is minimal with respect to some norm $|| \cdot ||$:

$$y^* = \arg\min_{y \in \mathcal{M}^n} \sum_{h=1}^{C} ||W\mu(y, E_h) - p_{E_h}||. \tag{6}$$

Note that for one channel the minimization problem is equivalent to (3) where the labeling is given by the attenuation values x, by setting $\mu(y, E_1) = x$ and $\mathcal{M}^n = \mathcal{R}^n$ and $p_{E_1} = p$:

$$y^* = \arg\min_{y \in \mathcal{M}^n} ||W\mu(y, E_1) - p_{E_1}|| \tag{7}$$

$$= \arg\min_{x \in \mathcal{R}^n} ||Wx - p||. \tag{8}$$

3   Algorithms

In this section the Multi-Channel DART (MC-DART) framework for solving the minimization problem of Eq. (6) is introduced. We first explain the DART algorithm as given in [4] by discussing the overall structure and its building blocks. We then describe each building block of the MC-DART algorithm separately in more detail. Note that ASTRA [2,15] provides an implementation for numerically computing all projection matrices in these algorithms, either by storing the full matrix or doing all necessary computation in a matrix-free way.

3.1   DART

The DART algorithm attempts to solve the optimization problem of Eq. (3) by iteratively alternating between continuous reconstruction steps and discrete segmentation steps. The number of materials in the object to be reconstructed and their attenuation values should be known beforehand, given by the function μ. The algorithm consists of several phases, which are indicated in the flow-chart in Fig. 2. The pseudocode of DART is given in Algorithm 1.

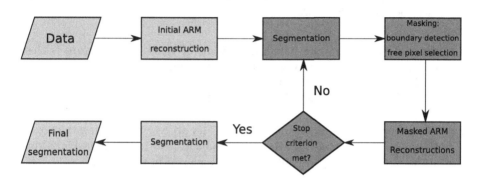

Fig. 2. Flow chart of the DART algorithm. The DART iteration activities are indicated in red and the initialization and post-segmentation activities are indicated in blue. (Color figure online)

Algorithm 1. DART

    Input: W, p, $\mathcal{R}$
1: $x^0 \leftarrow$ **Mask-ARM**$(W, p, 1_n, 0_n)$
2: **for** $k = 1$ to K **do**
3:     $y^k \leftarrow$ **Seg**$(x^k, \mathcal{R})$
4:     $M^k \leftarrow$ **Mask**(y^p)
5:     $x^k \leftarrow$ **Mask-ARM**(W, p, M^k, x^{k-1})
6: **Output:** $x^K, \mathbf{Seg}(x^K, \mathcal{R})$

Initialization. In the initialization phase, given the projection data p and the projection properties by means of W, an initial reconstruction x^0 is calculated using an Algebraic Reconstruction Method of choice (hereafter referred to as the ARM), for example ART, SART or SIRT [11]. With the initial reconstruction x^0 at hand, the main loop of the DART algorithm begins.

Segmentation. In this main loop, in iteration k the image x^{k-1} is segmented using a simple thresholding scheme, forming the image $y^k \in \mathcal{R}^n$, by computing for every voxel j the closest material attenuation value:

$$
\boldsymbol{y}_j^k =
\begin{cases}
\rho_1, & \boldsymbol{x}_j^{k-1} < \frac{1}{2}(\rho_1 + \rho_2) \\
\rho_2, & \frac{1}{2}(\rho_1 + \rho_2) \leq \boldsymbol{x}_j^{k-1} < \frac{1}{2}(\rho_2 + \rho_3) \\
\vdots & \\
\rho_m, & \frac{1}{2}(\rho_{m-1} + \rho_m) \leq \boldsymbol{x}_j^{k-1}
\end{cases}
\tag{9}
$$

$$
= \arg\min_{\rho \in \mathcal{R}} ||\boldsymbol{x}_j^{k-1} - \rho||_2. \tag{10}
$$

The second expression is easier to generalize to a higher-dimensional setting, which will be done in Sect. 3.2.

Boundary Detection and Masking. A set of voxels in the figure is then selected for a new reconstruction to refine the resulting image. First, the set $B^k \subset \{1, \ldots, n\}$ of boundary voxel indices is determined based on the segmentation. Various schemes can be applied for boundary detection. Additionally, a set $U^k \subset \{1, \ldots, n\}$ of free voxel indices is determined, where each voxel is included with a certain probability $1 - \beta$, with $0 \leq \beta \leq 1$. The process of selecting the voxels $U^k \cup B^k$ to be reconstructed and the voxels to be left out is called masking. Note that in the initialization phase all voxels are included in the mask.

Masked ARM Reconstructions. The set of free voxel indices $U^k \cup B^k$ are subjected to a new ARM reconstruction. This is done by computing the forward projection of the voxels $(\boldsymbol{y}_j^k)$ with $j \notin U^k \cup B^k$, and subtracting this from the input data $\boldsymbol{p}$ to obtain the residual sinogram $\overline{\boldsymbol{p}}^k$. The subproblem that has to be solved in this phase is:

$$
\overline{\boldsymbol{W}}^k \overline{\boldsymbol{x}}^k = \overline{\boldsymbol{p}}^k. \tag{11}
$$

In Eq. (11) matrix $\overline{\boldsymbol{W}}^k$ is defined by $\overline{\boldsymbol{W}}^k = (w_{ij})_{j \in U^k \cup B^k}$ and vector $\overline{\boldsymbol{x}}^k$ to be found has length $|U^k \cup B^k|$. Thus, the system of equations contains the same number of equations as Eq. (2) but has fewer unknowns. The system is solved using a fixed number of ARM iterations, taking the values of $(\boldsymbol{x}_j^{k-1})_{j \in U^k \cup B^k}$ as the starting condition. The complete reconstruction $\boldsymbol{x}^k$ at the end of iteration k is then formed by merging $\overline{\boldsymbol{x}}^k$ with $\boldsymbol{y}^k$.

Some DART implementations also include a smoothing step at this point. The entire loop is repeated a predefined number of times. After the loop ends, the image is segmented one more time. Note that the DART algorithm has many degrees of freedom. This includes the number of ARM iterations in the initialization phase, the number of DART iterations, the number of ARM iterations during these DART iterations, the fixing probability β, and possibly parameters in the smoothing operation. The quality of the reconstructions also depends on the tomographic setup, such as the number of projections and the number of projection angles, and on the complexity of the object, including the number of materials and different attenuation values. Despite the DART algorithm performing well in practice, it is a heuristic method for which no solution guarantees exist [3]. The DART algorithm is also highly modular. Approaches for segmentation, boundary detection, reconstruction (ARM) and possible smoothing can easily be changed without sacrificing the overall structure of the algorithm. For the multi-channel algorithm proposed in this paper the segmentation phase is adapted to using all multi-channel reconstructions as input.

The complexity of the framework depends on the algorithms that are used for reconstruction and segmentation. In this paper we use SIRT as the reconstruction algorithm and the thresholding segmentation as described above. Therefore, in this case, the DART algorithm has a time complexity of $O(Kn(m + l))$. The space complexity of our implementation is $O(ln)$.

3.2   Multi-channel DART

We now present the Multi-Channel DART (MC-DART) algorithm and outline its separate building blocks. Most focus will be on the multi-channel segmentation. Note that labeling single-channel images separately by attenuation values does not work here, since across multiple channels different materials can have the same attenuation. Therefore, there are some slight changes in the other blocks as well due to a new labeling mechanism. The algorithm structure is shown in the flow-chart in Fig. 3. The pseudocode of MC-DART is given in Algorithm 2.

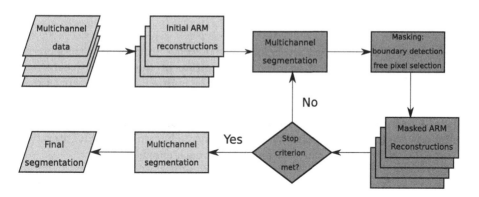

Fig. 3. Flow chart of the MC-DART algorithm. A stacked number of activities indicate that they are applied at different channels simultaneously.

Initialization. In the multi-channel setting we start out with a vector of projection data $\boldsymbol{P}$ at various channels and the matrix $\boldsymbol{W}$ as before. For each channel E_c a reconstruction $x^0_{E_c}$ is computed using the selected ARM. This results in C initial reconstructions for the MC-DART loop.

Multi-channel Segmentation. Given the reconstructions for all channels, similar to the DART segmentation, the multi-channel segmentation will determine a label image $\boldsymbol{y}^k \in \mathcal{M}^n$. Let $\boldsymbol{\mu}(s) = (\mu(s, E_1), \ldots, \mu(s, E_C)) \in \mathcal{R}_{E_1} \times$

Algorithm 2. MC-DART

    Input: W, $\mathcal{E}$, P, $\mathcal{R}$, $\mathcal{M}$, μ
1: for $c = 1$ to C do
2:    $x^0_{E_c} \leftarrow$ Mask-ARM$(W, p_{E_c}, 1_\mathrm{n}, 0_\mathrm{n})$
3: for $k = 1$ to K do
4:    $y^k \leftarrow$ MCSeg$(X^k, \mathcal{R}, \mathcal{M}, \mu)$
5:    $M^k \leftarrow$ Mask(y^k)
6:    for $c = 1$ to C do
7:        $x^k_{E_c} \leftarrow$ Mask-ARM$(W, p_{E_c}, M^k, x^{k-1}_{E_c})$
8: **Output:** X^K, MCSeg$(X^K, \mathcal{R}, \mathcal{M}, \mu)$

$\mathcal{R}_{E_2} \times \ldots \times \mathcal{R}_{E_C}$ be the vector of all attenuation values at each energy for material $s \in \mathcal{M}$, and let $X^k(\cdot, j) = (x^k_{j,E_1}, \ldots, x^k_{j,E_C})$ be the vector of all attenuation values of voxel j at each channel. We compute the segmented image by computing for each voxel $j \in \{1, \ldots, n\}$ the label using a basic thresholding scheme:

$$y^k_j = \arg\min_{s \in \mathcal{M}} ||X^k(\cdot, j) - \mu(s)||_2. \tag{12}$$

Essentially, this operation selects the material label for which the multidimensional difference between the material attenuation and voxel attenuations is smallest.

Masking and Boundary Detection. The masking works exactly the same as in the single-channel case. Given the segmentation y^k the masking produces a set $U^k \cup B^k$ of voxel indices to be included in the multi-channel reconstructions.

Multi-Channel Reconstructions. In the MC-DART algorithm the reconstructions are handled separately for each energy. Thus, in MC-DART iteration k the ARM is invoked C times to find $\overline{x}^k_{E_c}$ for each channel c in

$$\overline{W}^k \overline{x}^k_{E_c} = \overline{p}^k_{E_c}. \tag{13}$$

The resulting (merged) reconstructions are then given by $X^k := (x^k_{E_1}, \ldots, x^k_{E_C}) \in \mathbb{R}^{n \times C}$.

As with DART, the complexity of this framework depends on the reconstruction and segmentation methods that are chosen, as well as the extent of parallelization. If we use SIRT and the multi-channel segmentation method as described above and use a completely sequential implementation, the time complexity of MC-DART is $O(CKn(l + m))$. Because of the dependencies on the methods, we rather speak of a *relative complexity* of MC-DART to DART, which we define as the ratio of the sequential MC-DART complexity to that of DART, irrespective of the subroutines used. This relative time complexity is $O(C)$. The space complexity of this algorithm instance of MC-DART is $O(Cn)$, resulting in a relative space complexity of $O(C)$ as well.

4 Experimental Results

In this section the performance of the described MC-DART framework in terms of reconstruction and segmentation is presented. A series of experiments have been designed in which the number of channels C and different materials m are varied. For each experiment, multiple random phantoms are created. The size of these two-dimensional phantoms is 128×128 pixels, and each consists of a circular disk containing a random parcellation among m materials in such a way that the total surface is approximately equal for each material. An example of this random phantom is given in Fig. 1a, where $m = 3$. Given the number of materials and channels, random attenuation spectra are generated by assigning a random number $\mu(s, E_c) \sim \mathcal{U}(0,1)$ for each channel-material combination, where $s \in \{1, \ldots, m\}$ and $E_c \in \{E_1, \ldots, E_C\}$. With this way of generating spectra no dependencies between channels are established. Note that in most practical applications such dependencies do exist, as materials all have their own attenuation spectrum. For each phantom, reconstructions are made. The reference values for the tomographic setup and the parameter values of the MC-DART reconstruction algorithm for these reconstructions are summarized in Table 1. For multi-channel segmentation the method as described in Sect. 3.2 is used.

Table 1. Reference values for the parameters of the tomographic setup and the reconstructions algorithm for all experiments.

Parameter	Reference value
Angles	32 (equidistant)
ARM	SIRT
Start iterations	10
MC-DART iterations K	10
ARM iterations	10
Fix probability β	0.99

We vary the number of channels $C \in \{1, \ldots, 10\}$ and materials $m \in \{2, \ldots, 10\}$ independently. For each combination, a random phantom $\boldsymbol{y}_{\text{init}}$ is created, after which data $\boldsymbol{P}$ is generated by applying the forward projection as described in Sect. 2 on the phantom by applying μ and $\boldsymbol{W}$ on $\boldsymbol{y}_{\text{init}}$. In all experiments parallel-beam geometries are used and the detector size is 128 pixels. After this, the MC-DART algorithm as described in Sect. 3.2 is applied with $K = 10$ MC-DART iterations. The final segmentation is compared to the original phantom and the pixel error is computed, which is defined as the number of pixels in the final segmentation $\boldsymbol{y}^K$ that are labelled differently compared to the corresponding pixels in the original phantom $\boldsymbol{y}_{\text{init}}$. Only the pixels in the inner disk of the phantoms are taken into account. All experiments are repeated for and averaged over 100 runs with different phantoms.

The creation of random phantoms is implemented in MATLAB. The remainder of the experiment setup scripts are implemented in Python. The reconstruction algorithms, including the MC-DART algorithm, are implemented in Python, where the ASTRA Toolbox [2,15] is used to take care of the ARM invocations and forward projections, including the masking in each MC-DART iteration and the creation of matrices W and $\overline{W}^k$ based on the geometric properties.

Figure 4 shows the percentage of misclassified pixels with respect to the number of pixels in the inner disk. The percentage is lowest when the number of materials is low and the number of channels is high, while the percentage is highest when the number of channels is low and the number of materials is high. Given a number of channels, the percentage seems to scale logarithmically with the number of materials. On the other hand, given a number of materials, the percentage seems to scale exponentially with the number of channels for larger number of materials. Therefore, in this setup, the addition of only a few channels improves the reconstruction quality considerably. Figure 5 shows examples of the reconstructions at the corners of the curved plane of Fig. 4.

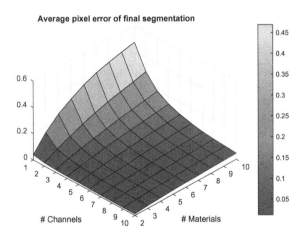

Fig. 4. Pixel error percentage for different number of material-channel combinations. (Color figure online)

We have investigated the effect of changing the parameters that are shown in Table 1. The number of starting iterations has no effect on the pixel error percentage curve. For these parameters, we found that increasing the number of MC-DART iterations further than 4 had no significant effect on the reconstructions. This threshold depends on the number of ARM iterations in each MC-DART iteration. Also, the quality of the reconstructions increases only marginally when β is increased. However, the pixel error percentage drops considerably as the number of ARM iterations during an MC-DART iteration increases. Also, when scanning data from many angles is available the reconstruction quality improvement with multiple materials become much better. For only 2 angles, the recon-

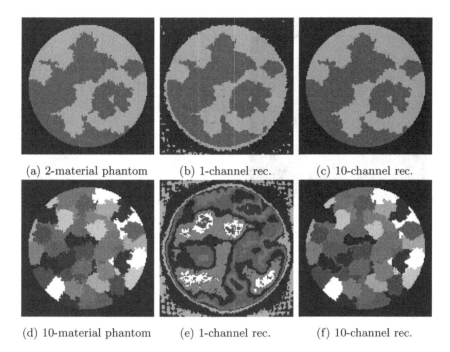

(a) 2-material phantom   (b) 1-channel rec.   (c) 10-channel rec.

(d) 10-material phantom   (e) 1-channel rec.   (f) 10-channel rec.

Fig. 5. Reconstructions for various setups. (a, d) Phantoms used with two and ten materials respectively. (b, e) Reconstructions using one channel. The mislabeled yellow pixels are because the attenuation of the yellow material is very close to zero. (c, f) Reconstructions using ten channels. (Color figure online)

struction between $C = 1$ and $C = 10$ channels improves from pixel error percentage 27% to 23% for two materials and from 55% to 41% for ten materials. In comparison, for as much as 128 angles the reconstructions between $C = 1$ and $C = 10$ channels improve by from 3% to less than 1% for two materials and from 46% to 4% for ten materials. We conclude that in all these cases the MC-DART algorithm gives better results when more channels are available.

Additionally, apart from the pixel error, we investigate how the number of assigned pixels per material class behave as the MC-DART reconstruction proceeds. The results are shown in Fig. 6. A random phantom with four different materials and background is used. The number of channels is set to $C = 10$, and for each channel c and material m a random attenuation value $\mu(s, E_c) \sim \mathcal{U}(0, 1)$ is generated. Then the MC-DART algorithm is applied to this phantom in two different experimental setups. In the first experiment, the number of MC-DART iterations is set to 10 and the number of ARM iterations per MC-DART iteration is set to 10. After each MC-DART iteration, the number of pixels assigned are calculated for each class. During the first four MC-DART iterations the number of assigned pixels is converging towards their real values. After this, the graphs enter an oscillatory phase in which for each class the number of assigned pixels

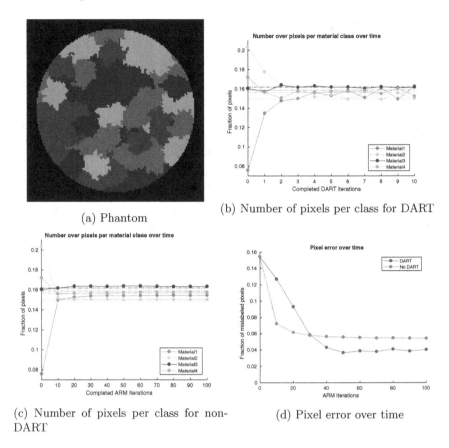

(a) Phantom

(b) Number of pixels per class for DART

(c) Number of pixels per class for non-DART

(d) Pixel error over time

Fig. 6. Convergence behavior for material classes with $C = 10$ channels. (a) Phantom that has been used with $m = 4$ materials (b) Graph showing the behavior for each material class in a DART routine for this phantom. The number of iterations for the initial reconstruction is set to 2, the number of DART iterations is 10, the number of ARM iterations is set to 10, the number of angles is 8, fixing probability is set to $\beta = 0.99$. The chosen ARM is SIRT. Shown are the number of pixels assigned per class during segmentation after each DART step, with the true value of these indicated by dashed lines. (c) Number of pixel assigned per class over number of ARM iterations. The number of DART iterations is 0, and instead we apply 100 ARM iterations with 2 initial iterations. The results are based on intermediate segmentations after each 10 ARM iterations, but these segmentations are not used in further iterations. Background pixels are excluded from the results (d) Pixel error over number of ARM iterations for both approaches. (Color figure online)

alternates between two values whose average is not necessary the real number of pixels for that class. For comparison, in the second experiment the same setup is used, but without using MC-DART iterations and applying the same ARM for 100 iterations instead. In this way the ARM is effectively invoked equally often.

After each 10 iterations a segmentation is made based on the current reconstruction and the pixels per class are measured, but no new forward projections are calculated from these segmentations and used in subsequent ARM iterations. In this case the number of pixels converges much more quickly for each class. Also, there is no oscillatory phase and the number of pixels are just as close to their true values as with the DART approach. However, plotting the total pixel error over time reveals that the pixel error in the non-DART case is higher. The pixel error for the MC-DART case needs more time to stabilize to its oscillatory phase, but the values are eventually lower than in the non-MC-DART case.

5 Conclusions

A new class of algorithms for solving discrete multi-channel reconstruction problems has been proposed. This framework uses the strength of DART regarding dealing with limited data in a multi-channel setting by using a multi-channel segmentation method. The experiments have shown that combining information from different channels by a multi-channel segmentation method increases the reconstruction quality compared to the single-channel DART algorithm. Therefore, we conclude that the MC-DART framework is a promising approach for dealing with multi-channel data.

6 Discussion

This paper presents the first steps to implement a multi-channel reconstruction technique using multi-channel segmentation. Currently, there are no standard approaches for the discrete multi-channel problem presented in Sect. 2. We propose a framework in which reconstruction and segmentation techniques can be exchanged. The modules in the framework can be adjusted to the problem to be solved. For instance, segmentation can be performed with neural network-based methods. The proposed method is not aimed at optimizing reconstructions with state-of-the-art ARMs or segmentation techniques but at presenting a framework to work with multi-channel data. If more data from different channels is available, this implementation outperforms DART but it does not mean that the problem is optimally solved. To further develop this technique and transfer it to real-world settings, real-data properties should be taken into account. These properties include the correlation of attenuation values between channels and noise contained in the projection data. In our study we only make use of the multi-channel data during segmentation. Another approach could be to use the multi-channel data during reconstruction, modeling the reconstruction problem as a large inverse problem where the unknowns are the material concentrations in each pixel (e.g. see [12, 16]). However, solving this problem is much more involved and the MC-DART framework presented in this paper provides a simple but effective alternative of separating materials using multi-channel data.

References

1. van Aarle, W., Batenburg, K.J., Sijbers, J.: Automatic parameter estimation for the discrete algebraic reconstruction technique (DART). IEEE Trans. Image Process. **21**(11), 4608–4621 (2012)
2. van Aarle, W., et al.: Fast and flexible X-ray tomography using the ASTRA toolbox. Opt. Express **24**(22), 25129–25147 (2016)
3. Batenburg, K.J., Fortes, W., Hajdu, L., Tijdeman, R.: Bounds on the quality of reconstructed images in binary tomography. Discret. Appl. Math. **161**(15), 2236–2251 (2013)
4. Batenburg, K.J., Sijbers, J.: DART: a fast heuristic algebraic reconstruction algorithm for discrete tomography. In: 2007 IEEE International Conference on Image Processing. ICIP 2007, vol. 4, pp. IV-133. IEEE (2007)
5. Batenburg, K.J., Sijbers, J.: DART: a practical reconstruction algorithm for discrete tomography. IEEE Trans. Image Process. **20**(9), 2542–2553 (2011)
6. Bleichrodt, F., Tabak, F., Batenburg, K.J.: SDART: an algorithm for discrete tomography from noisy projections. Comput. Vis. Image Underst. **129**, 63–74 (2014)
7. Buzug, T.M.: Computed Tomography: From Photon Statistics to Modern Cone-Beam CT. Springer, Heidelberg (2008). https://doi.org/10.1007/978-3-540-39408-2
8. Dabravolski, A., Batenburg, K.J., Sijbers, J.: A multiresolution approach to discrete tomography using DART. PloS one **9**(9), e106090 (2014)
9. Frank, J.: Electron Tomography. Springer, New York (1992). https://doi.org/10.1007/978-1-4757-2163-8
10. Hsieh, J., et al.: Computed Tomography: Principles, Design, Artifacts, and Recent Advances. SPIE, Bellingham (2009)
11. Kak, A.C., Slaney, M., Wang, G.: Principles of computerized tomographic imaging. Med. Phys. **29**(1), 107–107 (2002)
12. Kazantsev, D., Jørgensen, J.S., Andersen, M.S., Lionheart, W.R., Lee, P.D., Withers, P.J.: Joint image reconstruction method with correlative multi-channel prior for X-ray spectral computed tomography. Inverse Probl. **34**(6), 064001 (2018)
13. Maestre-Deusto, F.J., Scavello, G., Pizarro, J., Galindo, P.L.: Adart: an adaptive algebraic reconstruction algorithm for discrete tomography. IEEE Trans. Image Process. **20**(8), 2146–2152 (2011)
14. Midgley, P., Weyland, M.: 3D electron microscopy in the physical sciences: the development of Z-contrast and EFTEM tomography. Ultramicroscopy **96**(3–4), 413–431 (2003)
15. Palenstijn, W.J., Batenburg, K.J., Sijbers, J.: The ASTRA tomography toolbox. In: 13th International Conference on Computational and Mathematical Methods in Science and Engineering, CMMSE, vol. 2013, pp. 1139–1145 (2013)
16. Tairi, S., Anthoine, S., Morel, C., Boursier, Y.: Simultaneous reconstruction and separation in a spectral CT framework. In: Nuclear Science Symposium, Medical Imaging Conference and Room-Temperature Semiconductor Detector Workshop (NSS/MIC/RTSD), 2016, pp. 1–4. IEEE (2016)
17. Wilson, M., et al.: A 10 cm × 10 cm CdTe spectroscopic imaging detector based on the HEXITEC ASIC. J. Instrum. **10**(10), P10011 (2015)
18. Zhuge, X., Palenstijn, W.J., Batenburg, K.J.: TVR-DART: a more robust algorithm for discrete tomography from limited projection data with automated gray value estimation. IEEE Trans. Image Process. **25**(1), 455–468 (2016)

Evaluation of Chaos Game Representation for Comparison of DNA Sequences

André R. S. Marcal$^{(\boxtimes)}$ (iD)

Departamento de Matemática, Faculdade de Ciências, Universidade do Porto,
Porto, Portugal
`andre.marcal@fc.up.pt`
`http://www.fc.up.pt/pessoas/andre.marcal`

Abstract. Chaos Game Representation (CGR) of DNA sequences has been used for visual representation as well as alignment-free comparisons. CGR is considered to be of great value as the images obtained from parts of a genome present the same structure as those obtained for the whole genome. However, the robustness of the CGR method to compare DNA sequences obtained in a variety of scenarios is not yet fully demonstrated. This paper addresses this issue by presenting a method to evaluate the potential of CGR to distinguish various classes in a DNA dataset. Two indices are proposed for this purpose - a rejection rate (α) and an overlapping rate (β). The method was applied to 4 datasets, with between 31 to 400 classes each. Nearly 430 million pairs of DNA sequences were compared using the CGR.

Keywords: Chaos game representation · Discrete Fourier Transform
Fractals

1 Introduction

Comparison between DNA sequences of the same type from different organisms represents a subject of continuous interest for biology research [9]. As more and more genomes are being sequenced it has become possible to study evolutionary events by comparing whole genomes of closely related species and identifying differences [4].

A genetic DNA sequence can be treated formally as a string composed from the four letters 'A', 'C', 'G', and 'T', each corresponding to a nucleotide name adenine (A), cytosine (C), guanine (G) and thymine (T) [9]. Chaos Game Representation (CGR), proposed by Jeffrey [3], is a two-dimensional graphical representation of DNA sequences using iterated function systems [2]. CGR images of genetic DNA sequences originating from various species show rich fractal patterns [5,10]. CGR is particularly useful as images obtained from parts of a genome present the same structure as that of the whole genome [1]. However,

© Springer Nature Switzerland AG 2018
R. P. Barneva et al. (Eds.): IWCIA 2018, LNCS 11255, pp. 179–188, 2018.
https://doi.org/10.1007/978-3-030-05288-1_14

the robustness of the CGR method to compare DNA sequences obtained in a variety of scenarios is not yet fully demonstrated.

The goal of this paper is to present a methodology to evaluate the potential of CGR to distinguish between various classes in a DNA dataset. The following section of this paper includes a brief description of the CGR procedure, as well as a method for comparison of CGR sequences. The proposed method is presented in Sect. 3, followed by an experimental evaluation with 4 datasets (Sect. 4), and conclusions (Sect. 5).

2   Chaos Game Representation of a DNA Sequence

Consider a function f that maps the 4 elementary values of a DNA sequence, to 4 points in the complex plane, according to (1). The function domain is $D = \{A,C,G,T\}$.

$$f(x) = \begin{cases} 0 + 0i, & \text{if x = 'A'} \\ 0 + 1i, & \text{if x = 'C'} \\ 1 + 1i, & \text{if x = 'G'} \\ 1 + 0i, & \text{if x = 'T'} \end{cases} \tag{1}$$

A sequence $\mathbf{x}$, with N elements in D, is mapped to a sequence $\mathbf{z}$ with N elements in the complex domain C using (2), considering the initial position $z_0 = 0.5 + 0.5i$.

$$z_n = [z_{n-1} + f(x_n)]/2 \tag{2}$$

The values of z_n are contained in an open square in the complex plane, limited by the vertical lines $\text{Re}\{z\} = 0$ and $\text{Re}\{z\} = 1$, and the horizontal lines $\text{Im}\{z\} = 0$ and $\text{Im}\{z\} = 1$, where $\text{Re}\{z\}$ and $\text{Im}\{z\}$ are the real and imaginary components of a complex number z. The graphic representation of $\mathbf{z}$ results in a fractal image, with each of the 4 nucleotides associated with a corner in this square.

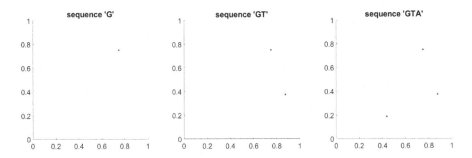

Fig. 1. CGR of very small sequences: 'G' (left), 'GT' (center) and 'GTA' (right).

A very simple case is presented next to clarify the process of converting a DNA sequence to the complex domain, using the CGR approach. Consider a sequence **x** with only 3 elements, **x** = 'GTA'. The computation of the first element (z_1) of the CGR of this sequence is presented in (3), using (2) and considering that $f(x_1) = f('G') = 1 + i$ (1). The location of z_1 is the midpoint between the center of the square (z_0) and the top right corner, which is the corner associated with the nucleotide G, as it can be seen in the graphical representation in Fig. 1 (left).

$$z_1 = [z_0 + f(x_1)]/2 = (0.5 + 0.5i + 1 + i)/2 = 0.75 + 0.75i \qquad (3)$$

A similar approach is used to compute z_2 ($0.875 + 0.375i$), from z_1, and then z_3 ($0.4375 + 0.1875i$). The location of z_2 is the midpoint between z_1 and the bottom right corner (T), and z_3 is the midpoint between z_2 and the bottom left corner (A), shown in Fig. 1 (center and right).

For longer DNA sequences the fractal nature of the images produced by the CGR is clearly noticeable. An example for 3 DNA sequences of mammals (Gorilla, Leopard, and Blue Whale [2]) is presented in Fig. 2. In [7] the CGR images of 10 different species of mammalian chromosomes DNA sequences are presented. Although some visual interpretations are possible [1], a quantitative approach is required to compare CGR of DNA sequences.

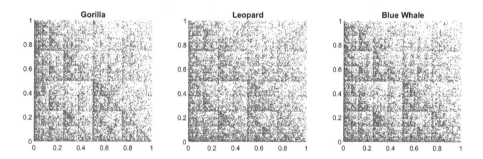

Fig. 2. CGR of 3 DNA sequences of mammals Gorilla, Leopard, and Blue Whale [2].

2.1   Comparison of Sequences in CGR

The comparison of two DNA sequences in the CGR is performed in the frequency domain, using the Discrete Fourier Transform (DFT). The DFT of a sequence **z** is computed using (4), resulting in a sequence **f** with the same number of elements of **z** [6].

$$f_k = \sum_{n=0}^{N-1} z_n e^{-2\pi kn/N} \qquad (4)$$

The distance d_{AB} between two sequences z_A and z_B is computed as the Euclidean distance between the power spectra of their DFT (f_A and f_B), excluding the constant component (f_0) [2]. In order to perform this task, the original sequences need to have the same length, which is accomplished by extending the shortest one with zeros.

As an illustration, the power spectrum (f^2) of the 3 DNA sequences of mammals is presented in Fig. 3. The distance between these sequences are: $d_{GW} = 7.98$, $d_{LW} = 8.38$, $d_{GL} = 8.81$ (x10^5). In this case the shortest distance is between Gorilla and Blue Whale.

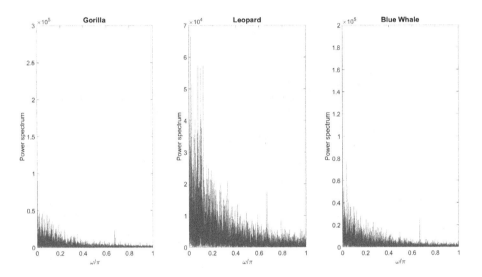

Fig. 3. Power spectrum of the DNA sequence CGR for Gorilla, Leopard and Blue Whale.

3   Methodology

Let us consider a set of DNA sequences of N classes, with S observations for each class (e.g. different species). These observations can be obtained from different individuals of the same class or, as an alternative, as different sub-sequences of the complete DNA sequence available in the dataset. This latter approach uses sub-sequences with slightly smaller length than the complete DNA sequence, which, for a robust representation, should be enough to characterize the class.

For a given distance, or metric, it is expected that sequences corresponding to the same class should be more similar to each other than those representing different classes. In an ideal case, the distance (d_{kl}) between any two sequences (k,l) of a given class (C_i) is smaller than the distance between any pair formed with one sequence from Ci and one sequence from another class (C_j), Eq. (5).

$$\forall k, l \in C_i, \forall m \neq k \in C_j, d_{kl} < d_{km} \tag{5}$$

However, it often happens that a pair of sequences from different classes have a lower distance than a pair of sequences from the same class. This can occur due to a variety of reasons, such as noise, insufficient length of the DNA sequences, differences in the regions covered in the DNA profiles, similarity between classes/species, etc.

3.1   Evaluation Strategy

The strategy proposed to evaluate a DNA sequence comparison methodology and dataset considers all pairs of species (classes) separately. For a set of DNA sequences with N classes, the number of pairs of classes (M) is $N(N-1)/2$.

For a given class pair, with S observation per class, there are $S(S-1)$ internal pairs of sequences, where both belong to the same class, and S^2 external pairs, where the two sequences belong to different classes. The distances between all pairs of sequences are computed, using the CGR approach, and grouped in internal (d^{int}) and external (d^{ext}) distances.

The total number of pairs of sequences compared (T) is obtained by Eq. (6), for a set of DNA sequences with N classes and S observations per class.

$$T = N(N-1)S(S-1)/2 \tag{6}$$

3.2   Evaluation Indices

Two indices are proposed to evaluate the potential to distinguish between the various classes in a dataset - a rejection rate (α) and an overlapping rate (β).

Rejection Rate (α). Each class pair is evaluated according to the maximum internal distance (d_{max}^{int}) and minimum external distance (d_{min}^{ext}). The class pair is rejected if $d_{max}^{int} > d_{min}^{ext}$, as a classification experiment could group two sequences from different classes before all pairs of sequences from the same class are paired. The rejection rate (α) is computed as the ratio between the number of class pairs rejected (M_r) and the total number of class pairs (M) - $\alpha = M_r/M$.

Overlapping Rate (β). A less restrictive approach is to perform the evaluation on a sequence pair basis. For a class pair, the distances $(d_{i,j})$ between all pairs of sequences (i,j) are computed using the CGR approach. The values of d_{max}^{int} and d_{min}^{ext} are established. The pairs of sequences from the same class with $d_{i,j} > d_{min}^{ext}$ are rejected, as well as the pairs of sequences from different classes with $d_{i,j} < d_{max}^{int}$. The safety region is thus established by d_{min}^{ext} for internal pairs $(d < d_{min}^{ext})$, and by d_{max}^{int} for external pairs $(d > d_{max}^{int})$. The overlapping rate (β) is computed as the ratio between the number of pairs rejected and the total number of pairs tested.

A slightly more favorable version for an overlapping rate (not used here) is to focus on each sequence individually. For a sequence i, an internal pairing (with sequence j from the same class) is considered valid if its distance $(d_{i,j})$ is smaller that all external distances computed for that sequence $(d_{i,k}$, for all k in the pairing class). This alternative overlapping rate is computed as the ratio between the number of non-valid internal pairs and the total number of internal pairs tested. It is worth noting that the sequence pair i,j needs to be evaluated separately from the pair j,i. Although the internal distances are the same $(d_{i,j} = d_{j,i})$, the corresponding external distances $(d_{i,k}$ and $d_{j,k})$ are not.

4   Results

4.1   Test Dataset

The experimental evaluation was made using 4 sets of DNA sequences provided by [2] - Mammals, Influenza, HRV and HPV. More details for the HRV dataset are available in [8], and for the HPV dataset in [11].

A summary of the characteristics of the DNA sequence datasets used is presented in Table 1, together with some experimental parameters. The number of species in each dataset varies from 31 (Mammals) to 400 (HPV), which correspond to between 465 (Mammals) to 79800 (HPV) pairs of species within a dataset. The lengths (L) of the DNA sequences are shortest in the Influenza dataset (1406 elements on average), and longest in the Mammals dataset (16696 elements on average).

Table 1. Characteristics and experimental parameters of the DNA sequence sets.

Sequence set	# classes	Average L	Min, max L	# class pairs	# runs	# pairs tested
Mammals	31	16696	16338,17447	465	10	4.2×10^6
Influenza	38	1406	1350,1467	703	10	6.3×10^6
HRV	116	7154	6944,7458	6670	10	60×10^6
HPV	400	7914	7814,10424	79800	5	359×10^6

4.2   Simplified Illustrative Case

A reduced experiment was carried out to illustrate in more detail the evaluation process. The following parameters were used: 4 classes (first 4 classes from the Influenza dataset), 5 sub-sequences extracted with lengths between 0.997 and 0.998 of the original size, 3 runs (repetitions). Some of the results obtained are presented in Table 2.

Each line in Table 2 corresponds to one run comparing two classes (I and II), with 5 sub-sequences extracted randomly from each class. These sub-sequences are used to compute 20 internal distances (d^{int}) and 25 external distances (d^{ext}). The table presents the average values $(<d^{int}>$ and $<d^{ext}>)$, the maximum internal distance (d^{int}_{max}) and minimum external distance (d^{ext}_{min}). For the class pair 1–2, $d_{max}^{int} < d_{min}^{ext}$ for all 3 repetitions carried out (lines 1 to 3 in Table 2). The same happens for all class pairs tested, except for the class pair 2–3, where $d_{max}^{int} > d_{min}^{ext}$ in 2 out of the 3 runs. The rejection rate (α) is thus $\alpha = 0.1111 = 2/18$ (2 rejected runs out of 18). The overlapping rate (β) is lower, $\beta = 0.0568 = 46/(45 * 18)$, as only 46 of the 135 pairs tested for the class pair 2–3 overlapped the safety region.

Table 2. Results from the reduced experiment with only 4 classes.

Class I	Class II	run #	$<d^{int}>$	d_{max}^{int}	d_{min}^{ext}	$<d^{ext}>$
1	2	1	1.4018	2.5169	10.479	10.813
1	2	2	1.2684	2.6650	10.290	10.606
1	2	3	1.6076	3.4362	10.324	10.516
1	3	1	1.7101	4.9201	10.519	10.688
1	3	2	1.7975	4.8891	10.498	10.721
1	3	3	2.1327	5.1003	10.481	10.841
1	4	1	3.1194	5.1055	13.204	13.954
1	4	2	1.5156	4.1469	13.006	13.758
1	4	3	3.0931	5.2504	13.367	13.989
2	3	1	2.1930	4.3070	3.2610	4.1491
2	3	2	1.0854	2.8174	3.8234	4.2078
2	3	3	2.1094	4.9513	3.1223	4.3344
2	4	1	3.4137	6.0912	13.200	14.217
2	4	2	3.4545	6.1764	13.106	14.161
2	4	3	2.1349	4.0524	13.763	14.214
3	4	1	3.2971	5.5625	14.152	15.054
3	4	2	4.2445	8.4573	13.682	15.033
3	4	3	4.5572	8.3713	13.692	15.184

It is worth noting that the lengths of the 4 DNA sequences used for this experiment are rather short, from 1398 to 1433 elements, so the sub-sequences extracted have in fact only 3 or 4 elements less than the original versions.

4.3   Full Dataset Evaluation

The 4 available DNA sequence datasets were evaluated separately. The experimental parameters are summarized in Table 1.

For each class pair (two species), 5 sub-sequences with a random length between L_{min} and L_{max} are extracted, with the values L_{min} and L_{max} referring to the ratio to the full length sequence (L). The initial position of a sub-sequence is also assigned randomly. The sub-sequences are then used to compute 20 internal distances (d^{int}) and 25 external distances (d^{ext}), and a procedure similar to that described for the reduced experiment is performed. The number of runs (repetitions) for each class pair is 10, except for dataset HPV with only 5 runs per class pair (due to the much larger number of class pairs in HPV).

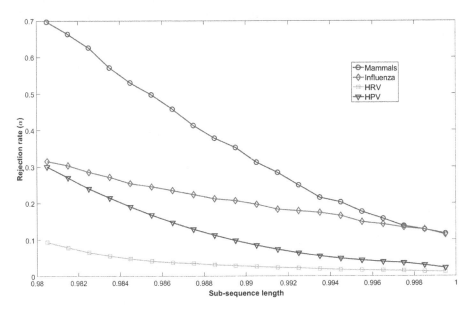

Fig. 4. Rejection rate (α) for the 4 DNA datasets, as a function of the sub-sequence length.

The experiment was repeated 20 times for each dataset, with different values of L_{min} and L_{max} (0.980 to 1.000, with $L_{max} - L_{min} = 0.001$ and increments of 0.001). The results are presented in Fig. 4 (rejection rate, α) and 5 (overlapping rate, β). The sub-sequence length displayed in the x-axis of these plots is mid point in the interval of lengths possible: $(L_{min} + L_{max})/2$. As expected, the values of β are consistently lower than the values of α, both decreasing as the sub-sequence length increases.

The highest values for both indices and for all sub-sequence lengths tested occur for the "Mammals" dataset, which has the longest average sequence length but the lowest number of classes. The dataset with second highest values is "Influenza", which has the DNA sequences with shortest lengths. The lowest values for both indices (α and β) occur for the HRV dataset, which has more than 3 times the number of classes than both the "Mammals" and "Influenza" datasets. These results suggest that the most relevant aspect is not the number of classes or the length of the original DNA sequences, but the actual similarity between the classes being compared.

Focusing on the overlapping rate (β), the values for the HRV dataset are rather low throughout. For sub-sequences of 99% or more of the original length, less than 1% of the internal pairs are more dissimilar than an external pair. On

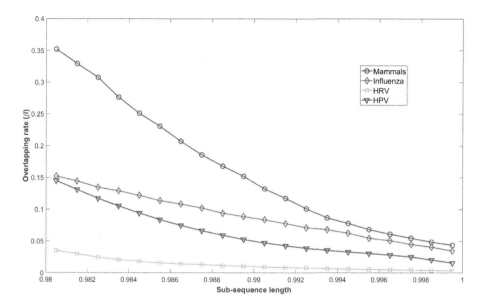

Fig. 5. Overlapping rate (β) for the 4 DNA datasets, as a function of the sub-sequence length.

the contrary, the "Mammals" dataset has high values of β, with 4.3% of the internal pairings being invalid, for sub-sequences of 99.9% of the original length. The value increases steadily as the sub-sequence length decreases, reaching a value of 35.2% for sub-sequences of 98% of their original length.

The results presented in Figs. 4 and 5 were produced from the comparison of a total of 429.6 million pairs of sequences, using the CGR approach. The number of pairs of sequences analyzed ranges from 4.2 millions ($465 \times 45 \times 10 \times 20$) for the Mammals dataset, to 359 millions for the HPV dataset (Table 1).

5   Conclusions

It can be concluded that although there is some robustness in comparing DNA sequences using CGR, the process is clearly dependent on the sub-sequence length and location within the original sequence. The high values of the rejection (α) and overlapping (β) rates obtained for the experiment with the "Mammals" dataset, with only 31 classes, clearly demonstrates this point. For other datasets, such as the HRV dataset with 116 classes, the values obtained were much more favorable. The ability to distinguish between classes in a DNA dataset depends not only on the length and location of the sub-sequence, but most importantly also on the similarity between the classes being compared.

The methodology proposed, including the indices α and β, can be used to evaluate different sets of DNA sequences. As the DNA sequences available are always pieces of the whole genome, the method can be used to evaluate the potential impact of the sub-sequence extracted on derived information such as matching, hierarchical structuring and other forms of grouping the data. The same methodology can be used, with slight modifications, to evaluate the impact of noise on the recognition and comparison of DNA sequences using the CGR approach.

References

1. Deschavanne, P.J., Giron, A., Vilain, J., Fagot, G., Fertil, B.: Genomic signature: characterization and classification of species assessed by chaos game representation of sequences. Mol. Biol. Evol. **16**(10), 1391–1399 (1999)
2. Hoang, T., Yin, C., Yau, S.S.T.: Numerical encoding of DNA sequences by chaos game representation with application in similarity comparison. Genomics **108**, 134–142 (2016)
3. Jeffrey, H.J.: Chaos game representation of gene structure. Nucleic Acids Res. **18**, 2163–2170 (1990)
4. Joseph, J., Sasikumar, R.: Chaos game representation for comparison of whole genomes. BMC Bioinform. **7**, 243 (2006)
5. Kari, L., et al.: Mapping the space of genomic signatures. PLoS ONE **10**(5), e0119815 (2015)
6. Mitra, S.K.: Digital Signal Processing: A Computer-Based Approach, 4th edn. McGraw-Hill, New York (2011)
7. Ni, H.M., Qi, D.W., Mu, H.B.: Applying MSSIM combined chaos game representation to genome sequences analysis. Genomics **110**(3), 180–190 (2018)
8. Palmenberg, A.C., et al.: Sequencing and analyses of all known human rhinovirus genomes reveal structure and evolution. Science **324**, 55–59 (2009)
9. Stan, C., Cristescu, C.P., Scarlat, E.I.: Similarity analysis for DNA sequences based on chaos game representation. Case study: the albumin. J. Theoret. Biol. **267**, 513–518 (2010)
10. Stepanyan, I.V., Petoukhov, S.V.: The matrix method of representation, analysis and classification of long genetic sequences. Information **8**(1), 12 (2017)
11. Tanchotsrinon, W., Lursinsap, C., Poovorawan, Y.: A high performance prediction of HPV genotypes by chaos game representation and singular value decomposition. BMC Bioinform. **16**, 71 (2015)

Image-Based Object Spoofing Detection

Valter Costa[1,2(✉)] [iD], Armando Sousa[1,3] [iD], and Ana Reis[1,2] [iD]

[1] FEUP - Faculty of Engineering of the University of Porto,
Rua Dr. Roberto Frias s/n Porto, Porto, Portugal
ee09115@gmail.com

[2] INEGI - Institute of Science and Innovation in Mechanical and Industrial
Engineering, Campus da FEUP, Rua Dr. Roberto Frias 400 Porto, Porto, Portugal

[3] INESC TEC - INESC Technology and Science (formerly INESC Porto),
Campus da FEUP, Rua Dr. Roberto Frias Edifício I, Porto, Portugal

Abstract. Using 2D images in authentication systems raises the question of spoof attacks: is it possible to deceive an authentication system using fake models possessing identical visual properties of the genuine one? In this work, an anti-spoofing method approach for a wine anti-counterfeiting system is presented. The proposed method relies in two different color spaces: CIE L*u*v* and YC_rC_b, to distinguish between a genuine instance and a spoof attack. To evaluate the proposed strategy, two databases were used: a private database, with photos/2D attacks of cork stoppers, created for this work; and the public Replay-Attack database that is used for face spoofing detection methods testing. The results on the private database show that the anti-spoofing approach is able to distinguish with high accuracy a real photo from an attack. Regarding the public database, the results were obtained with existing methods, as the best HTER results using a single frame approach.

Keywords: Replay-attack database · Cork-Print-Attack Database
Spoofing detection · Face spoofing detection · Object spoofing detection

1 Introduction

In biometric-based authentication systems, the challenge of discriminating between a genuine subject and a spoof attack has been a hard task to tackle. Face recognition systems are an example of a biometric-based authentication systems vulnerable to spoof attacks. In this context, two types of attacks can be identified: (i) 2D attacks, including print and videos attacks characterized by the use of a printed photo or a recorded video from an authorized person; (ii) 3D attacks, described by the usage of a mask from an authorized person. This work focuses on the detection of 2D spoofing attacks for a different application. An image-based wine anti-counterfeiting system has been proposed in previous work [16]. In that work, each wine bottle is individually recognized using a photo of the cork stopper. As in face recognition systems, a problem of circumventing

R. P. Barneva et al. (Eds.): IWCIA 2018, LNCS 11255, pp. 189–201, 2018.
https://doi.org/10.1007/978-3-030-05288-1_15

the authentication system using a fake replica possessing identical visual features arises. To overcome this issue, an anti-spoofing approach based on color space transformations (YC_rC_b and CIE L*u*v*) is proposed. The anti-spoofing method was tested in a private database – Cork-Print-Attack database – built in the context of this work. This database includes photos of cork stoppers and photos of printed images of cork stoppers. To test the generalization of the proposed method for spoofing detection and be able to compare the results with other researchers' works, a public database named Replay-Attack [13] from Idiap Research Institute was used. This database comprises over 1300 video clips of photo/video attacks and real access for face spoofing detection. In order to perform a fair comparison with other works on the public database, only static methods were considered (a detailed explanation defining a static method can be found in Sect. 4). The main contributions of this work are:

- Proposing a 2D spoofing detection strategy for a wine anti-counterfeiting system;
- Finding that CIE L*u*v* color space provides valuable information for spoofing detection (to the best knowledge of the authors, this is the first work that uses this conversion in the context of spoofing detection);
- Achieving a HTER of 0.59% in the Replay-Attack database, which is the best reported result using a static approach.

The remainder of this paper is organized as follows: background work is presented in Sect. 2; Sect. 3 details the proposed approach for spoofing detection; the results and discussion are shown in Sect. 4; finally, Sect. 5 draws the conclusions for this work.

2   Related Work

Since no references were found regarding object spoofing detection, this section presents some works for face spoofing detection using a single frame approach. The methods considered in this review are based on generic features (non specific characteristics of the face). To identify a spoof attack, some researchers [13,15,20,33] have used LBP – Local Binary Patterns – by assuming that the texture a 2D spoof attack is different from a real attempt. Other approach is the usage of different color space/models. Some methods successfully tested on public databases can be found in [10–12,31]. A different approach is the evaluation of the image quality, referenced in the literature as image quality measures. Galbally and Marcel proposed a face anti-spoofing method, by combining 14 different image quality measures [23]. Wen et al. used specular reflection, blurriness, chromatic moment and color diversity to distinguish a real access from a spoof attack [17]. Alotaibi and Mahmood used a non-linear diffusion method based on anisotropic diffusion to identify an attack attempt [3]. In the context of face spoofing detection, several strategies have been proposed. Regarding object spoofing detection, no references were found. In the next section, a method for object spoofing detection is presented.

3   Proposed Approach

This work focuses on the problem of detecting a printed attack of a previously registered cork in the RIOTA recognition system [16], analogous to face spoofing attacks in face recognition systems (e.g., circumvention of face recognition systems using attacks with printed or video materials of authorized persons). As mentioned in the related work, several researchers have used color-based approaches for face spoofing detection. In spite of the RGB color space being the most used in video acquisition and display devices, according to Li et al. [31], it is not the most suitable color space to detect spoofing attacks, due to the correlation between red, green and blue that obstruct the separation between the luminance and chrominance information. The anti-spoofing scheme proposed in this work takes advantage of the use of two different color spaces: YC_rC_b and CIE L*u*v*, see Fig. 1. For each input frame or image in the RGB color space, a conversion to YC_rC_b and CIE L*u*v* is made. Then, 6 histograms are calculated, corresponding to each component of these two color spaces. Next, the six histograms are concatenated into a Feature Vector $FV = (Y, C_r, C_b, L, u, v)$ of size 1536 (six normalized histograms in the range of 0–255) that serve as input for the Extra Trees Classifier - ETC. Finally, the classifier decides if the input feature vector corresponds to an image of a genuine sample or it is a spoofing attack.

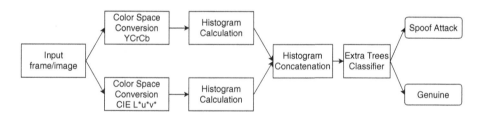

Fig. 1. Flowchart of the proposed anti-spoofing scheme.

The proposed approach is based on the idea that since two images of the same object (one of the real object and another of an attack; see Fig. 2) have different visual features, this information may be represented through its corresponding color histograms. Other works [11,12,22,31,35] demonstrated the effectiveness of combining different color spaces followed by a texture descriptor to detect a face spoof attack. In this work, only the histograms of YC_rC_b and CIE L*u*v* color spaces are used to train a classifier and identify an image spoof attack. The concept of this approach came from observing some regular distinctions in the YC_rC_b and CIE L*u*v* color histograms between two images (an image of a genuine sample and a printed attack) from the same cork stopper, as shown in Fig. 3. It can be seen that the luminance information in both color spaces has almost "regular shape" in the genuine photos (which does not happen in the print attack images); regarding the chrominance histograms, the "regular shape"

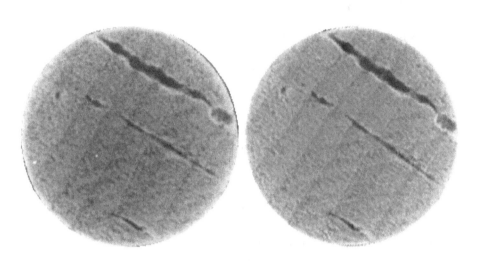

Fig. 2. Images of cork stopper examples: (left) an image of a printed cork stopper; (right) an image of a genuine cork stopper.

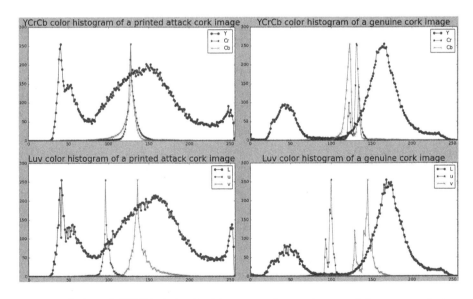

Fig. 3. YC_rC_b and CIE L*u*v* color histograms for two images of the same cork stopper: (left) column histograms of a printed attack cork image; (right) column histograms of a genuine cork image.

appears in the images from the print attacks. This behavior was detected in some pair image samples, which formulated the hypothesis of this work: is there enough information in the YC_rC_b and CIE L*u*v* color histograms to train a classifier to distinguish between an image of a genuine cork and a printed attack?

3.1   L*u*v* Color Space

The CIE L*u*v* color space was introduced by the International Commission on Illumination (also known as CIE from its French title, the Commission Internationale de l'Eclairage) in 1976 [9]. The RGB conversion to CIE L*u*v* is described in Eqs. (1), (2) and (3). Equations (4), (5) and (6) are intermediate steps and normalizations needed for this color space conversion.

$$L \leftarrow \begin{cases} 116 * \sqrt[3]{Y} & for \quad Y > 0.008856 \\ 903.3 * Y & for \quad Y \leq 0.008856 \end{cases} \tag{1}$$

$$u \leftarrow 13 \times L \times (u' - u_n) \quad where \quad u_n = 0.19793943 \tag{2}$$

$$v \leftarrow 13 \times L \times (v' - v_n) \quad where \quad v_n = 0.46831096 \tag{3}$$

$$u' \leftarrow 4 \times \frac{X}{X + 15 \times Y + 3 \times Z} \tag{4}$$

$$v' \leftarrow 9 \times \frac{X}{X + 15 \times Y + 3 \times Z} \tag{5}$$

$$\begin{bmatrix} X \\ Y \\ Z \end{bmatrix} \leftarrow \begin{bmatrix} 0.412453 & 0.357580 & 0.180423 \\ 0.212671 & 0.715160 & 0.072169 \\ 0.019334 & 0.119193 & 0.950227 \end{bmatrix} \cdot \begin{bmatrix} R \\ G \\ B \end{bmatrix} \tag{6}$$

To convert the L, u and v in a 8-bit image, these components need to be normalized. As such, $L \leftarrow 255 \times L/100$, $u \leftarrow 255/(354 \times (u + 134))$ and $v \leftarrow 255/(262 \times (v + 140))$.

3.2 YC_rC_b Color Space

This model is mostly used in compression for TV transmission and was defined by ITU - International Telecommunication Union in ITU-R BT.601 standard [27]. Y corresponds to the luminance or luma component obtained from RGB after gamma correction, C_r signifies how far the red component is from luma and C_b denotes how far the blue component is from luma.

$$Y \leftarrow 0.299 \times R + 0.587 \times G + 0.114 \times B \tag{7}$$

$$C_r \leftarrow (R - Y) \times 0.713 + \delta \tag{8}$$

$$C_b \leftarrow (B - Y) \times 0.564 + \delta \tag{9}$$

For 8-bit image representation $\delta = 128$.

To facilitate the development process[1], two public libraries were used: OpenCV[2] and scikit-learn[3] [39].

4   Performance Evaluation

The evaluation of the proposed anti-spoofing method is reported in this section. First, it presents the metrics used for the evaluation. Then, it gives details about the databases used in the tests. Next, it presents the results and compares the work with other researchers' works found in the literature. Finally, it discusses the results obtained.

4.1   Evaluation Metrics

The evaluation metric used in this work is the HTER - Half Total Error Rate [4], see Eq. (10). HTER is the mean value between the FAR - False Acceptance Rate, Eq. (11) and FRR - False Rejection Rate, Eq. (12). The effectiveness of an attack is measured by FAR. Analogously, FRR relates to the measure of a system to reject genuine instances.

$$HTER(\%) = \frac{FAR + FRR}{2} * 100 \tag{10}$$

$$FAR = \frac{FP}{FP + TN} \tag{11}$$

$$FRR = \frac{FN}{TP + FN} \tag{12}$$

In an ideal spoofing detection system, both FAR and FRR should be 0. Another metric commonly used to evaluate a biometric system is the EER - Equal Error Rate. This error rate is obtained at the threshold that provides the same FAR and FRR.

4.2   Cork-Print-Attack Database

The Cork-Print-Attack database was conceived to test and gauge the anti-spoofing method proposed in this work. It comprises 2200 photos from 200 cork stoppers, see Table 1. The photos were captured using 4 different smartphone rear cameras. Two types of paper were used to reproduce the visual aspect of a cork stopper: (i) photo paper, and (ii) printer paper. Two different printers were also used. The printed attacks have the correct correspondence in the genuine set and were printed at the same scale of the genuine sample. The diameter of the corks used ranges from 19 mm to 23.5 mm.

---

[1] The source code of this work is available at: https://github.com/ee09115/spoofing_detection.

[2] https://opencv.org/.

[3] http://scikit-learn.org/stable/index.html.

Table 1. Cork-print-attack database characterization.

Genuine			Print		
ID	#Photos	Camera	ID	#Photos	Camera
④	300	Xperia Z1 compact	①	300	Xperia Z3 compact
⑤	200	Xperia Z1 compact	②	300	Xperia Z3 compact
⑥	200	Xperia SP	③	300	Xperia Z1 compact
⑦	300	Asus Zenfone 2	⑧	100	Asus Zenfone 2
⑨	100	Asus Zenfone 2	⑩	100	Xperia Z3 compact

Table 2. Photos division of the cork-print-attack database into three distinct folds: training set, development set and testing set.

Train		Devel		Test	
#Photos	ID	#Photos	ID	#Photos	ID
200	①	100	①	100	⑨
200	②	100	②	100	⑩
200	③	100	③	-	-
200	④	100	④	-	-
100	⑤	100	⑤	-	-
100	⑥	100	⑥	-	-
200	⑦	100	⑦	-	-
-	-	100	⑧	-	-

The 2200 photos were divided in three different folds: training set, development set and testing set. The distribution of the photos is shown in Table 2. The corks stoppers used in the training and developments folds are not present in the testing set (in other words, there are no overlapping photos between the training/development sets and the test set).

4.3   Replay-Attack Database

The Replay-Attack database[4] consists of 1300 video clips of photo and video attacks recorded under different lightning conditions of 50 clients [13]. These clips are divided in four different folds: (i) training set – comprising 60 videos of real-accesses and 300 video attacks; (ii) development set – containing 60 videos of real-accesses and 300 attack videos; (iii) testing set – consisting of 80 videos of real-accesses and 400 attack videos; and (iv) enrollment set – including 100 videos of real-accesses. According to the protocol defined for this database, the train set is used to train the classifier, the development set is used to calibrate

---

[4] https://www.idiap.ch/dataset/replayattack.

the threshold (at the EER – Equal Error Rate point), and the testing set should be used to report the results of the proposed anti-spoofing approach.

4.4 Results

This subsection presents the results achieved exploring the private and public database. Table 3 presents the results obtained exploring the Cork-Print-Attack database.

Table 3. HTER on Cork-Print-Attack database.

Cork-print-attack database results		
Method	EER(%)	HTER (%)
	Dev	Test
Proposed approach: YC_rC_b+Luv+ETC	1.5	**2.5**

The results reached with the Replay-Attack database are exhibited in Table 4.

The authors would like to clarify that the HTER results in Table 4 only refer to static methods (i.e., methods using only a single image to detect spoof attack). When comparing to methods based on liveness detection and/or the use of time windows, there are some methods yielding better results than the proposed approach, like in [21,24,34,45,46] and some works achieving worse HTER results, such as in [7,8,22,26,30,37,38,42,51]. Naturally, these kind of methods cannot be applied in the cork-print-attack database because cork is a non-living organism and all the information available is a single image.

4.5 Discussion

The results presented in Table 3 suggest that the proposed cork spoofing detection approach is adequate for the wine anti-counterfeiting system. The tests on the private database were performed without embedding the spoofing detection approach in the wine anti-counterfeiting system. Since the wine authentication system relies on the match of local feature descriptors and not all of the print attacks are recognized as genuine, when incorporating this method in the wine authentication system, the FAR will most likely decrease. As such, the overall HTER will probably drop as well.

Regarding the Replay-Attack database, the results demonstrate that the combination of YC_rC_b and CIE L*u*v* is capable of challenging the state-of-art methods specifically designed for face spoofing detection. To enhance the performance, a texture descriptor may be used after the color space conversion. Some authors have exposed the gains of using a texture descriptor as in [11,12,22,31,35].

Table 4. HTER on Replay-Attack database.

Replay-attack database results		
Method	EER(%) Dev	HTER (%) Test
Radiometric transforms [19]	-	0.8
DEND-CLUSTERING-ensemble [1]	-	5.0
MAXDIST-ensemble [1]	-	5.0
CTMF [50]	-	4.4
Unicamp [14]	9.83	15.62
ATVS [14]	0.83	12.00
MUVIS [14]	0.00	1.25
PRA Lab [14]	0.00	1.25
Client specific MsLBP [28]	-	1.45
Client specific HOG [28]	-	3.58
Client specific LBP-TOP+SVM [15]	-	3.95
LBP+SVM [33]	-	13.87
LBP_{3x3}^{u2}+SVM [13]	14.84	15.16
HSV-YC_bC_r+C-SURF+PCA [10]	0.1	2.2
IQA+LDA [23]	-	15.2
CNN [2]	-	10
CNN [36]	-	0.75
CNN [25]	-	4.74
Radiometric transforms [18]	-	2.75
Kernel fusion (MBSIF-TOP+MLPQ-TOP) [5]	1.67	1.00
DPCNN [32]	-	4.3
LBP+DoG+HOG+IQA [20]	1.6	1.0
Multiscale (HSV+YC_bC_r)+SVM [12]	-	3.1
LSP+SVM [49]	13.72	12.50
IDA+SVM [17]	-	7.41
HSV+YC_bC_r+SVM [11]	-	2.8
YC_bC_r+HSV+SVM [31]	-	2.9
Non-linear Diffusion+CNN [3]	-	10
LBP + GS-LBP [41]	0.17	3.13
Color texture CNN + SVM [51]	0.1	0.9
CTMF [50]	4.0	4.4
CNN [6]	0.79	0.72
FDL-270 [44]	5.92	5.21
Skin blood flow + SVM [48]	-	4.92
FASNet [29]	-	1.2
ResNet-50[47]	1.16	1.28
GIF + IQA [40]	1.02	1.31
LiveNet [43]	7.68	5.74
Proposed approach: YC_rC_b+Luv+ETC	0.074	**0.59**

5   Conclusions

This work presented an anti-spoofing method based on two different color space transforms and histograms calculation using a single image for a wine anti-counterfeiting system. The results showed that the combination of YC_rC_b and CIE L*u*v have proved to be a reliable choice for cork spoofing detection. To test how good the proposed method can generalize, a public database named Replay-Attack database was used. The results achieved on the public database are able to compete with the state-of-art results. Moreover, using a single image/frame approach the reported HTER is the lowest found in the literature. Finally, the results confirm the hypothesis raised in this work: the combination of YC_rC_b and CIE L*u*v* color histograms provide enough discrimination for image spoofing detection applications.

Acknowledgments. Authors gratefully acknowledge the funding of Project NORTE-01-0145-FEDER-000022 - SciTech - Science and Technology for Competitive and Sustainable Industries, co-financed by Programa Operacional Regional do Norte (NORTE2020), through Fundo Europeu de Desenvolvimento Regional (FEDER).

References

1. Akhtar, Z., Foresti, G.L.: Face spoof attack recognition using discriminative image patches. J. Electr. Comput. Eng. 1–14 (2016). http://www.hindawi.com/journals/jece/2016/4721849/
2. Alotaibi, A., Mahmood, A.: Enhancing computer vision to detect face spoofing attack utilizing a single frame from a replay video attack using deep learning. In: 2016 International Conference on Optoelectronics and Image Processing (ICOIP), pp. 1–5. IEEE (2016). http://ieeexplore.ieee.org/document/7528488/
3. Alotaibi, A., Mahmood, A.: Deep face liveness detection based on nonlinear diffusion using convolution neural network. Signal Image Video Process. **11**(4), 713–720 (2017). https://doi.org/10.1007/s11760-016-1014-2
4. Anjos, A., Marcel, S.: Counter-measures to photo attacks in face recognition: a public database and a baseline. In: 2011 International Joint Conference on Biometrics (IJCB), pp. 1–7. IEEE (2011). http://ieeexplore.ieee.org/document/6117503/
5. Arashloo, S.R., Kittler, J., Christmas, W.: Face spoofing detection based on multiple descriptor fusion using multiscale dynamic binarized statistical image features. IEEE Trans. Inf. Forensics Secur. **10**(11), 2396–2407 (2015). http://ieeexplore.ieee.org/document/7163625/
6. Atoum, Y., Liu, Y., Jourabloo, A., Liu, X.: Face anti-spoofing using patch and depth-based CNNs. In: 2017 IEEE International Joint Conference on Biometrics (IJCB), pp. 319–328. IEEE (2017). http://ieeexplore.ieee.org/document/8272713/
7. Benlamoudi, A., Aiadi, K.E., Ouafi, A., Samai, D., Oussalah, M.: Face antispoofing based on frame difference and multilevel representation. J. Electron. Imaging **26**(4), 043007 (2017). https://doi.org/10.1117/1.JEI.26.4.043007
8. Bharadwaj, S., Dhamecha, T.I., Vatsa, M., Singh, R.: Computationally efficient face spoofing detection with motion magnification. In: 2013 IEEE Conference on Computer Vision and Pattern Recognition Workshops, pp. 105–110. IEEE (2013). http://ieeexplore.ieee.org/document/6595861/

9. Billmeyer, F.W.: Color Science: Concepts and Methods, Quantitative Data and Formulae, 2nd ed., by Gunter Wyszecki and W. S. Stiles, John Wiley and Sons, New York, 1982, 950 pp. Price: $75.00. Color Res. Appl. **8**(4), 262–263 (1983). https://doi.org/10.1002/col.5080080421

10. Boulkenafet, Z., Komulainen, J., Hadid, A.: Face anti-spoofing using speeded-up robust features and fisher vector encoding. IEEE Signal Process. Lett. 1 (2016). http://ieeexplore.ieee.org/document/7748511/

11. Boulkenafet, Z., Komulainen, J., Hadid, A.: Face spoofing detection using colour texture analysis. IEEE Trans. Inf. Forensics Secur. **11**(8), 1818–1830 (2016). http://ieeexplore.ieee.org/document/7454730/

12. Boulkenafet, Z., Komulainen, J., Xiaoyi Feng, Hadid, A.: Scale space texture analysis for face anti-spoofing. In: 2016 International Conference on Biometrics (ICB), pp. 1–6. IEEE (2016). http://ieeexplore.ieee.org/document/7550078/

13. Chingovska, I., Anjos, A., Marcel, S.: On the effectiveness of local binary patterns in face anti-spoofing. In: 2012 BIOSIG - Proceedings of the International Conference of Biometrics Special Interest Group (BIOSIG), pp. 1–7 (2012)

14. Chingovska, I., et al.: The 2nd competition on counter measures to 2D face spoofing attacks. In: 2013 International Conference on Biometrics (ICB), pp. 1–6. IEEE (2013). http://ieeexplore.ieee.org/document/6613026/

15. Chingovska, I., dos Anjos, A.R.: On the use of client identity information for face antispoofing. IEEE Trans. Inf. Forensics Secur. **10**(4), 787–796 (2015). http://ieeexplore.ieee.org/document/7031941/

16. Costa, V., Sousa, A., Reis, A.: Preventing wine counterfeiting by individual cork stopper recognition using image processing technologies. J. Imaging **4**(4), 54 (2018). http://www.mdpi.com/2313-433X/4/4/54

17. Wen, D., Han, H., Jain, A.K.: Face spoof detection with image distortion analysis. IEEE Trans. Inf. Forensics Secur. **10**(4), 746–761 (2015). http://ieeexplore.ieee.org/document/7031384/

18. Edmunds, T., Caplier, A.: Fake face detection based on radiometric distortions. In: 2016 Sixth International Conference on Image Processing Theory, Tools and Applications (IPTA), pp. 1–6. IEEE (2016). http://ieeexplore.ieee.org/document/7820995/

19. Edmunds, T., Caplier, A.: Face spoofing detection based on colour distortions. IET Biom. **7**(1), 27–38 (2018). http://digital-library.theiet.org/content/journals/10.1049/iet-bmt.2017.0077

20. Farmanbar, M., Toygar, Ö.: Spoof detection on face and palmprint biometrics. Signal Image Video Process. **11**(7), 1253–1260 (2017). https://doi.org/10.1007/s11760-017-1082-y

21. Feng, L., et al.: Integration of image quality and motion cues for face anti-spoofing: a neural network approach. J. Vis. Commun. Image Represent. **38**, 451–460 (2016). http://linkinghub.elsevier.com/retrieve/pii/S1047320316300244

22. de Freitas Pereira, T., et al.: Face liveness detection using dynamic texture. EURASIP J. Image Video Process. **2014**(1), 2 (2014). https://jivp-eurasipjournals.springeropen.com/articles/10.1186/1687-5281-2014-2

23. Galbally, J., Marcel, S.: Face anti-spoofing based on general image quality assessment. In: 2014 22nd International Conference on Pattern Recognition, pp. 1173–1178. IEEE (2014). http://ieeexplore.ieee.org/document/6976921/

24. Gan, J., Li, S., Zhai, Y., Liu, C.: 3D convolutional neural network based on face anti-spoofing. In: 2017 2nd International Conference on Multimedia and Image Processing (ICMIP), pp. 1–5. IEEE (2017). http://ieeexplore.ieee.org/document/8221060/

25. Gragnaniello, D., Sansone, C., Poggi, G., Verdoliva, L.: Biometric spoofing detection by a domain-aware convolutional neural network. In: 2016 12th International Conference on Signal-Image Technology and Internet-Based Systems (SITIS), pp. 193–198. IEEE (2016). http://ieeexplore.ieee.org/document/7907465/

26. Kim, I., Ahn, J.., Kim,D.: Face spoofing detection with highlight removal effect and distortions. In: 2016 IEEE International Conference on Systems, Man, and Cybernetics (SMC), pp. 004299–004304. IEEE (2016). http://ieeexplore.ieee.org/document/7844907/

27. ITU: ITU-R Recommendation BT.601-5: Studio encoding parameters of digital television for standard 4:3 and wide-screen 16:9 aspect ratios. Technical report, ITU, Geneva, Switzerland (1995)

28. Yang, J., Lei, Z., Yi, D., Li, S.Z.: Person-specific face antispoofing with subject domain adaptation. IEEE Trans. Inf. Forensics Secur. **10**(4), 797–809 (2015). http://ieeexplore.ieee.org/document/7041231/

29. Karray, F., Campilho, A., Cheriet, F. (eds.): Image Analysis and Recognition. LNCS, vol. 10317. Springer, Cham (2017). https://doi.org/10.1007/978-3-319-59876-5

30. Komulainen, J., Hadid, A., Pietikainen, M., Anjos, A., Marcel, S.: Complementary countermeasures for detecting scenic face spoofing attacks. In: 2013 International Conference on Biometrics (ICB), pp. 1–7. IEEE (2013). http://ieeexplore.ieee.org/document/6612968/

31. Li, L., Correia, P.L., Hadid, A.: Face recognition under spoofing attacks: countermeasures and research directions. IET Biom. **7**(1), 3–14 (2018). http://digital-library.theiet.org/content/journals/10.1049/iet-bmt.2017.0089

32. Li, L., Feng, X., Boulkenafet, Z., Xia, Z., Li, M., Hadid, A.: An original face antispoofing approach using partial convolutional neural network. In: 2016 Sixth International Conference on Image Processing Theory, Tools and Applications (IPTA), pp. 1–6. IEEE (2016). http://ieeexplore.ieee.org/document/7821013/

33. Maatta, J., Hadid, A., Pietikainen, M.: Face spoofing detection from single images using micro-texture analysis. In: 2011 International Joint Conference on Biometrics (IJCB). pp. 1–7. IEEE (2011). http://ieeexplore.ieee.org/document/6117510/

34. Manjani, I., Tariyal, S., Vatsa, M., Singh, R., Majumdar, A.: Detecting silicone mask-based presentation attack via deep dictionary learning. IEEE Trans. Inf. Forensics Secur. **12**(7), 1713–1723 (2017). http://ieeexplore.ieee.org/document/7867821/

35. Määttä, J., Hadid, A., Pietikäinen, M.: Face spoofing detection from single images using texture and local shape analysis. IET Biom. **1**(1), 3 (2012). http://digital-library.theiet.org/content/journals/10.1049/iet-bmt.2011.0009

36. Menotti, D., et al.: Deep Representations for iris, face, and fingerprint spoofing detection. IEEE Trans. Inf. Forensics Secur. **10**(4), 864–879 (2015). http://ieeexplore.ieee.org/document/7029061/

37. Asim, M., Ming, Z., Javed, M.Y.: CNN based spatio-temporal feature extraction for face anti-spoofing. In: 2017 2nd International Conference on Image, Vision and Computing (ICIVC), pp. 234–238. IEEE (2017). http://ieeexplore.ieee.org/document/7984552/

38. Pan, S., Deravi, F.: Facial action units for presentation attack detection. In: 2017 Seventh International Conference on Emerging Security Technologies (EST), pp. 62–67. IEEE (2017). http://ieeexplore.ieee.org/document/8090400/

39. Pedregosa, F., et al.: Scikit-learn: machine learning in Python. J. Mach. Learn. Res. **12**, 2825–2830 (2011)

40. Peng, F., Qin, L., Long, M.: POSTER: non-intrusive face spoofing detection based on guided filtering and image quality analysis. In: Deng, R., Weng, J., Ren, K., Yegneswaran, V. (eds.) SecureComm 2016. LNICST, vol. 198, pp. 774–777. Springer, Cham (2017). https://doi.org/10.1007/978-3-319-59608-2_49

41. Peng, F., Qin, L., Long, M.: Face presentation attack detection using guided scale texture. Multimed. Tools Appl. **77**(7), 8883–8909 (2018). https://doi.org/10.1007/s11042-017-4780-0

42. Pinto, A., Pedrini, H., Schwartz, W.R., Rocha, A.: Face spoofing detection through visual codebooks of spectral temporal cubes. IEEE Trans. Image Process. **24**(12), 4726–4740 (2015). http://ieeexplore.ieee.org/document/7185398/

43. Rehman, Y.A.U., Po, L.M., Liu, M.: LiveNet: Improving features generalization for face liveness detection using convolution neural networks. Expert Syst. Appl. **108**, 159–169 (2018). http://linkinghub.elsevier.com/retrieve/pii/S0957417418302811

44. Stuchi, J.A., et al.: Improving image classification with frequency domain layers for feature extraction. In: 2017 IEEE 27th International Workshop on Machine Learning for Signal Processing (MLSP), pp. 1–6. IEEE (2017). http://ieeexplore.ieee.org/document/8168168/

45. Tian, Y., Xiang, S.: Detection of video-based face spoofing using LBP and multiscale DCT. In: Shi, Y.Q., Kim, H.J., Perez-Gonzalez, F., Liu, F. (eds.) IWDW 2016. LNCS, vol. 10082, pp. 16–28. Springer, Cham (2017). https://doi.org/10.1007/978-3-319-53465-7_2

46. Tirunagari, S., Poh, N., Windridge, D., Iorliam, A., Suki, N., Ho, A.T.S.: Detection of face spoofing using visual dynamics. IEEE Trans. Inf. Forensics Secur. **10**(4), 762–777 (2015). http://ieeexplore.ieee.org/document/7047832/

47. Tu, X., Fang, Y.: Ultra-deep neural network for face anti-spoofing. In: Liu, D., Xie, S., Li, Y., Zhao, D., El-Alfy, E.S. (eds.) Neural Information Processing, vol. 10635, pp. 686–695. Springer, Cham (2017). https://doi.org/10.1007/978-3-319-70096-0_70

48. Wang, S.Y., Yang, S.H., Chen, Y.P., Huang, J.W.: Face liveness detection based on skin blood flow analysis. Symmetry **9**(12), 305 (2017). http://www.mdpi.com/2073-8994/9/12/305

49. Kim, W., Suh, S., Han, J.-J.: Face liveness detection from a single image via diffusion speed model. IEEE Trans. Image Process. **24**(8), 2456–2465 (2015). http://ieeexplore.ieee.org/document/7084662/

50. Zhang, L.B., Peng, F., Qin, L., Long, M.: Face spoofing detection based on color texture markov feature and support vector machine recursive feature elimination. J. Vis. Commun. Image Represent. **51**, 56–69 (2018). http://linkinghub.elsevier.com/retrieve/pii/S1047320318300014

51. Zhao, X., Lin, Y., Heikkila, J.: Dynamic texture recognition using volume local binary count patterns with an application to 2D face spoofing detection. IEEE Trans. Multimed. **20**(3), 552–566 (2018). http://ieeexplore.ieee.org/document/8030131/

Improvement of Measurement Accuracy of Optical 3D Scanners by Discrete Systematic Error Estimation

Christian Bräuer-Burchardt[1]([✉]), Peter Kühmstedt[1],
and Gunther Notni[1,2]

[1] Fraunhofer Institute for Applied Optics and Precision Engineering,
07745 Jena, Germany
christian.braeuer-burchardt@iof.fraunhofer.de
[2] Technical University Ilmenau, 98693 Ilmenau, Germany

Abstract. A new methodology is introduced which enables the improvement of measurement accuracy of optical 3D scanners. This improvement is based on geometric compensation of the systematic measurement error over the measurement volume. Possible sources for systematic measurement errors are introduced and discussed. Estimation of the systematic error is performed by determination of length measurement error of a ballbar in different positions in the measurement volume. Description of the systematic error may be done using polynomials or sampling points in an equidistant volumetric grid. Simulations as well as experimental measurements using real data were performed in order to evaluate the new methodology. The results show that a reduction of the systematic error to about half of the original error is possible. The method is discussed, and potential improvements are given as prospective future work.

Keywords: Computer vision · 3D reconstruction · Image analysis
Optical 3D scanner

1 Introduction

Contactless 3D reconstruction of objects is a sophisticated task in many applied fields such as industrial quality control, inspection tasks, rapid prototyping, medical diagnosis and surgery planning, architecture, arts and cultural heritage preservation, scientific research, forensics, and archaeology and paleontology. Additionally, there are also applications of 3D reconstruction under water, e.g., at volume determination of fish, digitization of sunken shipwrecks, or archaeological sites at the sea ground. Recently, applications that are also considering the temporal course of the 3D data of the observed object have gained importance. Such examples are object or person tracking, gesture detection and interpretation, and highly dynamic process supervision, e.g., car crash tests or documentation of airbag unfolding. Special 3D scanning devices have been developed for each of these applications. Besides, scanning systems based on ultrasound technology, laser scanning, or X-radiation, photogrammetric 3D scanners in conjunction with or without structured light illumination, etc., are a common class of devices for solving such tasks.

© Springer Nature Switzerland AG 2018
R. P. Barneva et al. (Eds.): IWCIA 2018, LNCS 11255, pp. 202–215, 2018.
https://doi.org/10.1007/978-3-030-05288-1_16

Structured light projection technique is a common method for contactless 3D reconstruction with a high accuracy potential. However, certain developments require a very high accuracy level. Here, a classical dilemma occurs. Random errors cannot be prevented but may be reduced by averaging. Systematic errors, however, determine the quality of the measurement system, and can be compensated if known. However, the problem is that systematic errors of photogrammetric 3D scanners are usually unknown.

The objective of this work was to develop a method for the estimation of the systematic measurement error of 3D scanning devices based on structured light projection technique and stereo camera observation. This method should be practically applicable for arbitrary optical 3D scanners based on structured light projection technique.

First, the state of the art in this topic is described. Then, the approach for the developed methodology is outlined. A simulation tool is described, which helps to evaluate the proposed method. Experiments are described and the results are discussed. After the summary, an outlook to future work is given.

2 State-of-the-Art

The compensation of systematic errors is a typical matter of different kinds of measurement techniques. Here, a lot of theoretic work has been done in the past. Error compensation methods have been developed also for 3D measurement systems, for example, for CT devices [16], laser-scanning systems [8, 12], or time-of-flight cameras (ToF) [7]. Kahlmann and Ingensand [10] proposed a method for range imaging cameras, especially for use in geodesy.

However, determination of measurement errors of photogrammetric 3D scanners with or without structured light illumination has not been performed very carefully in the past. Often, measurement accuracy is characterized by a certain value, which typically describes the measurement noise. However, this is not sufficient for a quality characterization of a scanning device. Hence, the "Verein Deutscher Ingenieure" developed certain guidelines for such devices [15]. These guidelines provide a helpful tool for the quality characterization of 3D scanners using structured light illumination. However, a systematic error determination can be performed only partly.

Several works can be found concerning calibration evaluation in the literature. Gu et al. performed calibration accuracy evaluation and compared two calibration methods [5]. Remondino and Fraser performed an analysis and comparison of calibration methods for off-the-shelf digital cameras [13]. Rieke-Zapp et al. analyzed the geometric stability and the accuracy potential of digital cameras by comparing mechanical stabilization and parameterization [14]. In a former work we performed systematic error compensation by sensor re-calibration [2]. Hastedt and Luhmann analyzed the quality of camera calibration using OpenCV [6]. Luhmann et al. gave an overview of camera calibration methods for close-range photogrammetry including calibration accuracy considerations [11].

Methods for geometric correction of 3D scanners based on photogrammetric stereo with or without structured light illumination after calibration improvement are not thoroughly studied. One reason is the high entire accuracy contingent on the measurement principle of such scanners. Additionally, the estimation of the systematic measurement error is not superficial and connected with high effort. In this work, we try to give a promising approach.

3 Approach

3.1 Error Treatment

Systematic and Random Measurement Errors. Before the new method is presented, some consideration concerning error analysis should be done. When a 3D object is measured, points will be captured on the surface of the object. The measurement error of each point is the deviation of the measured point to its true position in the world coordinate system. However, this true position is usually not known and even not determinable. In order to estimate the measurement error, certain characteristic parameters such as sphere-spacing error and flatness measurement error [15] have been defined. These parameters describe the systematic measurement error, whereas random error is characterized by the so-called noise of the measured 3D points.

In [9], the measurement error is defined as the difference of the measured quantity minus a reference quantity value, where a reference quantity value for a systematic measurement error is a true quantity value, or a measured quantity value of a measurement standard of negligible measurement uncertainty, or a conventional quantity value.

The systematic measurement error is a component of the measurement error that remains constant in repeated measurements or varies in a predictable manner. The random error is the component of the measurement error that varies in an unpredictable manner in repeated measurements [9].

For more definitions and notifications concerning errors in measurement technique, see, e.g., [1] or [9].

Systematic error estimation by sphere-spacing error (SSE) and flatness measurement error (FE) according to the VDI/VDE guidelines [15], however, is only an average case systematic error estimation. Worst-case error may be considerably higher. Additionally, SSE and FE tell something about the amount of the systematic error, but not about the actual error at a certain measurement position.

The idea of our new methodology is to estimate the systematic error depending on the position in the well-defined measurement volume, and consequently, subtraction of the determined systematic error from the 3D measurement values.

Error Sources. The most elegant way to improve measurement accuracy would be the prevention of error. However, this is almost impossible. In particular, the following error sources cannot prevented.

Photonic noise of the pixels of the image sensor is a random error source. This typically Poisson-distributed (approximately normally distributed) random error can only be reduced by averaging. Correspondence errors are also random and can occur due to different origins (image artifacts, reflections, and others) and have typically an uncertain distribution.

Origins of systematic errors are mainly inaccurate calibration and the deviation of the true camera ray geometry from the selected model description. The first error can be reduced by using of an expensively performed well-selected calibration procedure. The second error can be reduced only by selection of a more suitable camera model, which is closer to the reality. This may be, for example, the ray-based camera model instead of the pinhole camera model.

3.2 Global Error Compensation Approach

Because error prevention may be too complex or impossible, the global approach for error compensation should be the locally dependent estimation of the systematic measurement error in the measurement volume (MV). Let the MV be defined as a polyhedral region in the usual 3D world coordinate system (WCS) where the measurement objects (MO) are placed in and the scanner captures the 3D data of the MO. It is assumed that when measuring an object point at a certain position in the MV, always the same systematic measurement error occurs. This error should be determined and subsequently compensated.

Compensation should performed by application of a correction function in MV describing the systematic error depending on the three-dimensional position coordinates in the MV. The task is to find this correction function.

Representation of the correction function can be either continuous or discrete. In the second case, a number of well-distributed sampling points should be placed in the MV, preferably at equidistant points of a 3D grid. Additionally, an interpolation function is necessary for all points between the grid points.

3.3 New Methodology

Situation. Let the following situation be given. The considered device is a calibrated stereo camera-based 3D scanner supported by structured light illumination of the scene. A well-defined polyhedral measurement volume (MV) characterizes the valid three-dimensional measurement points. For simplification, the MV can described by a cuboid, but a frustum of a pyramid would be closer to the scanner's field of view. Our approach is the description of the systematic error as a 3D function f in the MV. The description may be realized by a polynomial in three variables or by a finite set of sampling points and a function, which realizes interpolation and extrapolation between the sampling points.

The approach of the new methodology can outlined as follows:

- Measurements of certain specimen(s) which allow the exact determination of a systematic error relative to a reference object
- Estimation of the systematic errors at many well distributed positions in the MV
- Construction of the error function f
- Subtraction of the systematic error from the 3D coordinates of the measurement values using f

The proposed specimens for the error estimation are ballbars with different distances between the center-points of the spheres as also proposed by the VDI/VDE guidelines [15]. The measurements of the specimens, however, are performed in a different way to [15] in order to get more information concerning the position of the occurring error (see Sect. 4). An exemplary specimen is shown in Fig. 1.

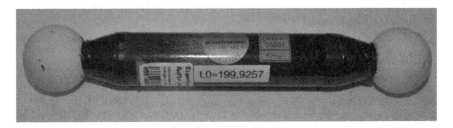

Fig. 1. Ballbar as specimen for systematic error determination

Construction of Systematic Error Functions. The general approach is the description of the systematic error in the MV. This can done, e.g., by a polynomial in three variables (the coordinate axis of the WCS). However, construction of such a polynomial with degree of at least three leads to numerous coefficients, namely 60 at degree three:

$$(\Delta x, \Delta y, \Delta z) = f(x, y, z) \text{ with}$$
$$\Delta x = a_1 x^3 + a_2 y^3 + a_3 z^3 + a_4 x^2 y + a_5 x^2 z + a_6 xy^2 + a_7 xz^2 + a_8 xyz + a_9 y^2 z + a_{10} yz^2$$
$$+ a_{11} x^2 + a_{12} y^2 + a_{13} z^2 + a_{14} xy + a_{15} xz + a_{16} yz + a_{17} x + a_{18} y + a_{19} z + a_{20}$$
$$\Delta y = b_1 x^3 + b_2 y^3 + b_3 z^3 + b_4 x^2 y + b_5 x^2 z + b_6 xy^2 + b_7 xz^2 + b_8 xyz + b_9 y^2 z + b_{10} yz^2$$
$$+ b_{11} x^2 + b_{12} y^2 + b_{13} z^2 + b_{14} xy + b_{15} xz + b_{16} yz + b_{17} x + b_{18} y + b_{19} z + b_{20}$$
$$\Delta z = c_1 x^3 + c_2 y^3 + c_3 z^3 + c_4 x^2 y + c_5 x^2 z + c_6 xy^2 + c_7 xz^2 + c_8 xyz + c_9 y^2 z + c_{10} yz^2$$
$$+ c_{11} x^2 + c_{12} y^2 + c_{13} z^2 + c_{14} xy + c_{15} xz + c_{16} yz + c_{17} x + c_{18} y + c_{19} z + c_{20}.$$
$$(1)$$

Unfortunately, the shape of the error function is usually unknown. This can mean that higher degree of polynomial is necessary and certain coefficients of the polynomial are vanishing. In order to analyze this, considerable effort is necessary. Restriction to certain coefficients may be useful, e.g., according to the following formula:

$$(\Delta x, \Delta y, \Delta z) = f(x, y, z) \text{ with}$$
$$\Delta x = a_1 x^3 + a_2 xy^2 + a_3 xz + a_4 x + a_5 y + a_6 z$$
$$\Delta y = b_1 y^3 + b_2 x^2 y + b_3 yz + b_4 x + b_5 y + b_6 z \qquad (2)$$
$$\Delta z = c_1 z^3 + c_2 x^2 + c_3 y^2 + c_4 x + c_5 y + c_6 z$$

with re-numbered coefficients (a_4 becomes a_2, a_7 becomes a_3, ...). Selection of the certain coefficients was done intuitively, but after visual inspection of real error data. However, this requires a kind of idea or assumption regarding the occurring systematic error. As we will see later, looking at the experimental data, the presence and absence of certain coefficients can be guessed by looking at error maps. Granted, this is a very heuristic strategy, but sometimes successful.

A second approach to the error function is the representation by sampling points and a suitable interpolation and extrapolation of the error function between the sampling points. The constant distance between neighboring sampling grid points and the interpolation function should be found "by instinct".

Method Description. As already mentioned, the idea of the new methodology is to find the distribution of the systematic error in the MV. A valid calibration of the scanner is assumed. First, the measurement volume is defined by a polyhedron in the WCS. A three-dimensional grid of sampling points in the MV together with an interpolation function for points of the MV being no sampling point or, alternatively, a continuous error function f in MV (by a polynomial in three variables) is defined.

Although ballbars with different distances between the spheres may be useful, the approach uses measurements of one ballbar only. The idea is to place the ballbar in as many orientations in the MV as possible.

The methodology (including variants V1 and V2) can be outlined as follows:

Part A: error function determination

- Measurements of ballbar length errors (ΔL) at as many positions of the spheres as possible
- Splitting of the length error (ΔL) into two vectors (Δv_1, Δv_2) of equal length with opposite orientation, allocated to the two positions of the spheres (center-points) – according to formula (4) with deliberate equal distribution of the error to both positions
- Storing the error vectors (Δv_1, Δv_2) or using (Δv_1, Δv_2) for estimation and averaging of the error at neighboring sampling points
- Variant V1: Estimation of the error polynomial f, or, alternatively
- Variant V2: Definition of the interpolation error function g

Part B: error compensation

- Performing measurement
- Correction of every measurement point $p_i = (x, y, z)_i$ by subtraction of error function f or g, respectively: $p'_i = p_i - f(p_i)$, (V1) or $p'_i = p_i - g(p_i)$, (V2)

The error function f can be found by estimation of the 18 polynomial coefficients $a_1, a_2, \ldots, c_6$ of Eq. (2) using three separated optimization tasks S_x, S_y, and S_z according to

$$S_x = \frac{\sum_{i=1}^{n} (a_1(x_i - \Delta x_i)^3 + a_2(x_i - \Delta x_i)(y_i - \Delta y_i)^2 + a_3(x_i - \Delta x_i)(z_i - \Delta z_i) +}{a_4(x_i - \Delta x_i) + a_5(x_i - \Delta x_i) + a_6(x_i - \Delta x_i))^2 \rightarrow min}$$

$$S_y = \frac{\sum_{i=1}^{n} (b_1(y_i - \Delta y_i)^3 + b_2(y_i - \Delta y_i)(x_i - \Delta x_i)^2 + b_3(y_i - \Delta y_i)(z_i - \Delta z_i) +}{b_4(y_i - \Delta y_i) + b_5(y_i - \Delta y_i) + b_6(y_i - \Delta y_i))^2 \rightarrow min} \quad (3)$$

$$S_z = \frac{\sum_{i=1}^{n} (c_1(z_i - \Delta z_i)^3 + c_2(x_i - \Delta x_i)^2 + c_3(y_i - \Delta y_i)^2 + c_4(x_i - \Delta x_i) +}{c_5(y_i - \Delta y_i) + c_6(z_i - \Delta z_i))^2 \rightarrow min}$$

which should be resolved by a suitable optimization algorithm [4]. Here, n is the double number of ballbar measurements.

Alternative error function g can be defined as follows. We distinguish between the error values at the predefined grid points $g(p_{gi})$ and the interpolated error values $g(p_i)$ at arbitrary positions (p_i) in the MV. For determination of g we use the observations of the ball positions (p_j) and the measured length error ΔL between two ball positions (p_{j1}) and (p_{j2}). The $\Delta v(p_i) = (\Delta x, \Delta y, \Delta z)_i$ with set $\Delta v(p_{j2}) = -\Delta v(p_{j1})$ are obtained by:

$$\begin{aligned}
\Delta x_1 &= (x_2 - x_1)\Delta L/2L_{ref}; \Delta x_2 = -\Delta x_1 \\
\Delta y_1 &= (y_2 - y_1)\Delta L/2L_{ref}; \Delta y_2 = -\Delta y_1 \\
\Delta z_1 &= (z_2 - z_1)\Delta L/2L_{ref}; \Delta z_2 = -\Delta z_1
\end{aligned} \quad (4)$$

Error function at the grid points is defined as:

$$g(p_{gi}) = k_c \frac{\sum_{i=1}^{n} w_i \Delta v_i}{\sum_{i=1}^{n} w_i} \quad (5)$$

with

$$w_i = \begin{cases} \left(\frac{d_{max}-d}{d_{max}}\right)^2; d < d_{max} \\ 0; otherwise \end{cases} \quad (6)$$

where d is the actual distance of the point to the grid point p_{gi}, d_{max} is a threshold for the maximum distance of influence, predefined by the user, and k_c is a correction factor ($k_c > 1.0$) which should compensate the averaging effects.

Analogously, for correction, the value of function g is obtained by

$$g(p_i) = \frac{\sum_{j=1}^{n} w_j g(p_{gi})}{\sum_{j=1}^{n} w_j} \quad (7)$$

where the weights are calculated analogously to (6). The amount of k_c can be determined experimentally by simulation (see Sect. 5).

The evaluation of the methodology was realized using simulated and real measurement data. Results are presented in Sect. 5.

Performance Automation. As the new method requires many measurements for achieving robustness, some of the necessary actions should happen automatically. This may concern the placement of the ballbars in the different orientations in the MV for the measurement data collection as well as the automated analysis of the measured 3D point clouds in order to obtain a robust distance measurement between the center points of the spheres.

The first demand was not yet realized, but can be achieved by various means, e.g., using a robot. The second demand was fulfilled using a self-made algorithm and implementation realizing the detection of two or more spheres in the scene, the automated fitting of spherical surfaces, and automatic outlier removal. This algorithm uses the known diameter for detection of the sphere positions. All points not belonging to a sphere surface are removed. Figure 2 shows an example of appropriate dataset reduction of a ballbar measurement.

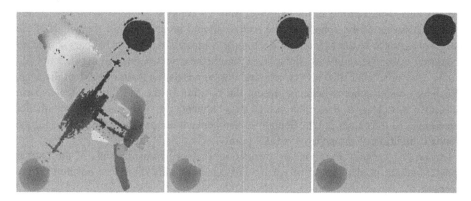

Fig. 2. Original 3D dataset (left), after background removal (middle), outlier extraction (right)

4 Evaluation Method

Evaluation of the new methodology must consider improvements of the 3D measurement results. Here, the framework of the VDI/VDE guidelines [15] may be used. We constructed an evaluation method, which is more robust than the technique proposed by VDI/VDE guidelines and already introduced before [3]. The main ideas of the evaluation method are briefly outlined here.

The characteristic parameters suggested by the VDI/VDE guidelines are flatness measurement error, sphere-spacing error (or length measurement error), and probing error. For systematic error characterization we use the mean length measurement error ΔL_{mn}, the standard deviation of ΔL_{mn}, and the span ΔL_S of the sphere-spacing error as a measure for the largest systematic error of the scanning system according to the following formulas:

$$\Delta L_{mn} = \sum_{i=1}^{n} \Delta L_i$$

with $\qquad\qquad \Delta L_i = L_i - L_{ref}(i = 1, \ldots, n)$ (8)

and $\qquad\qquad \Delta L_S = \Delta L_{max} - \Delta L_{min} = L_{max} - L_{min}$

where L_{max} is the largest and L_{min} the smallest measured length value of the ballbar, and L_i is the i-th measurement of the calibrated reference length L_{ref} of the ballbar.

Contrary to the VDI/VDE guidelines, the minimum number of ballbar measurements should be considerably higher than six (see Fig. 3) as proposed in [15]. We require at least 20 measurements (40 sphere positions). Additionally, at least one measurement should be involved touching every region of the MV. A region of the MV can be produced by equal separation of the MV, say two cuts in width, depth, and height. This would produce, for example, $3^3 = 27$ regions.

The distance of the spheres of the ballbar should be at least half the length of the maximal distance in the MV (room diagonal). Additionally, shorter ballbars should be measured, too. The radius of the spheres should be selected not too big and not too small, say not smaller than a twentieth and not bigger than a tenth of the ball distance. Whereas smaller spheres better represent the position in the MV by the center-point (the surface is closer to the center point), larger spheres provide larger surface (smaller uncertainty of the center point calculation) and hence more points of the surface for the robust estimation of the spheres' center points.

In order to obtain a convincing evaluation, distance measurements of the ballbar spheres' center points should be robust and accurate. This should be ensured by the operator.

5   Simulations, Experiments, and Results

5.1   Simulated Measurements

Several simulation experiments were performed using one single ballbar. A cuboid measurement volume of a certain size was defined. It was performed simulation of the systematic position error of a measured 3D point using an error function given by a polynomial of the form (2).

The coefficients of the polynomial were produced randomly in a meaningful range (leading to maximum error as observed by real measurements). A ballbar with well-defined sphere distance was assumed, and an arbitrary, random distribution in the MV was simulated in such a way, that both spheres always were completely inside MV (see an example in Fig. 3).

In the first simulation we tried to estimate the coefficients of the polynomial under the assumption of the knowledge of the degree of the polynomial. Random error at the determination of the spheres' center points was given by a normal distribution with a

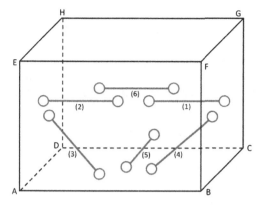

Fig. 3. Example of six placements of the ballbar in the MV

given standard deviation, called *noise*. For the distance, a constant reference length L_{ref} was chosen.

In our simulation, we set the sphere radius to zero and described the uncertainty of the determination of the center-point position by *noise*.

We choose the following parameters:

- Measurement volume (MV) size: 300 mm × 200 mm × 200 mm
- Reference length: L_{ref} = 200 mm (one single ballbar)
- Noise: variable, $noise_{min}$ = 0.0 mm, $noise_{max}$ = 0.01 mm (normal distribution)
- Parameters (randomly produced) for the polynomial coefficients:
  - Normal distribution, μ = 0 (for all parameters)
  - $\sigma = 10^{-4}$ (for a_4, a_5, a_6, b_4, b_5, b_6, c_4, c_5, c_6,)
  - $\sigma = 5 \odot 10^{-8}$ (for a_1, a_2, a_3, b_1, b_2, b_3, c_1, c_2, c_3,)

Simulated estimation of the polynomial coefficients was performed as follows:

1. Fixing of the noise level and maximal number of iterations
2. Random production of the polynomial coefficients
3. Random placements (n = 60) of the ballbar in the MV
4. Setting all coefficients of the estimated set of the polynomial coefficients *ESC* of *f* to zero
5. For each ballbar placement:
   a. measurement of the ballbar's length L, determination of the length measurement error $\Delta L = L - L_{ref}$ under consideration of *ESC*
   b. calculation of the error vector of both spheres' center points according to the placement in the MV (according to formula (4))
   c. (new) estimation of *ESC* using the set of error vectors *vec*
6. Determination of the test statistic according the finishing criterion, repeat step 5 or finish
7. Finishing criterion: mean length measurement error does not reduce or maximum number of iterations is reached

Step 5(c) was realized using the digital image analysis software tool DIAS developed by the Friedrich Schiller University Jena, Germany, which is not commercially available.

For determination of the characteristic quantities 500 random ballbar placements in the MV and consequently as many measurements were performed. Table 1 shows the averaged results of 20 simulations (±standard deviation). The characterizing quantities are:

- Remaining mean length measurement error ΔL_{mn},
- Standard deviation σ of ΔL_{mn}
- Remaining span of length measurement error ΔL_S

Table 1. Mean errors of simulated polynomial correction depending on noise

Noise [mm]	Uncorrected			Corrected		
	ΔL_{mn} [mm]	σ [mm]	ΔL_S [mm]	ΔL_{mn} [mm]	σ [mm]	ΔL_S [mm]
0.0	0.014 ± 0.066	0.077 ± 0.045	0.293 ± 0.154	−0.001 ± 0.001	0.005 ± 0.005	0.040 ± 0.044
0.001	0.011 ± 0.068	0.076 ± 0.042	0.286 ± 0.146	−0.001 ± 0.001	0.007 ± 0.003	0.051 ± 0.028
0.002	0.013 ± 0.069	0.074 ± 0.043	0.282 ± 0.151	−0.001 ± 0.001	0.008 ± 0.002	0.062 ± 0.024
0.005	−0.012 ± 0.068	0.073 ± 0.044	0.277 ± 0.148	−0.001 ± 0.002	0.010 ± 0.001	0.077 ± 0.016
0.01	−0.015 ± 0.062	0.075 ± 0.024	0.279 ± 0.081	−0.002 ± 0.004	0.020 ± 0.002	0.149 ± 0.027

The second simulation used the same scenario but the error determination and correction was based on sampling point (grid) representation of the measurement error. Error vectors were selected referring to an observed error distribution of a real data measurement. The variated quantity was the number of ballbar measurements for the grid production. We used nine, 30, 100, 300, and 1000 ballbar measurements for grid production. Noise was added with standard deviation of 1 µm. Best correction factor was found at $k_c = 1.8$. Results are given in Table 2. The mean absolute error was denoted by ΔL_{mn}, and the mean span of all 500 measurements was denoted by ΔL_S. Standard deviation σ represents the mean absolute length error.

The results show that using at least 100 ballbar measurements for grid production, mean absolute length error (represented by σ) can reduced by factor two, whereas maximum error (represented by ΔL_S) can be reduced by factor 1.5 using $n = 100$ and by factor two using $n = 1000$ initial measurements.

Table 2. Errors of simulated sampling point correction depending on number n of ballbar measurements for sampling point grid production, averaged values of 100 simulations

n	Initial			Corrected		
	ΔL_{mn} [mm]	σ [mm]	ΔL_S [mm]	ΔL_{mn} [mm]	σ [mm]	ΔL_S [mm]
9	0.036 ± 0.011	0.032 ± 0.010	0.252 ± 0.036	0.006 ± 0.009	0.027 ± 0.003	0.262 ± 0.023
30	0.035 ± 0.005	0.033 ± 0.005	0.211 ± 0.027	0.002 ± 0.006	0.021 ± 0.002	0.176 ± 0.020
100	0.036 ± 0.003	0.034 ± 0.003	0.201 ± 0.003	0.001 ± 0.003	0.016 ± 0.002	0.131 ± 0.018
300	0.037 ± 0.002	0.034 ± 0.001	0.215 ± 0.002	0.000 ± 0.002	0.014 ± 0.002	0.120 ± 0.013
1000	0.036 ± 0.001	0.034 ± 0.001	0.238 ± 0.001	0.000 ± 0.001	0.014 ± 0.001	0.118 ± 0.008

5.2   Experiments on Real Data

Experiments we performed on real data using a mobile, handheld 3D scanner (Fig. 4).

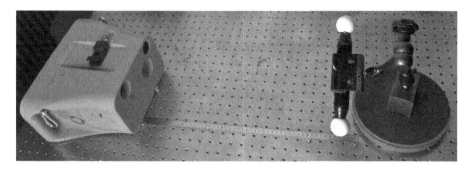

Fig. 4. Laboratory setup with 3D scanner, ballbar, and holding mechanism of the ballbar

Some specification of the scanners features are

- Measurement volume: 320 mm × 200 mm × 120 mm
- 3D frame rate: 3 Hz
- Measurement principle: triangulation between the images of the stereo camera pair
- Projection of structured light (sinusoidal fringes and Gray code sequence for phase value production)

Measurements of a single ballbar with sphere center distance of about 200 mm were performed analogously to simulations in two steps. First, a series of measurements (Set1) was used for determination of the error function. Second, a series (Set2) was used for correction. In the first series $m = 20$ measurements were performed, in the second one, $m = 10$. Both polynomial and sampling point model were applied. The results for the correction set are given in Table 3.

Table 3. Results of error correction by our new method using real data

Data	Uncorrected		Polynomial		Sampling points	
	$\Delta L_{mn} \pm \sigma$[mm]	ΔL_S[mm]	$\Delta L_{mn} \pm \sigma$[mm]	ΔL_S[mm]	$\Delta L_{mn} \pm \sigma$[mm]	ΔL_S [mm]
Set2	0.081 ± 0.087	0.328	0.001 ± 0.042	0.189	0.012 ± 0.030	0.131

The results show an improvement potential of about factor two. Sampling Points Algorithm gave a little bit better correction than the polynomial one. However, finding a better polynomial description by, e.g., other selection of the coefficients, may also improve the results of the polynomial correction. Appropriate experiments will also be part of the future work.

6 Summary, Discussion, and Outlook

We presented a new method to implement systematic error reduction of optical 3D scanners, preferably using structured light illumination. The method can be applied to other (passive) photogrammetric scanners, too. However, a robust length measurement is necessary.

Results of simulations and real measurements show the potential and the limitations of the new technique. The potential can be detected looking at the significant reduction of the systematic measurement error both at simulation results and at real data measurements. Using the polynomial approach, the mean length measurement error can be reduced significantly in the simulation by factor four and on real data by a factor of about two assuming center point detection uncertainty of about 1 µm. Experiments with the scanner used showed that position uncertainty of the spheres' center points had actually a standard deviation below 1 µm.

Using grid representation of sampling points, even better results can be achieved. However, many, well-distributed ballbar placements and measurements in different positions are necessary.

Unfortunately, a complete compensation of the systematic error could not be reached using this method as it has several origins. Although the degree and the number of coefficients of the polynomial is set and consequently known in the simulation experiment, the randomly produced coefficients cannot be found by the optimization even if the noise is suppressed completely. This is due to the high number of coefficients and the partial correlation between them. Additionally, rounding effects always occur.

For practical application, it is important, that the kind of error of real data is typically not known. Additionally, using ballbars for length measurement errors, there must be found a compromise between high measurement accuracy because of the high number of measured surface points and the deviation of the sphere center and the locations of measurement (surface).

Real data results imply to use sampling point representation of the error function. The disadvantage of missing sampling points in some regions of the measurement volume using this method must be overcome by suitable interpolation.

However, despite of the ambitious challenges the authors think that a significant improvement of the method is possible.

Future work will address several tasks. First, automation of the data capturing should be realized in order to obtain numerous well-distributed data observations. Second, more different scanning devices should be involved into the experiments. Third, extension of the data acquisition can provide more information concerning the depth error. This is due to the fact, that ballbar center points have typically larger lateral distance than longitudinal. Here, measurement of plane surfaces could provide the necessary information.

References

1. Brinkmann, B.: Internationales Wörterbuch der Metrologie: Grundlegende und allgemeine Begriffe und zugeordnete Benennungen (VIM) Deutsch-englische Fassung ISO/IEC-Leitfaden 99. Beuth, Berlin (2012)
2. Bräuer-Burchardt, C., Kühmstedt, P., Notni, G.: Error compensation by sensor re-calibration in fringe projection based optical 3D stereo scanners. In: Maino, G., Foresti, G.L. (eds.) ICIAP 2011. LNCS, vol. 6979, pp. 363–373. Springer, Heidelberg (2011). https://doi.org/10.1007/978-3-642-24088-1_38
3. Bräuer-Burchardt, C., Ölsner, S., Kühmstedt, P., Notni, G.: Comparison of calibration strategies for optical 3D scanners based on structured light projection using a new evaluation methodology. In: Videometrics, Range Imaging, and Applications XIV. Proceedings of SPIE, vol. 10332, pp. 103320F1–103320F10 (2017)
4. Griva, I., Nash, S.G., Sofer, A.: Linear and Nonlinear Optimization, 2nd edn. George Mason University, Fairfax (2009)
5. Gu, S., McNamara, J.E., Johnson, K., Gennert, M.A., King, M.A.: Calibration accuracy evaluation with stereo reconstruction. In: IEEE Nuclear Science Symposium Conference Record, San Diego, CA, pp. 3242–3246 (2006)
6. Hasetedt, H., Luhmann, T.: Analyse der Kamerakalibrierung mit OpenCV. In: Luhmann, T., Müller, C. (eds.) Photogrammetrie, Laserscanning, Optische 3D-Messtechnik, Proceedings of Oldenburger 3D-Tage 2015, pp. 259–268 (2015)
7. He, Y., Liang, B., Zou, Y., He, J., Yang, J.: Depth errors analysis and correction for time-of-flight (ToF) cameras. Sensors 17(92), 1–18 (2017)
8. Isheil, A., Gonnet, J.-P., Joannic, D., Fontaine, J.-F.: Systematic error correction of a 3D laser scanning measurement device. Opt. Lasers Eng. 49, 16–24 (2011)
9. JCGM 200: International vocabulary of metrology—basic and general concepts and associated terms (VIM), 3rd edn. (2012). https://www.bipm.org/utils/common/documents/jcgm/JCGM_200_2012.pdf. Accessed 02 Aug 2018
10. Kahlmann, T., Ingensand, H.: Calibration and development for increased accuracy of 3D range imaging cameras. J. Appl. Geod. 2(2008), 1–11 (2008)
11. Luhmann, T., Fraser, C., Maas, H.-G.: Sensor modelling and camera calibration for close-range photogrammetry. ISPRS J. Photogramm. Remote. Sens. 115, 37–46 (2016)
12. Muralikrishnan, B., et al.: Volumetric performance evaluation of a laser scanner based on geometric error model. Precis. Eng. 40, 139–150 (2015)
13. Remondino, F., Fraser, C.: Digital camera calibration methods: considerations and comparisons. Int. Arch. Photogramm., Remote. Sens., Spat. Inf. Sci. XXXVI(5), 266–272 (2006)
14. Rieke-Zapp, D., Tecklenburg, W., Peipe, J., Hastedt, H., Haig, C.: Evaluation of the geometric stability and the accuracy potential of digital cameras – comparing mechanical stabilisation versus parameterization. ISPRS J. 64(3), 248–258 (2009)
15. VDI/VDE 2634: Optical 3D-measuring systems. VDI/VDE guidelines, Part 2. Beuth, Berlin (2008). https://m.vdi.de/uploads/tx_vdirili/pdf/1456386.pdf. Accessed 02 Aug 2018
16. Wang, B., Pan, B., Tao, R., Lubineau, G.: Systematic errors in digital volume correlation due to the self-heating effect of a laboratory x-ray CT scanner. Meas. Sci. Technol. 28, 055402 (2017)

Defect Detection in Textiles with Co-occurrence Matrix as a Texture Model Description

Karolina Nurzynska[1,2]([✉]) [iD] and Michał Czardybon[1]

[1] Future Processing Sp. z o.o., ul. Bojkowska 37A, 44-100 Gliwice, Poland
Karolina.Nurzynska@polsl.pl
[2] Institute of Informatics, Silesian University of Technology, ul. Akademicka 16, 44-100 Gliwice, Poland

Abstract. Automatized inspection at textile production lines becomes very important. However, there is still a need to design methods which meet not only demands concerning accuracy of defect detection, but also ones related to the processing time. In this work, a novel approach for defect model definition is presented. It is derived from the idea of co-occurrence matrix. Due to scale incorporation and binarization of the model content it proved to be a very powerful descriptor of the novelties. Moreover, it also satisfies the requirements of short processing time. The defect mask achieved with the introduced method was compared visually to other popular solutions and show a very high accuracy and quality of defect description. The processing time is real-time as the response for a 1MP (megapixel) image is reached within tens of milliseconds.

Keywords: Defect detection · Image segmentation
Co-occurrence matrix

1 Introduction

Defect detection based on image processing techniques becomes more popular in the industry every year, because of the product quality demands and the growing cost of complaints. Traditional and new emerging methods find various applications from automotive part manufacturing, through customer electronics assembly, print verification, surface inspection to textile novelty description. In all the cases, the goal is the same: to find an anomaly in the image when a defect appears or to state that the object under inspection is correct otherwise.

When analysing the available data for such system implementation one notices that the class of correct samples is characterised by large representation, while defects usually are described by few elements, if any. In consequence, the system is taught to correctly recognize one class and raise notification when anything else appears as an input. In the literature, complex methods designed to novelty detection (another name for defect, anomaly, or outlier detection) exploit

© Springer Nature Switzerland AG 2018
R. P. Barneva et al. (Eds.): IWCIA 2018, LNCS 11255, pp. 216–226, 2018.
https://doi.org/10.1007/978-3-030-05288-1_17

one of the following approaches [3,5,16]: k-nearest neighbourhood method, k-means model, Gaussian Mixture Model (GMM), and one-class support vector machine [19]; while improved thresholding or local features calculation represents much simpler approaches.

In works [21,22], a system based on a pyramid of GMMs trained with small texture patches – texems – is introduced. The model consists of the mean texem and a covariance matrix used to build a multivariate Gaussian distribution. In order to keep the texem size small and enable it to work with multi-scale data, an image pyramid is created. The resulting image is a combination of responses generated by each level of the pyramid. Some improvements to the original method for large texture scale variation were achieved by using the method of compressed sensing additionally [4].

Simple techniques start with an application of Otsu thresholding method [10] and introduce some improvements addressing the problem of thresholding of unimodal histograms as well [23]. Others calculate the autocorrelation coefficient in the vertical and horizontal directions to find out the pattern size, and compute the quality in order to detect defects [8]. A thorough review [17] of filtering techniques applied for texture segmentation shows deficiencies of these approaches in texture segmentation and thus are not applicable for defect detection. Finally, there is also a bunch of methods which are based on wavelets analysis [6,12,18,20] or Gabor filters [9]. It is interesting to point out that features extracted from co-occurrence matrices computed for sub-band images of wavelet transform prove good texture recognition [7,11].

The aim of this paper is to present a novel system for defect detection in textile images, where the main assumption was to work in a real-time with satisfactory accuracy. Since the timing restrictions in the industry are severe the number of operations performed on each pixel needed to be reduced significantly. Moreover, it was expected to train such system with a limited number of training data, preferably with one, defect-less picture only.

2   Materials and Methods

The proposed system works in two modes: training and testing. During the training stage, a sample image of correct material should be supplied to prepare a model of the texture. Moreover, it is necessary to decide how to parametrize the program. The computed model with the parameters is then passed to the testing module, which for each image on the input generates a defect mask. A detailed description of the elaborated method is given below while Fig. 1 presents a system overview.

2.1   Texture Model

Texture is a complex composition of pixels values featuring some set of fixed spatial relationships. Thus, in several texture operators those relations are considered as a means of texture description [1,2,7,15]. In the case of the presented

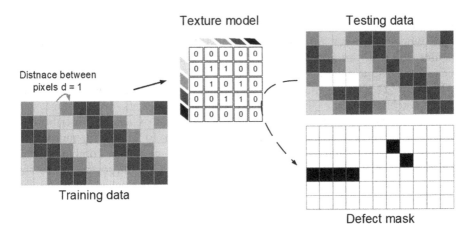

Fig. 1. Presentation of the idea of the proposed method.

system, it was necessary to design a model which on one hand enabled storing the diverse texture characteristics, while on the other hand was as simple as possible, since the number of performed operations was restricted to obtain high performance. Therefore, a relation of illumination changes between adjacent pixels was chosen as a metric, and the co-occurrence matrix introduced in [7] was used to build the model.

The co-occurrence matrix in the original definition stores probabilities of co-appearances of pixel values, where the values are given as the indices of the matrix columns and rows. Hence for given G illumination levels, the matrix size is $G \times G$. The distance d between considered pairs of pixels is parametrized, and $d > 0$. The co-occurrence can be observed in any direction θ, but usually, the angles $\alpha = 0°, 45°, 90°, 135°$ are sufficient in practice. The matrices are normalized, and then 14 features are derived to describe a texture [7]. Calculation of these features is the most costly element of this algorithm but as was presented in other research [13,14] applying only the matrix is sufficient.

Having in mind the constraints and capabilities for texture description, the co-occurrence matrix is chosen to become the specification of a texture model. In the presented realization, the problem of texture rotation is neglected, as for instance in industrial textile inspection it should not take place, and therefore only the matrix for $\alpha = 0°$ and/or $\alpha = 90°$ is computed. That also reduced the computational load up to four times. The presented solution enables the user to choose whether the full intensity space is exploited or should the pixel values be quantized.

2.2   Scale Incorporation

Defining the model with only one possible distance between pixels considered as co-appearing proves correct for uniform textures and for input data without noise. However, such data is rather rare and it would be better to prepare the system to deal with more demanding inputs. Therefore, except smoothing for noise removal, the scale information was included.

Scale in the proposed algorithm is understood as a changeable distance between co-occurring pixels defined already as d. The user supplies the initial distance used on the basic level l_0, while next levels recalculate the distance according to the formula:

$$d_{l_h} = d_{l_0} + 2^{h-1}, \qquad (1)$$

where $h = 1 \ldots H - 1$, and H is the number of considered levels and $H > 1$. This simple change in the distance enables storing in the model not only the very local information but also looking at the texture more globally. As a result that leads to efficient handling of more sophisticated texture themes.

Each entry of a co-occurrence matrix holds information about a probability that two pixel values co-occure in the input image. When an entry is larger than zero, it means that such a pair of pixels belongs to the model, while zero defines an outlier. Thus, a defect mask could be a map of probability of the pixel belonging to the original image. Yet, due to a large number of possibilities, each entry has very low probability and since it does not give much information, it was decided to set zero for correct answers and one for outliers in a defect mask. When several levels H are calculated, the final response becomes a novelty if that is stated by results computed at all the scale levels.

Another possibility to preserve the scale information would be by application of Gaussian image pyramid (as it is applied in [21,22]). In this case, the step in the co-occurrence matrix is set constant, but the image is rescaled. This idea was also evaluated but proved less accurate in the performed experiments.

3   Results and Discussion

In order to verify the quality of the proposed solution, several tests on various image examples have been performed. Some of the results are presented below. Additionally, to have better insight into the capabilities of the presented method, its outputs are compared to those achieved for the TEXEM method [21,22], which is based on Gaussian Mixture Model analysis of the texture. Both methods were implemented in C++ making all efforts to optimize the implementation regarding time performance of the algorithms.

3.1   Case 1: Simple Background

In these experiments a database of textiles with simple structure was used. This database consisted of 12 images presenting typical defect classes on various fabrics. Therefore, from each image a faultless area of 200×200 pixels was cut for training, while in a testing stage the whole image was considered (its resolution was 627×472 pixels). During the training, the mode of two directions was applied (horizontal and vertical distances were considered), a Gaussian smoothing filter, which had a window size of 3×3, was applied and two matrix levels were calculated. In the case of first four images presented in Fig. 2 the step parameter was

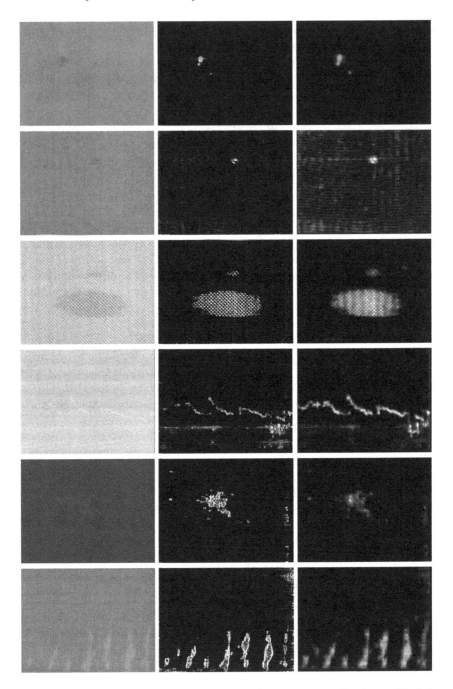

Fig. 2. Examples of achieved defect detection performances on a database with defects presented on a simple background. The original image on the left. The output of the introduced method in the middle, while on the right the result of the TEXEM method is given for comparison. The white colour depicts the defect area.

set to one, while in the further two examples it was set to two. The TEXEM method was trained with texems of resolution 3×3 pixels, the pyramid height was set to 4 with Gaussian smoothing of size 3×3 applied at each pyramid level. Figure 2 in the first column presents the original images, which grey-scale versions were transformed with the presented method and the outcomes are given in the middle column while the results achieved with TEXEM approach are depicted on the right. As one can observe, the new method detects defect regions very well. Its quality is comparable with the more sophisticated TEXEM method. The outcome is binary (in the TEXEM method the distance from the correct class is given), but there are fewer false positives (please refer to the second row in Fig. 2). The improvement in noise reduction is especially visible in the example in the second row, while in the other cases if the noise exist, it is presented similarly. It is worth to point out, that the defect regions correspond to each other, however their contours are more precisely marked with the introduced method, what is well visible on the sample presented in the fourth row, where the defect line in case of TEXEM method is blurred due to the application of a pyramid.

3.2   Case 2: Knitwear

The knitwear dataset consists of 8 samples presenting a correct case of material and 26 samples depicting various types of defects. The resolution is 614×455 pixels of a monochromatic image. In the experiment one correct image was used for training, while other 33 images constituated the testing set. Figure 3 presents achieved results. The original input data is on the left. The outcomes of the introduced method are in the middle. The distance for calculation was set to 1, there were 2 matrix levels, Gaussian smoothing was applied in 5×5 window and the co-occurrence matrix was filled using both horizontal and vertical directions. For comparison the output of the TEXEM technique is presented on the right. It was achieved for a texem size 3×3, with a pyramid height equal to four and smoothed with Gaussian kernel of 3×3 size. As it is easily seen, defects are detected very well with the introduced method. The type of defect does not influence much the quality of detection, what seems to be problematic in the case of the TEXEM method, where the big outliers are well detected, while minor novelties are less visible. Moreover, some slight changes in lighting conditions are also not problematic, while are clearly visible when TEXEM was applied, which forces application of further processing of the defect map image. Moreover, in some cases (see the samples in the third and fourth rows), the TEXEM system response for a defect and lighting change is on the similar level, which makes the correct anomaly description impossible. Finally, there were no false alarms for the correct input data in the case of presented method.

3.3   Time Performance

During the design of a method for anomaly detection, the time constraints had to be considered too. Table 1 summarizes achieved performances in presented

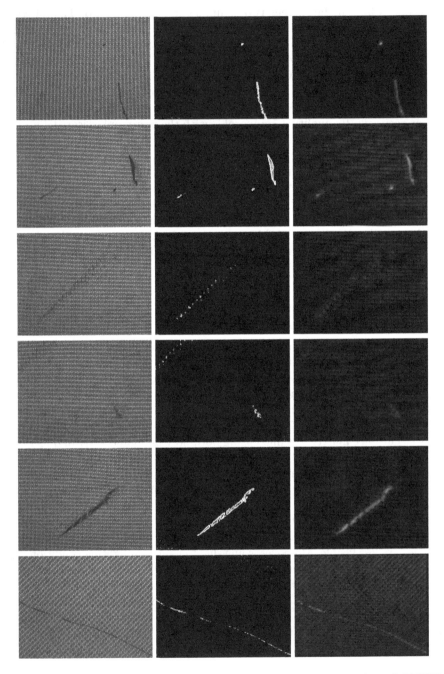

Fig. 3. Comparison of defect detection with the proposed approach and TEXEM method. Parameters for the method Step = 1, Matrix Level = 2, Gaussian window size = 5, Method = 2.

Table 1. Time performance comparison

	Experiment	Image resolution	Method	Time [ms]
Training	Case 1	200×200	Introduced	10
			TEXEM	8875
	Case 2	614×455	Introduced	14
			TEXEM	99216
Testing	Case 1	627×472	Introduced	6
			TEXEM	3728
	Case 2	614×455	Introduced	5
			TEXEM	3541

experiments, which were performed on the computer with processor Intel i7-4710HQ 2.5 GHz and 16 GB RAM. In all the cases, the time is an average taken from 10 experiments run with the same settings. Although the results of the introduced method and the TEXEM approach in many cases were very similar to each other, the time necessary to achieve the goal differs remarkably. As one can see, the training time used by the introduced method needed tens of milliseconds to compute the model, while it took seconds when the TEXEM method was applied. Moreover, the scalability in relation to the size of input data is linear and does not depend on the settings significantly in the novel approach, while the TEXEM method needs much more time for model preparation and additionally squarely depends on the texem size. Yet, when training was done off-line, for both solutions performance of this phase could still be considered reasonable. However, much more important is the time needed for the testing phase. Here the introduced method needs 5–6 ms to compute the response, while the TEXEM approach used more than 3.5 s. This is an enormous advantage of the proposed method: it not only gives good accuracy with low false detection rate but also features real-time performance.

Table 2. Hardware and software settings for performance tests.

Operating system	Processing unit	RAM
Windows 7	Intel Atom E3845 @1.91 GHz	4 GB
Windows 10	Intel Core i5-7500 @3.4 GHz	16 GB
Ubuntu Xenial 16.04 <small>(kernel tegra-ubuntu 4.4.38-tegra)</small>	NVidia Tegra TX2@~2 GHz	8 GB

In order to have better insight into the introduced method performance, its implementation (in C++) has been tested on some hardware and software platforms, which description is gathered in Table 2. Additionally for NVidia separate tests were run using only Cortex-A57 or Denver2 processors or both of them. In all the cases 64 bits platform was used. For Windows systems the program was compiled using the Microsoft Visual Studio 2015 with following flags: /Gy /Oi /MD /openmp /Ot /O2 and was placed on the system drive, while on Linux the gcc 5.4 with -O3 -fopenmp flags was applied and the binary files were copied on tmpfs (a temporary file storage facility on RAM). The experiments were performed for an image of resolution 512×512 pixels with following settings of introduced method parameters: Step $= 1$, Method $= 2$, and Matrix Level $= 1$ (Exp. 1) or Matrix Level $= 2$ (Exp. 2). Figure 4 presents average results obtained for 40 runs of the experiment with (MT) and without (NoMT) multi-threading. As an experiment, the image testing phase of the system is understood. In the case of NVidia Tegra (Both); we resigned from experiments with NoMT because here one thread is running anyway.

As it is depicted in the figure using the multi-threading improved the performance in all the experiments; particularly around 2× improvement is noticeable for NVidia and 3× for Intel processors. Additionally, the multi-threading shortens the executions time better in the case of Exp. 2. The longer execution times recorded in Exp. 2 are due to the higher number of matrix levels. The best performance was achieved on the platform running Intel Core.

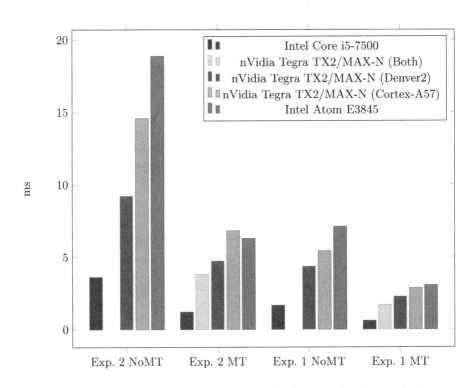

Fig. 4. Results of performance test on various hardware and software platforms.

4 Conclusions

This work presents a novel method for defect detection which derives its basic idea form the co-occurrence matrix and expands its descriptive possibilities by scale incorporation at various levels of the pyramid. The proposed technique was evaluated using samples of data gathered from the industry. Its accuracy was compared to the TEXEM method, and proved to be of the same sensitivity, but with lower false detection rate. The assumed time constraints are met as it is possible to process a 1MP image within tens of milliseconds.

Acknowledgements. This work has been based on the results of the project "Opracowanie systemu do efektywnej integracji aplikacji wizyjnych przez użyt- kowników końcowych" co-financed by the European Regional Development Fund under Operational Programme Innovative Economy 2007–2013, based on the Agreement no. UDA-POIG.01.04.00-24-067/11-00.

References

1. Ahonen, T., Hadid, A., Pietikäinen, M.: Face recognition with local binary patterns. In: Pajdla, T., Matas, J. (eds.) ECCV 2004. LNCS, vol. 3021, pp. 469–481. Springer, Heidelberg (2004). https://doi.org/10.1007/978-3-540-24670-1_36
2. Amadasun, M., King, R.: Textural features corresponding to textural properties. IEEE Trans. Syst. Man Cybern. **19**(5), 1264–1274 (1989)
3. Blanchard, G., Lee, G., Scott, C.: Semi-supervised novelty detection. J. Mach. Learn. Res. **11**, 2973–3009 (2010)
4. Böttger, T., Ulrich, M.: Real-time texture error detection on textured surfaces with compressed sensing. Pattern Recogn. Image Anal. **26**(1), 88–94 (2016)
5. Ding, X., Li, Y., Belatreche, A., Maguire, L.P.: An experimental evaluation of novelty detection methods. Neurocomputing **135**, 313–327 (2014)
6. Han, Y., Shi, P.: An adaptive level-selecting wavelet transform for texture defect detection. Image Vis. Comput. **25**(8), 1239–1248 (2007)
7. Haralick, R.M., Shanmugam, K., Dinstein, I.: Textural features for image classification. IEEE Trans. Syst. Man Cybern. SMC **3**(6), 610–621 (1973)
8. Hoseini, E., Farhadi, F., Tajeripour, F.: Fabric defect detection using autocorrelation function. Int. J. Comput. Theory Eng. **5**, 114–117 (2013)
9. Hu, G.H.: Automated defect detection in textured surfaces using optimal elliptical gabor filters. Optik - Int. J. Light Electron Opt. **126**(14), 1331–1340 (2015)
10. Iyer, M., Janakiraman, S.: Defect detection in pattern texture analysis. In: 2014 International Conference on Communication and Signal Processing, pp. 172–175, April 2014
11. Latif-Amet, A., Ertüzün, A., Erçil, A.: An efficient method for texture defect detection: sub-band domain co-occurrence matrices. Image Vis. Comput. **18**(6), 543–553 (2000)
12. Navarro, P., Fernandez-Isla, C., Alcover, P., Suardiaz, J.: Defect detection in textures through the use of entropy as a means for automatically selecting the wavelet decomposition level. Sensors (Bassel) **16**, 1178 (2016)
13. Nurzynska, K., Kubo, M., Muramoto, K.: Snow particle automatic classification with texture operators. In: 2011 IEEE International Geoscience and Remote Sensing Symposium, pp. 2892–2895, July 2011

14. Nurzynska, K., Kubo, M., Muramoto, K.: Texture operator for snow particle classification into snowflake and graupel. Atmos. Res. **118**, 121–132 (2012)
15. Ojala, T., Pietikäinen, M., Mäenpää, T.: Gray scale and rotation invariant texture classification with local binary patterns. In: Vernon, D. (ed.) ECCV 2000. LNCS, vol. 1842, pp. 404–420. Springer, Heidelberg (2000). https://doi.org/10.1007/3-540-45054-8_27
16. Pimentel, M.A.F., Clifton, D.A., Clifton, L., Tarassenko, L.: A review of novelty detection. Signal Process. **99**, 215–249 (2014)
17. Randen, T., Husoy, J.H.: Filtering for texture classification: a comparative study. IEEE Trans. Pattern Anal. Mach. Intell. **21**(4), 291–310 (1999)
18. Sari, L., Ertüzün, A.: Texture defect detection using independent vector analysis in wavelet domain. In: 2014 22nd International Conference on Pattern Recognition, pp. 1639–1644, August 2014
19. Schölkopf, B., Williamson, R., Smola, A., Shawe-Taylor, J., Platt, J.: Support vector method for novelty detection. In: Proceedings of the 12th International Conference on Neural Information Processing Systems, NIPS 1999, pp. 582–588. MIT Press, Cambridge (1999)
20. Vaidelienė, G., Valantinas, J.: The use of Haar wavelets in detecting and localizing texture defects. Image Anal. Stereol. **35**(3), 195–201 (2016)
21. Xie, X., Mirmehdi, M.: TEXEMS: texture exemplars for defect detection on random textured surfaces. IEEE Trans. Pattern Anal. Mach. Intell. **29**(8), 1454–1464 (2007)
22. Xie, X., Mirmehdi, M.: Texture exemplars for defect detection on random textures. In: Singh, S., Singh, M., Apte, C., Perner, P. (eds.) ICAPR 2005. LNCS, vol. 3687, pp. 404–413. Springer, Heidelberg (2005). https://doi.org/10.1007/11552499_46
23. Yuan, X., Wu, L., Peng, Q.: An improved Otsu method using the weighted object variance for defect detection. Appl. Surface Sci. **349**(Suppl. C), 472–484 (2015)

Multiscale Graph-Cut for 3D Segmentation of Compact Objects

Miroslav Jirik[1,2]([✉]) [ID], Vladimir Lukes[2] [ID], Milos Zelezny[2] [ID],
and Vaclav Liska[3] [ID]

[1] Biomedical Center, Faculty of Medicine in Pilsen, Charles University,
Pilsen, Czech Republic
miroslav.jirik@gmail.com
[2] Faculty of Applied Sciences, NTIS - New Technologies for the Information Society,
Pilsen, Czech Republic
[3] Biomedical Center and Department of Surgery, University Hospital and Faculty
of Medicine in Pilsen, Charles University, Pilsen, Czech Republic

Abstract. The article is a step forward towards improving image segmentation using a popular method called Graph-Cut. We focus on optimizing the algorithm for processing data, in which the target object occupies only a small portion of the total volume. We propose a two-step procedure. At the first step, the location of the object is determined roughly. At the second step, Graph-Cut segmentation is performed with a special multi-scale chart structure. Two different graph construction methods are suggested. The calculation time of both variants is compared with the original Graph-Cut method. The msgc_lo2hi method has been shown to provide a statistically significant time reduction of the computational costs.

Keywords: Graph-Cut method · Multiscale · Medical imaging
Image segmentation

1 Introduction

The Graph-Cut Algorithm, originally developed for combinatorial optimization, has long time been applied for image segmentation. First, it was employed to segment black and white images [7]. Later, Boykov suggested some major improvements in the usage of Graph-Cut Algorithm for image segmentation [1,3].

Currently, Graph-Cut Algorithm is a popular method in computer vision. Under certain conditions, a global minimum of the critical function can be found. With other segmentation methods, it is very difficult to determine a critical function, and the results often differ significantly from the global optimum.

An advantage of the Graph-Cut algorithm is the possibility to employ it in the N-D space. This allows using the method for processing data of 3D medical images [6]. However, the size of the data processed in the diagnostic procedure is enormous and the computational time can easily take several minutes. While,

© Springer Nature Switzerland AG 2018
R. P. Barneva et al. (Eds.): IWCIA 2018, LNCS 11255, pp. 227–236, 2018.
https://doi.org/10.1007/978-3-030-05288-1_18

it could be tolerable for offline computation, this is not acceptable for interactive tasks required, for example, for segmentation of parenchymatous abdominal organs (such as a liver, for example) in CT scans. In this paper, we aim to decrease the time required for such type of tasks.

To reduce the computational costs of the Graph-Cut segmentation, Kang and Wan proposed a segmentation procedure described in [10]. It uses a rectangular area of interest limiting the extent of the calculations. However, this method does not allow the reduction of computational costs for objects with complex shape.

In order to increase the efficiency of the algorithm, we propose multi-scale segmentation using the Graph-Cut method. It is based on detection of discontinuities in the 3D image and the unique construction of the corresponding graph. We introduce in the sequel two different methods of graph construction.

2   Methods

The data in three-dimensional medical imagery contain a large number of voxels and thus, their processing requires large amount of memory. Despite the efficiency of the algorithm used to calculate the Graph-Cut segmentation, the calculation time and the memory cost are considerable. The fact that the target volume is rather compact and the segmentation boundary occupies a small area of the total volume of the input data can be explored for improvement of the segmentation procedure.

The method described in [10] for an application in the bright-field of microscope images is based on performing Graph-Cut algorithm on a subset of the input image. In this case, rectangular areas are determined based on the Bhattacharyya distance for exploration on a fine scale. A local calculation is then performed on these areas. Output of the Graph-Cut segmentation is then transformed back to the coordinate system of the original image.

2.1   Graph-Cut for Computer Vision

The image segmentation approach described by Boykov in reference [2] is a well-known algorithm. It was used in our experiments as a baseline: To distinguish it from our modifications, we call it Single Scale Graph-Cut (SSGC). We use selection of a few foreground and background voxels as an input of the algorithm. Foreground and background intensity models are composed of three-component Gaussian mixtures which are set up by using the EM algorithm [4]. This model is used for assigning weights of the graph components.

The graph contains the same number of nodes as the number of pixels (see Fig. 1).

The edges connecting neighboring nodes (e.g., p and q) are called N-links. In addition, there are two nodes (terminal nodes) that represent the foreground and the background. The edges connecting the terminal nodes with the other graph nodes (e.g., S and v) are called T-links. The N-links weights correspond to local

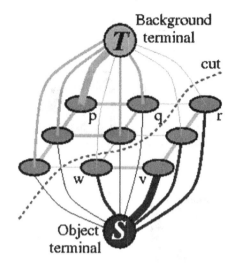

Fig. 1. Simple 2D example of a graph. The nodes corresponding to image pixels (p, q, r, v and w) are connected by N-links, the terminal nodes S and T are connected to other nodes with T-links [2].

discontinuities in the image. The T-links weights correspond to the likelihood with the foreground and background model. An algorithm max-flow/min-cut is run after the graph is constructed.

2.2   Multiscale Graph-Cut Segmentation

The main idea of multiscale segmentation is to work with high resolution only close to the border between the foreground and the background of the object and in low resolution in other parts of the data, i.e., those that are far from the border. The idea is shown in Fig. 2. The approach proposed here differs from the algorithm described in [10], because we explore the full volume of data. In addition, it is able to simplify the graph structure even inside of the bounding box area of the segmented object. The high resolution area may not be rectangular or even convex. This makes the algorithm more efficient.

All steps of the algorithm are shown in Table 1. The first step is the feature modeling. Although our implementation allows us to use wider range of feature descriptors (e.g., textures), we choose to use intensity modeling in this paper. As with the Single Scale Graph-Cut, the Gaussian mixture is used to model the foreground and the background.

The second step in the process is to locate discontinuities in the image. This is implemented by performing rough segmentation on the resampled data. The reduced resolution is determined by the block size. Similarly, the seed is over-sampled. In this case, interpolation by a nearest neighbor is used. In places near the border, controversial cases may arise, where pixels representing foreground and background segments may be within the block. In our implementation, we

Multiscale Graph-Cut

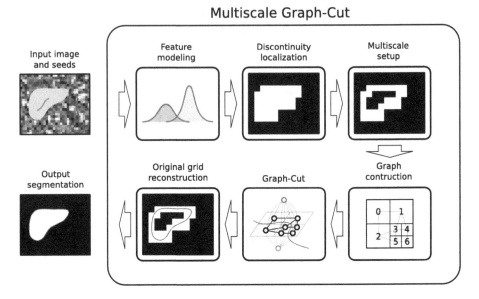

Fig. 2. Multiscale Graph-Cut scheme. Discontinuity localization is used for selection of voxels close to the border of segmentation.

Table 1. Algorithm of Multiscale Graph-Cut segmentation

Step	Name	Description
1	Feature modeling	Gaussian mixture intensity model
2	Discontinuity localization	Low resolution segmentation
3	Multiscale setup	Set the distance of high resolution area from the border
4	Graph construction	Low-to-High algorithm or High-to-Low algorithm
5	Graph-Cut	Perform max-flow/min-cut algorithm
6	High resolution grid reconstruction	Extract segmentation from the graph

perform decision-making based on the rule of the closest neighbor. An alternative approach is the removal of the inbred seed. Subsequently, the segmentation is performed in a conventional manner. Because of the low resolution of the image data, this process is very fast.

The next step is to identify the areas that will be calculated with the fine resolution. The multiscale idea is shown in Fig. 3 The fine resolution area it along the edge of the rough segmentation from the previous step. One of the parameters of our method is then the width of this edge. This may include blocks that are close to the boundary but do not touch it directly. This parameter is then selected taking into account the expected shape richness of the segmented

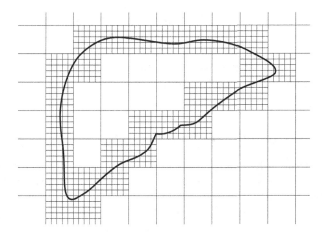

Fig. 3. Multiscale pixel schema. Discontinuity localization is used for selection of voxels close to the border of segmentation.

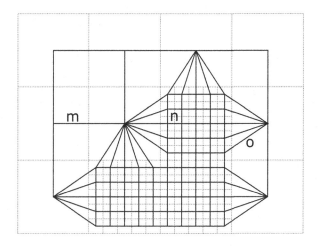

Fig. 4. 2D multiscale graph example with 3×4 blocks and 15×20 pixels. Green color is used for blocks and high resolution pixels (Color figure online)

object. In the example given in Fig. 3 the border width is set to 1. It means that only blocks located on the border are processed with high resolution.

The graph construction step is the most complex part of the multiscale segmentation procedure. We have proposed two different algorithms. The High-to-Low (hi2lo) algorithm builds the graph by simplifying the high resolution structure. The other one is called Low-to-High and it starts from low resolution structure. Both of them will be discussed later in Sects. 2.3 and 2.4. The main goal of this step is to build the graph structure with all the weights. Figure 4 shows an example with a multiscale structure. There are three types of N-links. In the high resolution grid, the weight of an edge n is set to w_n according to the N-link rule from the SSGC. The weight w_o between the high resolution pixel and the low resolution pixel is set the same as the weight w_n. The weight m between two low resolution pixels is set to $b \cdot w_n$.

The final step is reconstruction of the high resolution grid. In this step the graph structure and the Graph-Cut output is transformed into the original resolution.

2.3 High Resolution to Low Resolution Algorithm

The creation of the N-link multi-scale graph begins with the graph of the high resolution grid. The nodes are indexed ascendingly in the grid and the edges are represented by paisr of indexes of adjacent nodes. The node indexes in low resolution block areas are replaced by a new low resolution node index. One low-resolution node replaces multiple high-resolution nodes in the entire block. The edges inside of this block are searched and removed. The two adjacent low resolution blocks then create a series of edges connecting the same nodes. These duplicate edges are also removed. Now, some nodes are not used in the edge list anymore. The list of node indexes is rearranged to avoid unused nodes.

2.4 Low Resolution to High Resolution Algorithm

The multidimensional graph is made up of graphs of low resolution grids. In each high resolution block a high-resolution grid is created. It is then connected to the surrounding blocks. If a neighboring block is of high resolution, high-resolution border nodes are attached directly to each other. Otherwise, all border nodes are connected to one neighboring low-resolution node. During the reconnection, nodes and edges designated for removal are marked. This is then done at the end of the whole process.

3   Results

We performed experiments on artificial three-dimensional images (see Fig. 5). Every image contains a compact object with different brightness and the image is affected by Gaussian noise. This is a typical situation in the case of CT images of parenchymatous organs. The image has cubic shape. The size of the image, defined by the number of the pixels on the cube edge, varies and the volume of the object is constant. The seeds of one type are located within this object, the second type segments are located on the outside of the object.

We used 74 images for the experiments and an extended dataset with 151 images to produce some of the figures in this paper. We used compact objects because it is a typical situation for this type of medical images. The goal of the experiment was to verify the ability of the Multi-Scale Graph-Cut algorithm (MSGC) to reduce the computational and memory requirements.

Figure 7 shows the comparison of the calculation time of the SSGC methods.

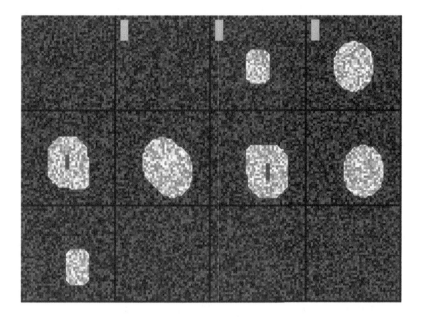

Fig. 5. Sample of test data with seeds

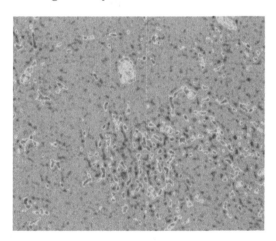

Fig. 6. One slice of porcine liver corrosion cast from Micro-CT

In the second experiment, we used Micro-CT porcine liver corrosion cast data [6]. Segmented veins on the image cover the whole area of 3D data. The measure times for SSGC, MSGC_hi2lo ad MSGC_lo2hi are 19.18[s], 617.4[s] and 71.48[s], respectively. All experiment scripts are publicly available [8].

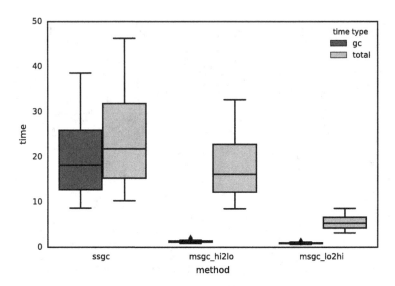

Fig. 7. Comparison of computation time of Single Scale Graph-Cut(SSGC) and Multi-scale Graph-Cut (with variants lo2hi and hi2lo). With green color (labeled as "total") the total time of whole segmentation process is visualized. The purple boxes (labeled as "gc") show time for max-flow/min-cut algorithm (Color figure online)

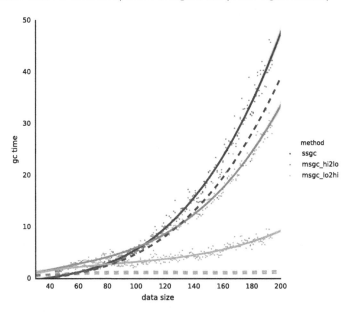

Fig. 8. Data size to time dependency. Time used for max-flow/min-cut algorithm is show by dashed line. Extended dataset was used to produce this figure.

4   Discussion

Based on the measurements, there is an evidence that after reaching some critical limit of data size the proposed MSGC method starts to be faster than SSGC. The larger the data area, the more the measured times are in favor of MSGC. The critical limit is affected by the size and the shape of the object. The smaller the surface, the more complexity reduction is achieved by the MSGC method (Figs. 7 and 8).

In our experiments we used 74 images with size higher than 130. On this dataset both MSGS variants are faster than SSGC for larger segmented image sizes. The one-sided paired T-test proves it. MSGV_hi2lo is faster than SSGC with $p = 1.896 \times 10^{-22}$ and MSGC_lo2hi with $p = 4.882 \times 10^{-29}$. The lo2hi variant overperforms both SSGC and MSGC_lo2hi (with $p = 9.359 \times 10^{-32}$. This is mainly due to the economical algorithm of chart construction.

5   Conclusion

The Graph-Cut method, when used on large data, has large computational demands. That's why we designed and verified a method improving its performance through increasing its speed. We showed experimentally that our Multiscale Graph-Cut method allows reducing the computational cost on data containing compact objects. We introduced two graph construction methods. The implementation is available as a Python module called imcut [8]. The segmentation is used in applications for computer aided liver surgery LISA [9].

Acknowledgements. This work has been supported by Charles University Research Centre program UNCE/MED/006 "University Center of Clinical and Experimental Liver Surgery" and Ministry of Education project ITI CZ.02.1.01/0.0/0.0/17_048/ 0007280: Application of modern technologies in medicine and industry and Erasmus+ project MedTrain3DModsim, nr. 2016-1-TR01-KA203-034929 provided by the Turkish National Agency. The research is also supported by the project LO 1506 of the Czech Ministry of Education, Youth and Sports. The authors appreciate the access to computing and storage facilities owned by parties and projects contributing to the National Grid Infrastructure MetaCentrum provided under the program "Projects of Large Research, Development, and Innovations Infrastructures" (CESNET LM2015042).

References

1. Boykov, Y., Veksler, O., Zabih, R.: Fast approximate energy minimization via graph cuts. IEEE Trans. Pattern Anal. Mach. Intell. **23**(11), 1222–1239 (2001)
2. Boykov, Y., Funka-Lea, G.: Graph cuts and efficient N-D image segmentation. Int. J. Comput. Vis. **70**(2), 109–131 (2006)
3. Boykov, Y., Kolmogorov, V.: An experimental comparison of min-cut/max-flow algorithms for energy minimization in vision. IEEE Trans. Pattern Anal. Mach. Intell. **26**(9), 359–374 (2001)
4. Dempster, A., Laird, N., Rubin, D.: Maximum likelihood from incomplete data via the EM algorithm. J. R. Stat. Soc. **39**(1), 1–38 (1977)

5. Eberlova, L., et al.: Porcine liver vascular bed in Biodur E20 corrosion casts. Folia Morphologica **75**(2), 154–161 (2016)
6. Gotra, A., et al.: Liver segmentation: indications, techniques and future directions. Insights Imaging **8**(4), 377–392 (2017)
7. Grieg, D.M., Porteous, B.T., Scheult, A.H.: Exact maximum a posteriori estimation for binary images. J. R. Stat. Soc. **51**(2), 271–279 (1989)
8. Jirik, M., Lukes, V.: imcut - 3D multiscale Graph-Cut segmentation module for python (2018). https://github.com/mjirik/imcut
9. Jirik, M., Lukeš, V.: LISA - Liver Surgery Analyser. https://github.com/mjirik/lisa
10. Kang, S.M., Wan, J.W.L.: A multiscale graph cut approach to bright-field multiple cell image segmentation using a Bhattacharyya measure. In: Proceedings of SPIE 8669, Medical Imaging 2013: Image Processing, p. 86693S (2013)

Author Index